HEALTH PROMOTION of the ELDERLY in the COMMUNITY

Estelle F. Heckheimer, R.N., M.A.
Discharge Planning Coordinator,
St. Joseph's Medical Center, Yonkers, New York

1989

W.B. SAUNDERS COMPANY

Harcourt Brace Jovanovich, Inc.

Philadelphia ■ London ■ Toronto ■ Montreal ■ Sydney ■ Tokyo

W. B. SAUNDERS COMPANY
Harcourt Brace Jovanovich, Inc.

The Curtis Center
Independence Square West
Philadelphia, PA 19106

89000.16964

Library of Congress Cataloging in Publication Data
Heckheimer, Estelle.
Health Promotions of the Elderly in the Community.
Includes index.
1. Aged—Health and Hygiene—United States.   2. Health Promotion—United States.   I. Title.
RA564.8.H46   1989   362.1′9897 00973   89–6236
ISBN 0-7216-2136-8

*RA
564.8
· H46
1989*

Editor: Ilze Rader
Designer: Terri Siegel
Cover Designer: Michelle Maloney
Production Manager: Peter Faber
Manuscript Editor: Ellen Thomas
Illustration Coordinator: Lisa Lambert

Health Promotion of the Elderly in the Community   ISBN 0-7216-2136-

Copyright © 1989 by W. B. Saunders Company

Printed in the United States of America.

Last digit is the print number: 9   8   7   6   5   4   3   2   1

*To my husband Charles for his encouragement,
support, and patience.*

*To my mother, Gertrude Popovsky, and the memory
of my mother-in-law, Beatrice Heckheimer,
two feisty women who taught
me so much about aging.*

PREFACE

Health Promotion of the Elderly in the Community is a concise and practical reference for providing holistic services to the rapidly growing geriatric population in the community. This handbook supplies health care providers with current, easily accessible information in outline form concerning primary and secondary changes, common health problems, and chronic health problems of the elderly in the community. Normal physiology has been reviewed briefly in many chapters to help the practitioner recognize how primary and secondary changes presented by the elderly differ from the responses of the so-called adult norm. Surgical treatments for primary aging changes (e.g., surgery for cataracts) are briefly described, as an understanding of these procedures is essential for the health care provider to effectively counsel the elderly client who is considering, anticipating, or recovering from such a surgical procedure. Assessment guidelines, practical provider strategies, and self-care strategies for promoting and maintaining the health of the elderly in the community are presented throughout.

In response to the desire of the elderly to live at home as independently as possible, there is a growing commitment to assist the geriatric client in maintaining a preferred lifestyle in the community. In this handbook, the nature of stressful interactions between the elderly and family is recognized, and ways to promote positive changes within the family system are emphasized, because such changes can allow the client to remain within the community. Resources for information, services, and group support are provided at the end of most sections or chapters. Generally, information may be obtained from the resources free of charge upon request by postcard. The locations of national headquarters of organizations are provided in the text, but local chapters are listed in area telephone directories. Chapter 17, "Making It in the Community," provides comprehensive information on the network of support services available in the community that may enrich the lives of the elderly and their families.

In the text, the pronoun "he" is used for clients except when the data require differentiating, as in discussions of "caregivers," who are usually female members of the family.

v

Because there is a paucity of data on the bicultural aspects of aging in the United States, this book is mostly concerned with the developmental aspects and problems of the white middle and lower socioeconomic class elderly and their families. When materials were available, such as concerning nutritional patterns and response to pain, bicultural behaviors or concerns were addressed. Although more research on aging and culture is needed, health care providers may continue to provide quality care by developing sensitivity to the adaptations to aging by a culturally diverse population.

I hope that *Health Promotion of the Elderly in the Community* will provide a reference for health care providers that will strengthen and enrich their practice in promoting and maintaining the health of the elderly in the community.

ESTELLE F. HECKHEIMER

ACKNOWLEDGMENTS

I thank Ilze Rader, nursing editor at W. B. Saunders, for her belief in this project; Dr. Ellen Hirsch for her encouragement; Dr. John Zimmerman for his guidance; and my informal reviewer Alice Champagne for her enthusiasm.

To Fairleigh Dickinson University and Frances Schervier Home and Hospital I express my appreciation for making their library facilities available to me for necessary research.

I am obliged to Ellen Thomas and her associates in Production at W.B. Saunders for their guidance in the final shaping of this work.

I also recognize the contribution of the following individuals who reviewed the manuscript:

Roberta P. Bartee, MS, BS
School of Nursing
Linfield College
Portland, Oregon

Beverly H. Bowns, DrPH
Department of Family Nursing and Community Health
College of Nursing
Rutgers University
Newark, New Jersey

Willie Mae Brown, MS
Home Health Coordinator
UT Home Health and Hospice
Knoxville, Tennessee

Sheron Chisholm, RNC, MSN
Director, Michigan Home Health Care
Traverse City, Michigan

Loretta G. Copple, BSN, MSN
School of Nursing
University of Indianapolis
Indianapolis, Indiana

Honore Fontes, PhD
School of Nursing
Mercy College
Dobbs Ferry, New York

Patricia A. Hoen, MPH
School of Nursing
Daemen College
Amherst, New York

Cheryl McCahon, MSN, RN
School of Nursing
Cleveland State University
Cleveland, Ohio

Jane McCormick, PhD, EdD, RN
Research Fellow, Rockefeller University
Reno, Nevada

A special thank you is in order for the Adjunct Nursing Faculty and Staff of the New York State Regents Program for their concern, input, and support that helped make this book a reality.

CONTENTS

Chapter 1

Chapter 2

Chapter 3

Chapter 4

Chapter 5

Chapter 6

Chapter 7

Chapter 8

Chapter 9

Chapter 10

Chapter 11

Chapter 12

Chapter 13

Chapter 14

Chapter 15

Chapter 16

Chapter 17

Appendix

Primary Aging in the Physical Dimension

CHARACTERISTICS OF PRIMARY PHYSICAL CHANGES
PRIMARY PHYSICAL CHANGES
STRATEGIES FOR HEALTH PROMOTION

1. There is no one unified theory that fully explains the cascade of events that characterize the aging process, but gerontologists agree that biologic, cultural, and historical conditions influence individuals as they experience important life changes and universal developmental stages.
2. Neither *chronological age* nor so-called *physiologic indices* are found to be reliable predictors of the performance of the individual adult. Aging is a highly individualized process, with large differences in the rates of change among individuals and within different systems in the same individual.
3. Distinguishing between normal aging changes *(primary changes)* and pathologic changes reflecting disease *(secondary changes)* is often difficult but nevertheless important for the development of strategies to effectively promote and maintain health.
4. *Average life span* may be extended by prevention or cure of specific diseases, but the *maximum life span* (the age reached by the longest-lived survivors of a large population, 110 to 115 years for humans) can be extended only by slowing the basic biologic processes of aging.
5. As gerontologic research has been of concern only in recent years, much more work must be done until we more fully understand how the individual ages.

CHARACTERISTICS OF PRIMARY PHYSICAL CHANGES

1. Primary physical changes occur gradually over time.
2. Usually, progressive decline in function is demonstrated.
   a. About 1% of function that an individual had at age 30 is lost each succeeding year.
   b. Function may be totally lost (e.g., female ability to reproduce is lost at the time of menopause).
   c. Units of function may be structurally lost, but the remaining units function as before unless stress occurs (e.g., the number of nephrons is reduced, but the kidney continues to function at a slower rate).
   d. Organ function may be diminished in proportion to the number of units lost (e.g., skeletal muscle loses strength in proportion to the number of fibers lost).
   e. Reduced functional efficiency may occur without anatomic loss (e.g., nerve fibers demonstrate reduced conduction velocity).
   f. There is a reduction in reserve of function available for coping with activity or challenge above that of resting state (e.g., cardiac reserve for response to stress is reduced).
3. Cellular changes occur.
   a. A gradual loss of cells occurs by attrition or by decrease in cell volume in nonreplenishing tissue (brain, kidney, and heart).
   b. Tissues demonstrate increasing irregularity in appearance.
   c. Lipofuscin (fatty brown pigment) accumulates in cells as nonfunctioning debris.
   d. T cells are reduced in the immune system.
   e. Loss of division potential occurs after mitotic cells reproduce 50 ± 10 generations. Either division stops, or reproduction occurs with chromosomal abnormalities.
   f. Colloid material accumulates in various tissues.
4. Control systems alter in function.
   a. Negative feedback systems take longer to trigger; however, once action is initiated, the response tends to be excessively prolonged (e.g., the heart rate increases more slowly in response to stress, but takes longer to return to a normal rate after stress is relieved).
   b. Interruption of a control may occur (e.g., follicle-stimulating hormone [FSH] and luteinizing hormone [LH] levels rise for 5 years after menopause even when estrogen levels are low).
   c. Increased function may occur, but rarely (e.g., increased secre-

tion of antidiuretic hormone occurs in response to hyperosmo-
larity).

PRIMARY PHYSICAL CHANGES

Body Configuration and Composition

1. Increased adipose tissue
   a. Increased distribution appears in central sites (omentum, peri-
      nephric area, and functioning areas of organs).
   b. Amount of subcutaneous fat decreases, thus decreasing insula-
      tion.
   c. The body appears heavier, with long thin arms and legs.
2. Decreased lean body mass
   a. Muscles, liver, and kidneys slowly atrophy (diminished in weight
      by 20 to 30% by age 70).
   b. Decreased oxygen-consuming mass reduces total body metabo-
      lism.
3. Decreased percentage of water
   a. Increased intracellular water loss occurs as cell mass is decreased.
   b. Extracellular water remains at about 20% of total body water.
4. Decreased stature
   a. A decrease of 1 cm (0.4 inch) per decade begins after age 40 and
      accelerates after age 70, owing to loss of foot arches, curvature
      of spine, drying out of intervertebral discs, and decrease in ver-
      tical size of vertebrae.
   b. Long bones of extremities do not shorten.
   c. Measurement of arm span is true height.
5. Posture
   a. Gradual stooping, slight bending forward, some flexing of knees
      and hips, bending of arms to raise hands, and tilting back of the
      head result as bone mass is reduced and muscle tissue atrophies.
   b. Decrease in shoulder width, increase in pelvic width, and de-
      crease in depth of the abdomen occur.
6. Decrease in weight after age 60 years
   a. For men, ideal weight is 106 pounds for the first 5 feet of height,
      and 6 pounds for each additional inch above 5 feet (±10%).
   b. For women, ideal weight is 100 pounds for the first 5 feet of
      height and 5 pounds for each additional inch above 5 feet
      (±10%).
7. Decreased bone mass
   a. Loss of bone mass is accelerated in postmenopausal women.

8. Face
   a. Loss of dermal tone.
   b. Increase in pigmented spots.
   c. Drooping look accentuates the jowls, lengthens ears, adds to bagginess of lower eyelids, and for some contributes to formation of a double chin.
   d. Nose lengthens.
   e. Loss of teeth may result in "loss of lip look."
   f. Fatty deposits increase in eyelids.
   g. Eyes appear sunken as a result of loss of orbital fat pads.
   h. Decreased size of lower face resulting from bone loss in mandible accentuates size of upper mouth, nose, and forehead.
9. Thorax
   a. Increased anterior-posterior diameter as lung elasticity decreases.
   b. Kyphosis and scoliosis often develop as bone mass is lost in the ribs and vertebrae and calcification of the costal cartilages increases.

The Integumentary System

1. Skin
   a. Epidermal atrophy leads to fine wrinkling, laxity, fragility, translucence, dryness, itchiness, thinning, decreased elasticity, decreased tensile strength, and decreased extensibility of skin. Wound healing is about four times slower.
   b. Increased collagenous support for dermal vessels results in senile purpura from even minor skin injury. Senile purpura is more likely to occur on extensor surfaces of the forearms.
   c. Blemishes and growths (skin tags and warts) are more frequent. Lentigo senilis (dark brown, flat lesions with an irregular outline) may appear in areas exposed to the sun.
   d. Subcutaneous loss of protective fat cushions increases vulnerability of skin to external physical trauma and development of pressure sores.
   e. Less insulation against cold results in susceptibility to hypothermia.
   f. Sebaceous gland activity decreases in men after age 80. In women, sebaceous gland activity decreases after menopause and remains relatively unchanged after age 60. Ability of the skin to keep itself moist decreases.
   g. Decreased ability of eccrine glands to produce sweat and a de-

crease in the number of sweat glands lessen tolerance to excessive heat.

h. Perception of pressure and touch decreases.

i. Decreased sensitivity to thermal stimulus leads to susceptibility to thermal injury.

j. Less vibratory sense in toes increases ambulation problems.

2. Hair

a. Loss of hair in frontal regions and vertex of scalp in men and women. Androgenetic alopecia or *male pattern alopecia* (baldness) exists to some degree in all the population.

b. Decrease in daily rate of hair growth.

c. Decrease in diameter of hair shaft. Coarse terminal hairs are replaced by vellus hairs that are thin and light in color.

d. Graying, beginning in the third decade for most people and progressing. By the fourth decade about 40% of people have some gray scalp hair. Body and facial hair tends to gray later.

e. Decrease in body and facial hair of men. Growth of coarse hair in external ear canals may increase.

f. Increase in facial hair in women.

3. Nails

a. Rate of growth decreases.

b. Nails may become brittle after menopause.

c. Longitudinal ridging occurs.

d. Fingernails fragment at tips.

e. Toenails are more likely to thicken and become dull and opaque with longitudinal ridging.

The Neurologic System

1. Brain

a. Weight decreases to about 10% of maximum weight in young adulthood.

b. Size of ventricles and sulci increases, as gray and white matter decrease.

c. Number of neurons, dendritic branches, and synapses decreases.

d. Neuritic plaques (degraded dendrites and axons), neurofibrillary tangles (degenerate microtubules), and lipofuscin accumulate.

e. Changes are not consistent in all persons, and no one factor accounts for decline in brain function.

2. Peripheral nervous system

a. Decreased number of motor neurons and demyelinization of nerve fibers slow reaction time.

b. Decreased somatic sensation is related to degenerative changes.

    c. Increased muscle tone is demonstrated by mild rigidity.

    d. Tremor (not noted in a majority of elderly) appears to be an exaggeration of physiologic tremor and may be in head, face, voice, hands, and legs. Tremors in the resting state are more likely to be due to pathology.

3. Reflexes
    a. Hypotonia or loss of distal reflexes (e.g., diminution of ankle jerks).
    b. Superficial abdominal reflexes often absent.
    c. Suck and grasp reflexes sometimes present.

4. Sensory perception
    a. Increased threshold for sensations of light, touch, sight, hearing, pain, and vibratory sense.

5. Vision
    a. The lens becomes opaque and rigid, with decreased ability to focus on near objects (presbyopia) occurring during the fourth decade.
    b. Yellowing of lens causes difficulty in discriminating colors in the blue end of the spectrum.
    c. Pupillary responses are decreased. The ability to recover from glare decreases.
    d. Visual acuity decreases. Distance vision decreases usually by age 70.
    e. Visually evoked responses are centrally delayed, possibly as a result of slowing in the visual pathways.
    f. Ocular motility is decreased, and upward gaze is limited.
    g. Visual field is decreased, with a decrease in peripheral vision.

6. Hearing
    a. Decrease in hearing acuity beginning about age 50, probably as a result of ossification and change in auditory nerve function.
    b. Lower perception of high-frequency tones.
    c. Dichotomic auditory stimuli less often correctly identified simultaneously.
    d. Decrease in central processing of auditory information.

7. Smell
    a. Sense of smell begins to lessen after age 70 as olfactory bulbs atrophy.
      (1) Less interest in eating and less sensitivity to personal hygiene may occur as olfactory sensation decreases.
      (2) Greater vulnerability to asphyxia occurs as ability to smell presence of natural gas lessens.

8. Touch

    a. Decrease in sense of touch as nerve conduction velocity slows and latency period for sensory and motor nerves increases.

    b. Decrease in fine touch as Pacini and Meissner corpuscles are reduced in the skin.

    c. Greater sensitivity to light touch after age 70 as a result of thinning of skin.

9. Mental status

    a. Relationship of cortical atrophy and cognitive losses not clear.

10. Sleep

    a. Time from the decision to sleep to sleep onset increases to 10 minutes (sleep latency).

    b. More awakenings (3 to 4 times a night) occur, with more recall for awakenings. Lower sleep efficiency (ratio of total sleep time to time in bed) results.

    c. Sleep time either stays the same or is decreased. Sleep averages 6½ to 7 hours per night.

The Musculoskeletal System

1. Bone changes (See "Body Configuration and Composition," earlier).

    a. Loss of bone mass.

    b. Loss of 1 to 3 inches in height owing to drying out of intervertebral discs.

    c. Bony spurs (osteophytes) occur in the spinal column as a result of aging and use.

    d. Degenerative progressive changes occur in the articular surfaces of the hip joint and knee joint.

    e. Loss of cartilage and bony thickening in the finger joints is more common in women and may be hereditary.

    f. In some joints, such as the ankle, little change may occur.

    g. The scapula acquires a moth-eaten appearance, and progressive calcification occurs in the shoulder joint.

2. Muscle changes

    a. Decrease in muscle mass reportedly begins in the third decade in men and in the fifth decade in women.

    b. Muscle fibers shrink, connective tissue proliferates, and fat infiltrates.

    c. Muscle changes are progressive and genetically determined.

The Cardiovascular System

1. Heart

    a. Slight increase in left ventricular wall thickness occurs, but overall size of heart does not increase.

   b. Overall mechanical performance is not affected except under conditions of extreme stress or pharmacologic stimulation.

   c. Slight decreases in heart rate, stroke volume, and cardiac output occur.

   d. Time to reach peak heart rate with exercise increases, and maximal heart rate that can be attained with exercise decreases.

   e. Maximal stroke volume, cardiac output, and oxygen uptake decrease in response to exercise.

   f. Myocardial responsiveness to adrenergic stimuli is reduced.

   g. As the pulse rate responds more slowly to movement and cardiac output decreases, there is greater susceptibility to dizziness, falling, and loss of consciousness when moving from a recumbent to an upright position.

2. Major arteries

   a. Decreased distensibility of arteries leads to increased systolic blood pressure.

   b. Blood pressure by age 70 may be 150 mm Hg systolic and 90 mm Hg diastolic with persistent arterial hypertension.

   c. Increase in fatty deposits in the intima of arteries increases vessel rigidity and circulatory insufficiency.

   d. Decreased circulation to liver, kidneys, and periphery occurs.

The Respiratory System

1. Breathing

   a. Changes are gradual, so that in the absence of illness the elderly are capable of effortless breathing.

   b. Decrease in diffusing capacity of the lung is associated with a decrease in alveolar surface area and capillary bed.

   c. Increased rigidity of the thorax due to skeletal changes causes decreases in ventilation and maximal breathing capacity.

   d. Decreased strength of the diaphragm and intercostal muscles and decreased elasticity of the lung lead to difficulty in expiring air. Increase in depth of respiration occurs to compensate and to increase amount of oxygen.

   e. Capacity for exercise decreases.

   f. Respiratory control may be disturbed during sleep.

   g. Performance ability in high altitudes decreases.

2. Respiratory defense mechanisms

   a. Decreased cough reflex, ciliary action, and secretory immunoglobulin A (IgA) of nasal and respiratory passages, which neutralizes viral activities, occur.

b. Activity of alveolar macrophages (phagocytic cells that ingest foreign material) decreases.
3. Larynx
   a. Although changes in the larynx affect pitch, loudness, and quality, the voice remains capable of effective communication and emotional expression for most of the adult life.
   b. The voice is characterized by a slight hoarseness and decreased pitch in women and increased pitch in men. These changes trouble the elderly, who may be sensitive to the loss of appeal or effectiveness of the voice.
   c. Use of the voice tends to maintain overall vocal performance.

The Gastrointestinal System

1. Mouth
   a. Teeth become worn, develop caries, and are lost through gum disease.
   b. The periodontal membrane thins, and resorption of roots and alveolar bone occurs.
   c. Oral mucosa becomes thinner.
   d. Saliva production decreases.
   e. Degenerative changes occur in the maxilla, mandible, and temporomandibular joints.
   f. Muscles of mastication decrease in bulk and strength.
   g. Deterioration of the taste buds results in decreased sensation for salt and sweet tastes; sensation for bitter and sour tastes remains functional longer.
2. Esophagus
   a. Disturbed motility of the esophagus results in a disorganized response to swallowing and delayed transit time.
   b. Slowed esophageal emptying causes maldigestion and increases susceptibility to aspiration by the elderly, who must maintain a horizontal position during feeding when incapacitated.
   c. The lower esophageal sphincter often becomes incompetent, and reflux esophagitis occurs.
3. Stomach
   a. Decreased gastric motility leads to delayed emptying and maldigestion.
   b. Decreased gastric secretion is usually associated with atrophic mucosa and with increased pepsin and acid concentration. Increased hydrochloric acid production may impair absorption of iron and vitamin B_{12}.
4. Liver

   a. Size, weight, and functional capacity decrease.
   b. Hepatic blood flow and capacity for liver regeneration decrease.
   c. Decreased hepatic protein synthesis reduces concentrations of serum albumin.
   d. Decreased activity of various drug-metabolizing enzymes delays drug breakdown by the liver.
5. Pancreas
   a. Slight decrease in size and function has negligible impact.
   b. Fibrosis and fat infiltration with progressive ductal dilatation occurs, but there is no significant decline in secretory capacity for bicarbonate or digestive enzymes.
   c. Age-related decline in glucose tolerance is attributed mainly to decrease in tissue sensitivity rather than to decreased insulin release by the pancreas.
6. Small intestine
   a. Subclinical degrees of malabsorption of nutrients occur partially as a result of atrophy of tissue, development of fibrous tissue, and lower amounts of lipase.
7. Colon
   a. Colonic motor disorder inhibits transit of stool.
   b. Muscle function and tone decrease.
   c. Increased threshold for perception of rectal distention and for initiation of defecation reflex occurs.
   d. Vasculofibrotic changes in the appendix predispose to rapid extension and earlier perforation in acute appendicitis.

The Genitourinary System

1. Kidney
   a. Decreased mass with fewer number of nephrons.
   b. Variable sclerotic changes in the walls of the larger renal vessels.
   c. Decreased glomerulofiltration rate.
   d. Homeostasis maintained under normal conditions, but decrease in efficiency occurs under stress.
2. Male reproductive system
   a. Prostate.
      (1) Decreased secretion of bactericidal fluid predisposes elderly men to higher incidence of bladder infections.
      (2) Glandular atrophy and fibrosis interfere with urination.
   b. Decreased frequency of erection and ability for repetitive ejaculations.
   c. Lower serum levels of testosterone. (See No. 7 under "The Endocrine System," next.)
   d. Fertility varies.

3. Female reproductive system
   a. Vagina
      (1) Generalized atrophy of the tract.
      (2) Vaginal vault shortened.
      (3) Disappearance of rugae.
      (4) Less vaginal elasticity and thinning of the lining.
      (5) Secretions scant and watery with mixed flora.
      (6) Greater susceptibility to atrophic vaginitis associated with decreased estrogen production and lack of stimulation.
      (7) Cervix and uterus decrease in size.
      (8) Distal part of urethra becomes rigid and inelastic as the epithelium thins. Urethral outflow obstruction may result.
      (9) Pubic relaxation with prolapse of urethra and vaginal tissue may lead to urinary obstruction.
     (10) Decrease in number of oocytes by atresia until menopause, when few remain.
   b. Fertility
      (1) Reproductive capacity lost after menopause.
   c. Breasts
      (1) Breast tissue and mammary ducts decrease.
      (2) Breasts flatten and sag.
      (3) Nipple may invert.
   d. Body hair
      (1) Pubic and axillary hair thins. (See No. 8 under "The Endocrine System," next.)

The Endocrine System

1. Decrease in secretory rate of hormones.
2. Decrease in metabolic degradation rate of hormones.
3. Decrease in sensitivity of target tissue to hormonal stimulation.
4. Greater thyroid nodularity. Decrease in production of thyroxine (but results of thyroid function tests usually are within normal limits).
5. Androgen cortisol secretion continuing to peak from 6 to 8 A.M.
6. Decreased glucose tolerance with a minimal increase in serum glucose, probably as a result of reduction of number of insulin receptors at target tissue. For each decade of life, after the fifth, the fasting blood glucose rises by 10 mg/dl ± 4. Insulin production appears to continue at normal levels.
7. Decrease in testosterone serum levels. Volume of ejaculate remains the same with a decrease in living sperm.

8. Decreased production of estradiol and circulating estrogen levels after menopause. Increased pituitary FSH and LH for 5 years after menopause, then secretion is decreased.

The Immune System

1. Modest decrease in immunologic capabilities occurs.
   a. Decreased ability to make protective antibodies after immunization.
   b. Disturbances in immunoregulation lead to increase in autoimmune phenomena.
   c. Decrease in ability for surveillance against malignant cells.
2. Decrease in capabilities of immune system place the elderly more at risk for infection and cancer.

STRATEGIES FOR HEALTH PROMOTION

1. Explain to the client that there are no known "anti-aging" treatments, drugs, or supplements that will affect the rate of biologic aging, but *health may be improved and maintained longer by pursuing an active healthy lifestyle.*

Resource

NIH Publication No. 85-2682, January 1985
Clinical Center Office of Division of Public Information
Clinical Reports and Inquires
National Institutes of Health (NIH)
Building 10, Room 1C-255
9000 Rockville Pike
Bethesda, MD 20205
(301) 496-2563
Behavior Patterns and Health

Presents information on the effect of lifestyle on health.

2. Utilize the following recommendations to guide the elderly client toward a healthy lifestyle that will help prolong functional capability and reduce the risk of disease and premature death. Teach the client to:
   a. Quit smoking or at least cut down.

(1) Avoid smoking, and limit exposure to an atmosphere of smoke.

(2) If you choose to continue smoking, decrease the number of cigarettes smoked; switch to a low-tar, low-nicotine brand; and do not smoke the cigarette down to the end.

Resources

Check the telephone directory for local chapters of national associations.

American Cancer Society
4 West 35th Street
New York, NY 10001
(212) 736-3030

American Heart Association
7320 Greenville Avenue
Dallas, TX 75231
(214) 373-6300

American Lung Association
1740 Broadway, P.O. Box 596
New York, NY 10019
(212) 315-8700

Office on Smoking and Health
5600 Fishers Lane
Park Building, Room 1-10
Rockville, MD 20857
(301) 443-1690

Office of Cancer Communications
National Cancer Institute
Bethesda, MD 20205
(301) 496-5583

Call Cancer Information Service
  (800) 4-CANCER
  In Alaska: (800) 638-6070
  In Hawaii: (808) 524-1234
  In Washington, DC: (202) 636-5700

b. Limit alcohol consumption.
  (1) Drink only in moderation if at all.

(2) Do not drink and drive.

Resources

Alcoholics Anonymous
468 Park Avenue South
New York, NY 10163
(212) 576-8400

See Chapter 5, under "Alcoholism in the Elderly."

c. Practice safety habits.
   (1) Avoid overexposure to sun, heat, and cold.
   (2) Prevent home accidents, such as burns and falls.
   (3) Wear seat belts when you are driving and when you are a passenger.

Resources

U.S. Consumer Product Safety Commission
Washington, DC 20207
Safety for Older Consumers: Home Safety Check List

See Chapter 3, under "Staying Warm and Keeping Cool."

See Chapter 16, "Accident, Crime, and Abuse Prevention."

d. Practice good nutritional habits.
   (1) Eat nutrient-dense foods.
   (2) Use food high in fiber and low in sugar, saturated fats, and salt.
   (3) Include adequate amounts of fluids, calcium, and vitamin D in the diet.
   (4) See Chapter 4, "Meeting the Nutritional Needs of the Elderly."
e. Exercise regularly.
   (1) Consult with the health care provider (doctor or nurse practitioner) before undertaking any physical activity program.
   (2) Take stress test to gauge your individual tolerance for exercise and to identify your target heart rate.

(3) Engage in an exercise program of regular moderate aerobic activity from 20 to 30 minutes at least three times a week.

Resources

NIH Publication No. 81-1677, May 1981
National Heart, Lung, and Blood Institute
Department of Health and Human Services
Building 31, Room 4A-21
9000 Rockville Pike
Bethesda, MD 20205
(301) 496-4236
Exercise and Your Heart

Presents information on the effects of physical activity on the heart and practical guidelines for starting and staying on an exercise program.

National Institute on Aging
Building 31, Room 5C-35
9000 Rockville Pike
Bethesda, MD 20205
(301) 496-1752
Don't Take It Easy—Exercise

Presents importance and benefits of exercise for older persons. Lists general precautions to take when initiating an exercise program and discusses how to choose an appropriate exercise program.

Arthritis Information Clearinghouse
P.O. Box 9782
Arlington, VA 22209
(703) 588-8250
Exercises for People with Arthritis

Reference list. Focus is on arthritis, but most materials are geared to older Americans.

Local chapter of American Heart Association.
"E" Is for Exercise

Describes exercise as one of several factors preventing cardiovascular disease. Prepares individuals of all ages for selecting and committing to a regular program.

American Association of Retired Persons
1909 K Street, N.W., Fifth Floor
Washington, DC 20049
(202) 872-4700
Pep Up Your Life

Outlines different levels of exercise for strength, flexibility, and endurance. Illustrated.

See Chapter 11, Figures 11–2 though 11–6, for range of motion exercises for the elderly.

   f. Allow time for rest and recreation.
      (1) Get enough sleep (7 to 8 hours a night).
      (2) Continue to socialize.
      (3) Maintain contact and involvement with family and friends.
      (4) Stay active through work, recreation, and community activities.

Resources

American Association for Retired Persons
1909 K Street, N.W., Fifth Floor
Washington, DC 20049
(202) 872-4700

Provides services for people age 50 or older, including a bimonthly magazine *(Modern Maturity)*, a travel service, a lobby on behalf of senior citizens, and a mail-order pharmacy service for members.

Widowed Persons
1909 K Street, N.W.,
Washington, DC 20049

Support group for widows and widowers.

See Chapter 17, "Making It in the Community."

   g. Avoid excessive stress.
      (1) Become involved with other people and groups.

(2) Use stress-reduction techniques as needed (e.g., meditation, yoga, biofeedback, imagery, and exercise).

Resources

U.S. Department of Health and Human Services
Public Health Service
Alcohol, Drug Abuse and Mental Health Administration
5600 Fishers Lane
Rockville, MD 20857
(301) 443-3783
Plain Talk Series
Handling Stress, DHHS Publication No. (ADM)85-502
Biofeedback, DHHS Publication No. (ADM)83-1273
Mutual Health Groups, DHHS Publication No. (ADM) 83-1138

Children of Aging Parents
2761 Trenton Road
Levittown, PA 19056

Offers materials to help people interested in forming support groups.

Information Officer
National Institute on Aging
Building 31, Room 5C-35
9000 Rockville Pike
Bethesda, MD 20205
Self-Care and Self-Help Groups for the Elderly: A Directory

Family Service Association of America
44 East 23rd Street
New York, NY 10010
(212) 674-6100

Offers counseling services.

h. Maintain regular health supervision. (See Chapter 17, "Making It in the Community.")
   (1) Do not attribute all problems to aging and thus assume that nothing will help.
   (2) Seek help from your physician when a problem is noticed.

(3) Assume responsibility for self-care. Keep a close watch on what is happening as a result of a chronic condition (e.g., test for blood glucose with diabetes, monitor blood pressure for hypertension).

(4) Carry out self-screening and testing in conjunction wth health supervision (e.g., breast screening for cancer [Table 1–1]).

(5) Use informed judgment in complying with a medication regimen.

(6) Ascertain vaccination status and bring up to date.

Table 1–1. Recommendations for the Early Detection of Cancer in Asymptomatic People*

Test or Procedure	Population		
	Sex	*Age*	*Frequency*
Sigmoidoscopy	M, F	Over 50	After two negative exams, 1 year apart, perform every 3–5 years
Stool guaiac slide test	M, F	Over 50	Every year
Digital rectal examination	M, F	Over 40	Every year
Pap test	F	All women who are, or who have been, sexually active, or have reached age 18, should have an annual Pap test and pelvic examination.	
Pelvic examination	F	After a woman has had three or more consecutive satisfactory normal annual examinations, the Pap test may be performed less frequently at the discretion of her physician.	
Endometrial tissue sample	F	At menopause, women at high risk†	At menopause
Breast self-examination	F	20 and over	Every month
Breast physical examination	F	20–40 Over 40	Every 3 years Every year
Mammography	F	35–39 40–49 50 and over	Baseline Every 1–2 years Every year
Chest x-ray	—	—	Not recommended
Sputum cytology	—	—	Not recommended
Health counseling and cancer checkup‡	M, F M, F	Over 20 Over 40	Every 3 years Every year

*From Summary of Current Guidelines for the Cancer-Related Checkup: Recommendations. American Cancer Society, 1988.

†History of infertility, obesity, failure to ovulate, abnormal uterine bleeding, or estrogen therapy.

‡To include examination for cancers of the thyroid, testicles, prostate, ovaries, lymph nodes, oral region, and skin.

(a) Obtain a diphtheria/tetanus vaccination every 10 years.
(b) Obtain immunization with pneumococcal vaccine by age 65.
(c) Obtain annual influenza vaccination.

Resources

See Table 1–1.

See Chapter 17, "Making It in the Community."

i. Avoid illicit drugs.

Resources

Narcotics Anonymous
P.O. Box 622
Sun Valley, CA 91352

For narcotic addicts; peer support for recovered addicts.

See Chapter 5, under "Drug Misuse and the Elderly."

References

Albert M: Health screening to promote health for the elderly. Nurse Practitioner 12(5):42, 48, 50–51, 55–56, 1987.

Burggraff V, Donlon B: System by system. American Journal of Nursing 85:973–988, 1985.

Burnside IR: Nursing and the Aged. New York: McGraw-Hill, 1976.

Cohen RC: Aging and the skin. Geriatric Medicine Today 5(1):26–29, 32, 37, 1986.

Cohen S: Sensory changes in the elderly. American Journal of Nursing 81:1851–1880, 1981.

Covington TR, Walker JI: Current Geriatric Therapy. Philadelphia: WB Saunders Co, 1984.

Drachman DA: An approach to the neurology of aging. In Birren J, Sloan RB, eds: Handbook of Mental Health and Aging. Englewood Cliffs, NJ: Prentice-Hall, 1977.

Duke DJ, Giaguzzi RA: Exercise for the elderly. Diabetes Self-Management January/February 1987, pp 10–14.

Forbes EJ, Fitzsimons VM: The Older Adult. St. Louis: CV Mosby, 1981.

Gardner ID: Relationship between aging and susceptibility to infection. Geriatric Medicine Today 5(3):29–32, 41, 1986.

Geokas MC: The aging process. Clinics in geriatric medicine. Philadelphia: WB Saunders Co, 1985.

Gullo L, Labo G: Age related changes in the exocrine pancreas. Geriatric Medicine Today 4(12):56, 59–62, 1985.

Hazzard WR: Preventive gerontology. Postgraduate Medicine 74:279–287, 1983.

Henderson ML: Altered presentations. American Journal of Nursing 81:104–1106, 1985.

Jacobs R: Physical changes in the aged. In O'Hara-Devereaux M, Andrus LH, Scott CD, eds: Eldercare. New York: Grune & Stratton, 1981.

Kohrs MB: Age-related changes in taste acuity. Geriatric Medicine Today 4(5):88–93, 1985.

Lakulta EG: Age-related changes in the heart. Geriatric Medicine Today 4(7):86, 91–97, 1985.

Leventhal EA, Prohaska TR: Age, symptom interpretation, and health behavior. Journal of the American Gerontologic Society 34(3): 185–191, 1986.

Mueller PB: The senescent voice. Geriatric Medicine Today 4(4):50–57, 1985.

Ory MG: Health promotion strategies for the aged. Journal of Gerontological Nursing 10(10):31–35, 1984.

Rock RD: Effects of age on common laboratory tests. Geriatrics 39(6):57–60, 1984.

Rossman I: What is normal aging? Geriatric Medicine Today 3(4):37–43, 1984.

Rothschild BM: Age-related changes in skeletal muscle. Geriatric Medicine Today 5(4):87, 89–90, 93, 94–95, 1986.

Scoggins CH: The cellular, biochemical, and genetic basis of aging. In Schrier RW, ed: Clinical Internal Medicine in the Aged. Philadelphia: WB Saunders Co, 1982.

Sloane PD: How to maintain the health of the elderly. Geriatrics 39(10):93–104, 1984.

Zoler M: What is aging? Highlights of a 25-year study. Geriatrics 39(8):85–87, 1984.

Primary Aging Changes in the Psychosocial Dimensions

THE EMOTIONAL DIMENSION
THE INTELLECTUAL DIMENSION
THE SOCIAL DIMENSION
THE SPIRITUAL DIMENSION

1. Regardless of socioeconomic status and cultural heritage, the elderly person faces a number of stresses in the psychosocial dimensions that are largely characterized by loss.
2. In response to the stresses of later life, personality traits become more pronounced as the individual becomes more of what he was before.
3. For the elder with a negative view of the future, his situation, and self, cognitive distortion is greater and emotional reaction is heightened. As a result, *depression*, the most common functional psychiatric disorder in the elderly, may occur.
4. The elder with an optimistic outlook is likely to experience a sense of subjective well-being and adapt to conditions that objectively may be considered less than optimal.
5. The following crises severely tax the coping mechanisms of the elderly, their families, and significant others:

   • Death of family and friends
   • Sexual problems
   • Retirement
   • Limited economic resources
   • Sensory, mobility, and memory losses

- Disease
- Illness
- Hospitalization
- Death and dying

THE EMOTIONAL DIMENSION

1. Because of the limited energy of the elderly, expression of feelings in response to loss may be more subtle. The exception is the elderly person with organic brain disease, who shows an increased response.
2. In an attempt to deal with conflicting and overwhelming needs and stresses, elderly people may resort to defense mechanisms.
3. By using defense mechanisms, the elderly often seem disagreeable and alienate themselves from family and friends; this may occur at a time when the elderly person is most in need of support.
4. As the elder may have alienated others with anger, hostility, and projection, establishment of a trusting positive relationship is of value in raising self-esteem, ameliorating loneliness, and reducing the use of negative coping mechanisms.
5. The senior who develops a sense of self, an understanding of personal motivations, and a realization of the human life cycle is able to accept assistance when needed and is able to substitute available satisfaction for losses experienced.
6. The nurse should recognize *behaviors that are valid responses to social pressures,* such as discrimination, crime, and abuse, and assist the elder to take appropriate action.

Emotional Reactions in Response to Loss

1. *Grief* may be expressed by somatic distress, preoccupation with image of the deceased, feelings of guilt, and behavioral changes.
   a. Postponement of grief with associated distortions in behavior and depression with suicidal signs indicate a morbid grief reaction.
   b. Chronic grief is demonstrated by extension and intensification of acute grief well beyond the 6- to 12-month period in which grieving is normally completed.
   c. After the death of a loved one, enshrinement may occur as the survivor attempts to keep the physical surroundings unchanged and also deliberately avoids new associations that may replace the role of the deceased.
   d. Ongoing emotional support is essential during this crisis, as the

loss of a loved one is the most important event foreshadowing decline both physically and emotionally.

2. *Anxiety* may be expressed as intensification of free-floating feelings of apprehension, rigid thinking, fear of being alone, suspiciousness to the point of paranoia, somatization, fatigue, insomnia, pacing back and forth, restlessness, wandering, isolation, preoccupation, hostility, dependency, changes of posture and motion, and talking too much or too fast.

3. *Anger* is usually repressed and manifested as depression. Feelings of anger are discussed only indirectly. However, some elderly are more likely to express anger because inhibition is gone.

4. *Rage* may be expressed in response to seemingly uncontrollable situations, indignities, and neglect.

5. *Guilt* may result in the elderly after reminiscence about previous events in their lives in which they believe that they did not live up to strict rules they set for themselves.

6. *Loneliness* is characterized by the fear of having no one to relate to. However, high valuation of independence and self-reliance may interfere with ability to accept living in communal settings. In group-oriented cultures this is less of a problem.

7. *Depression* is characterized by lack of hope and feelings of despair.
   a. There is a tense expression on the face and deep central furrows on the brow.
   b. Somatization is predominant and may become a hypochondriacal preoccupation and the beginning of somatic delusions.
   c. Nocturia occurs unaccompanied by daytime urgency.
   d. Depression associated with organic brain syndrome is characterized by forgetfulness, poor judgment, and confusion.

8. *Impotence* and *helplessness* are most keenly felt among white men who were leaders and decision makers. These feelings are reflected in the high suicide rates of white men in their eighties.

Defense Mechanisms as Used by the Elderly

1. *Denial* may be used for maintaining a sense of stability and equilibrium, but it becomes pathologic when it interferes with the accomplishment of developmental tasks (e.g., interference with acceptance of aging by failing to accept physical limitations).

2. *Projection* is used to reject and impute to others disowned aspects of the self; intolerable wishes, feelings, and motivations are attributed to others.
   a. The elder appears suspicious and fearful.

   b. Legitimate fears should be recognized as realities and not pro-
      jections.
   c. Projection occurs as a result of *internal* stress rather than external
      stress.
3. *Regression* may be a realistic attempt of the elder to adjust to *external*
   stressors rather than a return to earlier behaviors because of internal
   stress.
4. *Displacement* may assist the elder in disguising feelings of anxiety by
   the use of a less threatening object on which to release feelings.
5. *Idealization of a loss*—whether it is a person, place, or lifestyle—is an
   attempt by the elder to give meaning to life so that it will not seem
   meaningless.
6. *Counterphobia* occurs when the elder feels compelled to convince
   himself that a danger can be overcome by facing it. This can be life-
   threatening, particularly when he attempts physical activities that
   he realistically should assess as dangerous.
7. *Somatization* occurs as the senior attempts to cope with psychosocial
   problems by complaining about physical symptoms, which seem to
   create more interest in care givers.
8. *Selective memory* is used to remember pleasurable events in the distant
   past rather than more painful recent memories. This mechanism
   may be responsible at times for what has been attributed to loss of
   memory caused by arteriosclerotic change.
9. *Selective sensory response* aids the elder in blocking off input that he
   feels unable to deal with.
10. *Exploitation of age and disability* is used to obtain secondary gains, such
    as freedom from what is socially expected.
11. *Busyness* may be used as a defense against depression, anxiety, and
    other painful conditions.

Strategies

1. The nurse should provide opportunity for the elder for reminiscence, thinking about himself, "mirror gazing," and reconsideration
   of previous experiences and their meaning.
   a. The process of life review may be ongoing during several visits,
      completed in one visit, completed in written form, or conducted
      in a group setting.
   b. The elderly client has the opportunity to reassess his life as he
      consciously looks at past experiences and unresolved conflicts,
      which he may now resolve.
   c. Personality reorganization may be achieved with increased self-
      awareness, wisdom, and serenity.

d. Ego integrity may develop as the elder accepts that his life as he lived it was inevitable, appropriate, and meaningful.

e. For the negative personality, life review may result in depression, guilt, and rumination. If the decision is made that life was a waste, suicide may result.

f. The role of the health professional in life review is active listening, acknowledging past achievements, and giving positive feedback to reduce unhappy feelings and increase insight.

g. Acknowledging the bad times but pointing out the positive accomplishments promotes a sense of satisfaction and self-esteem.

h. Family members and significant others should be alerted to the beneficial effects of life review and the importance of listening to and recognizing accomplishments.

2. Recognize the client's personality traits and past coping mechanisms as revealed during life review. Utilize this information in assisting him to cope with changes and losses.

3. Assure the survivor experiencing grief that his feelings are normal and that he is not going "crazy." Provide opportunities for expressing grief. Repression of grief may lead to a morbid grief pattern.

4. Encourage the lowering of defense mechanisms by:
   a. Establishing a trusting relationship.
   b. Using behavior modification.
   c. Providing minimal attention to somatization and projection.
   d. Recognizing and praising positive interaction.

5. Increase self-esteem by inviting the elder to assume the consultant role (by sharing his opinion) when his wisdom and experience will be a recognized contribution.

6. Foster the development of a relationship with a confidant with whom the elder can relate and share his problems and feelings.

7. Assist the elder in continuing to satisfy his basic physiologic needs (food, clothing, and shelter) and the needs for safety, security, love, belonging, and self-esteem.

8. Encourage the use of relaxation techniques, such as deep breathing, progressive relaxation, and visualization.

THE INTELLECTUAL DIMENSION

1. The intellectual dimension is concerned with the ability to understand, communicate, and care for oneself.

2. Physical and psychosocial factors are influential, but the dimension is primarily influenced by the intellectual functions: perception, memory, cognition, and communication.

3. The brain experiences cortical atrophy, but the relationship between cortical atrophy and cognitive loss is not clear.
4. The relationship between initial levels of intellectual ability, age-related decline, and the role of physical illness has not yet been clarified.

Intellectual Changes

1. Perception of the world is affected by the loss of primary sensory input characterized in aging by changes in vision, hearing, taste, and smell. Sensory deprivation accelerates normal degenerative changes in central nervous system functioning.
2. Memory and learning are affected by accidents, major illness, and physical stressors. A high degree of anxiety leads to forgetfulness and inability to learn.
   a. Long-term memory on the whole is unaffected and appears resistant to aging.
   b. Short-term memory, involved in acquisition, retention, and retrieval of information, is impeded later in life.
3. Cognitive decline in men over 70 years of age has been observed in The Baltimore Longitudinal Study of Aging.
   a. At about 70 years of age, a noticeable reduction in the individual's ability to respond to specific, infrequent, and unpredictable events was noted.
   b. The ability to receive information and promptly interpret it is impaired.
   c. There is a slowing of response to verbal instruction.
   d. Less cognitive loss is experienced by individuals with more education and by professionals who are involved in thinking and reasoning.
   e. As older persons are less prone to risk taking, they may be less likely to respond in a cognitive learning or task situation. Thus, response inhibition related to fear of failure may affect learning.
4. Communication in normal aging is affected by a slight decrease in verbal ability and changes in pitch, loudness, and quality of the voice.
   a. Elderly persons in good physical condition appear to have vocal performance superior to less active peers. Clinical and research efforts are under way to develop skills for preserving the senescent voice.
   b. The older person with dementia demonstrates a general decline in vocabulary and range of expression with the occurrence of repetitious and concrete speech.

   c. Physical impairment may increase the need for nonverbal communication.
5. Although the typical elderly are likely to be somewhat slower at intellectual tasks and somewhat hindered in mastering new problems, they are relatively unimpaired in ordinary intellectual functioning and easily master the daily aspects of living.

Strategies

1. Consider identification of persons with severe short-term memory loss to be a first priority, as they are most at risk of not being able to care for themselves successfully.
2. Assess sensory status before assessing mental status because sensory losses interfere with the client's ability to respond during an interview or during a test.
3. When sensory loss is identified prior to initiating the assessment, do the following:
   a. Provide the client with eyeglasses or a hearing aid if equipment is available.
   b. Position yourself with the light behind you when assessing the visually impaired.
   c. Position yourself in appropriate relation to the hearing-impaired.
   d. Exclude extraneous stimuli such as the radio or television.
   e. Limit the number of other persons in the room.
4. Assess the intellectual dimension by using appropriate interviewing techniques to determine how the elderly understand, communicate, and care for themselves.
   a. The Set Test may be used to evaluate motivation, alertness, concentration, memory, and problem solving (Hays, 1985).
   b. The Set Test may be administered in a short time and may be helpful in identifying early manifestations of cognitive problems.
5. Recognize the impact of the physical, social, emotional, and spiritual dimensions on the elder's intellectual dimensions.
6. When teaching the elderly, do the following:
   a. Stress the benefit of learning the material presented in terms of improved health and lifestyle.
   b. Provide older persons with average cognition more slowly paced learning situations.
   c. Encourage the use of mnemonics for remembering.

THE SOCIAL DIMENSION

1. The social dimension is characterized by losses in relationships, environmental changes, and shifts from independence to dependence.

2. The following theories have been advanced in an attempt to explain how the older person copes with changes in the social dimensions:
   a. *The disengagement theory* proposes that there is a mutual phenomenon that occurs when people and society mutually disengage from each other. This disengagement starts at midlife with the realization of the inevitability of death. The individual looks over priorities and reorders them so that he may be free for expressivity and individuation. The disengagement theory has been supplanted and is no longer well accepted. Individuals who appear to be disengaging should be evaluated for possible withdrawal or depression, since pathology rather than disengagement may be presenting.
   b. *The activity theory* recommends that older adults remain active and engage in societies and activities, make new friends, assume new roles, and develop hobbies to replace discontinued activities. The rationale supporting this theory is that activity promotes well-being and life satisfaction. However, this seems most relevant for the extroverted personality.
   c. *The continuity theory* proposes that personality does not change and that a person's activities become more predictable as he develops his own system of relationships that he can turn to as he ages. The continuity theory, midway between the disengagement theory and activity theory, is becoming more widely accepted.

Factors Affecting the Social Dimension

1. *The Enduring Personality.* Research from The Baltimore Longitudinal Study of Aging suggests that the enduring personality disposition provides continuity to life, enabling the individual to make choices and to adapt to the events that influence aging. This continuity accounts for more stability than change and is predictive of the style that the elder will choose in the aging process.
2. *Social Relationships with Significant Others.* Social relationships change with the decline in the number of significant persons (as a result of death or relocation) and loss of mobility. Often the meaning and value of remaining relationships are increased.
   a. The spousal relationship and the level of satisfaction with the relationship usually continue into old age.
      (1) Some couples experience renewed closeness. A role reversal may occur in the relationship (e.g., husband may assume a more passive role and the wife may assume a more assertive role with increased initiative and responsibility).

(2) For other couples, the stress of retirement, financial concerns, health problems, and disagreement about moving result in increased stress in the relationship.
    b. Widowhood with associated loneliness may occur. The person becomes more introspective and concerned with her own needs. In addition to adjusting to the loneliness, the survior may have to make drastic changes in living arrangements because of physical limitations or financial need.
    c. Since the percentage of female survivors is greater than that of males, there is much greater opportunity for a single man to develop a romantic relationship with a widow that may result in a couple living together or in marriage.
    d. Relationships with children are primarily influenced by personalities and past familial relationships. Proximity, frequency of contact, cultural expectations, degree of dependency, other family responsibilities, health, and financial resources all have their effect.
3. *Finances.* Reduced income will necessitate changes in how the aged provide for basic needs (food, clothing, and shelter) and leisure activities.
4. *Relocation.* Living in their own homes positively influences the well-being and lifestyle of the majority of the elderly.
    a. Moving out of the established home often involves giving up treasured possessions, nearness to familiar meaningful places, independence, privacy, and control. When relocation is necessary, attempts should be made to minimize these losses to promote a more positive social adjustment.
    b. The elder's decision about whether to live alone, in a senior citizen setting, with children, or in an extended care facility is largely dependent on personality, state of health, financial status, availability of housing, and the existence of support systems.
5. *Dependency.* When the shift from independence to dependence is gradual, the accommodation is easier and less threatening for both the provider and the recipient of the care.
    a. Most often the elder is extremely reluctant to give up the independent role valued by our culture, as giving up independence admits to new losses and reduces personal control and choice while placing additional strain on the caretakers.
    b. For an elder with a basic lack of trust in himself and others, the need to assume a dependent role is especially threatening.
    c. Sensory losses, failing memory, or a major environmental change may trigger suspiciousness, mistrust, and eventually paranoia.

Strategies

1. Provide the elder with emotional support and understanding as he reacts to the factors that impinge upon him in the social dimension.
2. Work with the elder, the family, and significant others toward resolution of dependency needs.
3. Help families to recognize and respond appropriately to feelings, defense mechanisms, and adaptive techniques of the elderly.
4. Refer to local community activities or agencies that will assist the older person to meet all his needs. Help the elder to seek information on financial assistance, assistive or adaptive equipment, alternative living arrangements, and community agencies.

THE SPIRITUAL DIMENSION

1. The aged usually have more time to think of spiritual matters, particularly if greater involvement with family, employment, or peer groups is not available.
2. Many of the aged population today were raised in a period when the religious group one belonged to was of primary importance.
3. Memberships in religious organizations are the longest ones maintained by the elderly.

Changes in the Spiritual Dimension

1. The spiritually healthy have identified personal goals and values and spend time and energy in reaching these goals. They make moral and ethical decisions based on these beliefs and values.
2. Those who have not achieved this spiritually healthy state have adapted poorly to life's stresses. They express wishes to undo, redo, or relive the past as they admit shame, regret, or guilt for failing to meet some standard of conduct. Unable to forgive themselves or receive forgiveness, they project blame on others and engage in self-destructive behavior.
3. Older persons who have had ties with a formal religious organization or faith are likely to attempt to strengthen them.
4. Other aged people may not identify themselves with a formal religious group, but they reveal spiritual convictions when discussing inner thoughts and when practicing private rituals.
5. Some individuals who have not yet achieved ego integrity see themselves as worthless, unloved, and abandoned by God.
6. Most older people fear not death itself, but, rather, the process of

dying. They fear loss of control and being unable to obtain help when needed.

7. Many of the elderly, while striving to incorporate their religious outlook and philosophy into their life practices, still attempt to incorporate broader religious views and philosophy into their thinking and are more accepting of variation. These elderly try to understand new spiritual views motivating younger generations.

8. Transcending illness and preoccupation with the body, the elder may enjoy satisfying relationships and creative activity.

9. Peck theorizes that in achieving the final stage of ego transcendence versus ego preoccupation, the elder, through his contributions to society, children, and friendships, is able to achieve a sense of the significance of his actions that will endure beyond his life.

Strategies

1. Arrange access to formal religious services for those elderly who wish to attend.

2. Facilitate listening to religious ceremonies on radio or television if an individual is unable to attend the desired place of worship.

3. Provide for desired observance of dietary laws or other religious or cultural rituals.

4. Encourage the elder to find pride in his accomplishments and those of his generation as he works to establish ego integrity and healthy spirituality.

5. Provide seniors with opportunity for meditating, practicing Hatha Yoga, reciting poetry, singing, or playing a musical instrument to promote release and renewal. (See Chapter 17, under "Community Resources.")

6. Assist elders in regaining feelings of self-worth and self-esteem through altruistic activities.

7. Encourage mentor relationships such as "grandparenting" that provide opportunity for sharing their love, wisdom, and caring.

8. Facilitate sharing that will be rewarding to the elder. Sharing may be through some kind of legacy, such as memories, teaching skills, monetary belongings, or organ donation.

Resource

See Chapter 17, "Making It in the Community."

References

Beck CM, Rawlins RM, Williams SR: Mental Health Psychiatric Nursing. St. Louis: CV Mosby, 1984.

Burggraff V, Donlon B: System by system. American Journal of Nursing 85:973–988, 1985.

Burnside IR: Nursing and the Aged. (2nd ed.) New York: McGraw-Hill, 1987.

Busse EW, Pfeiffer E: Behavior and Adaptation in Late Life. (2nd ed.) Boston: Little, Brown & Co, 1977.

Butler RB, Lewis MI: Aging and Mental Health. (3rd ed.) St. Louis: CV Mosby, 1982.

Cohen S: Sensory changes in the elderly. American Journal of Nursing 81:1851–1880, 1981.

Costa PT Jr, McCrae RR: Aging, the life course, and models of personality. In Normal Human Aging, NIH Pub No. 84-2450. Washington, DC: US Government Printing Office, 1984a.

Costa PT Jr, McCrae RR: Concurrent validation after 20 years: the implications of personality stability for its assessment. In Normal Human Aging, NIH Pub No. 84-2450. Washington, DC: US Government Printing Office, 1984b.

Costa PT Jr, McCrae RR: Personality as a lifelong determinant of well-being. In Normal Human Aging, NIH Pub No. 84-2450. Washington, DC: US Government Printing Office, 1984c.

Costa PT Jr, McCrae RR, Arenberg A: Enduring dispositions in adult males. In Normal Human Aging, NIH Pub No. 84-2450. Washington, DC: US Government Printing Office, 1984a.

Costa PT Jr, McCrae RR, Arenberg A: Recent longitudinal research on personality and aging. In Normal Human Aging, NIH Pub No. 84-2450. Washington, DC: US Government Printing Office, 1984b.

Covington TR, Walker JI: Current Geriatric Therapy. Philadelphia: WB Saunders Co, 1984.

Cummings E, Henry WE: Growing Old: The Process of Disengagement. New York: Basic Books, Inc, 1961.

Erickson EH: Childhood and society. (2nd ed.) New York: WW Norton & Co, 1963.

Forbes EJ, Fitzsimons VM: The Older Adult. St. Louis: CV Mosby, 1981.

Gutman D: The cross-cultural perspective. In Birren J, Schaie W, eds: Handbook of the Psychology of Aging. New York: Van Nostrand Reinhold, 1977.

Havighurst RJ, Munnichs JMA, Neugarten B, Thomas H: Adjustment to Retirement. Netherlands: Royal VanGorcum Ltd, 1972.

Hays A, Borger F: A test in time. American Journal of Nursing 85:1107–1111, 1985.

Hazzard WR: Preventive gerontology. Postgraduate Medicine 74:279–287, 1983.

Henderson ML: Altered presentations. American Journal of Nursing 85:1104–1106, 1985.

Kimmel DC: Adulthood and Aging. New York: John Wiley & Sons, 1974.

Levenson AJ, Santos JF, Hubbard RW: Psychological aspects of aging. In Levenson AJ, ed: An Introduction to Gerontology and Geriatrics. Springfield, Ill: Charles C Thomas, 1984.

Lindemann E: Symptomatology and management of acute grief. American Journal of Psychiatry 101:141–148, 1944.

Maslow A: Toward a Psychology of Being. New York: Van Nostrand Reinhold, 1962.

Murray R, Huelskotter MM, O'Driscoll DL: The Nursing Process in Later Maturity. Englewood Cliffs, NJ: Prentice-Hall, 1980.

Neugarten BL: Personality and aging. In Birren J, Schaie W, eds: Handbook of the Psychology of Aging. New York: Van Nostrand Reinhold, 1977.

O'Hara-Devereaux M, Andrus LH, Scott CD, eds: Eldercare. New York: Grune & Stratton, 1981.

Peck RC: Psychological developments in the second half of life. In Neugarten B, ed: Middle Age and Aging. Chicago: The University of Chicago Press, 1968.

Quilter RE, Giambra LM, Benson PE: Longitudinal age changes in vigilance over an eighteen-year interval. In Normal Human Aging, NIH Pub No. 84-2450. Washington, DC: US Government Printing Office, 1984.

Robertson-Tchabo R, Arenberg D, Costa P Jr: Temperamental predictors of longitudinal change in performance on the Benton Revised Visual Retention Test among seventy-year-old men: An exploratory study. In Normal Human Aging, NIH Pub No. 84-2450. Washington, DC: US Government Printing Office, 1984.

Rossman I: What is normal aging? Geriatric Medicine Today 3(4):37–43, 1984.

Sloane PD: How to maintain the health of the elderly. Geriatrics 39(10):93–104, 1984.

Zoler M: What is aging? Highlights of a 25-year study. Geriatrics 39(8):85–87, 1984.

3

Common Problems

COPING WITH SKIN, HAIR, AND NAIL CHANGES
CONSTIPATION
THERMAL REGULATION
SLEEP DISTURBANCES

1. The elderly experience common health problems as a result of primary aging changes.
2. Appropriate self-care health practices may in many instances delay or minimize these problems.
3. Recognition of the problem, education about the cause, and appropriate intervention to alleviate the problem may markedly improve the quality of life for an elderly client.
4. Failure of response to appropriate interventions should alert the health provider to assess further for underlying diseases that may be intensifying the problems associated with primary aging.

COPING WITH SKIN, HAIR, AND NAIL CHANGES

1. The skin's aging process is the result of a combination of normal physiologic changes and exposure to ultraviolet rays.
2. As the aging skin becomes more vulnerable to dryness, wrinkling, pressure, and trauma, preventive and supportive care become more essential.
3. The appearance of wrinkles and the graying and loss of hair are often threatening to self-esteem in our youth-oriented society.
4. Changes in facial and body hair may be especially threatening to the elder's concept of his sexual identity.

5. With strategies geared toward addressing aging changes in the skin, hair, and nails, the elderly may prevent further damage while maintaining and improving these structures and thereby may strengthen their own self-concept.
6. Dry skin (xerosis) is the most common dermatologic problem experienced by the elderly (see below).

The Skin

PHYSIOLOGY AFFECTING SKIN HYDRATION

1. Skin hydration is determined by the rate of evaporation from the epidermal surface.
2. Loss of moisture from the stratum corneum is retarded by the sebaceous gland secretion of sebum, which coats the epidermal surface by forming an emulsion with sweat.

FACTORS PREDISPOSING TO DRY SKIN

1. Diminished sebaceous secretion as the number and activity of sebaceous glands are reduced with aging.
2. Reduction in the rate of perspiration.
3. Excessive bathing.
4. Exposure to hot water.
5. Use of harsh detergent.
6. Dry indoor heated air. (Dryness occurs when relative ambient humidity falls below 30%.)
7. Forced-air heating currents.
8. Exposure to cold wind.
9. Cumulative effects of exposure to ultraviolet rays.

SIGNS AND SYMPTOMS OF DRY SKIN

1. Skin may appear rough, scaly, flaky, chapped, cracked, and occasionally erythematous.

2. Dry skin is most apparent on extremities and also occurs on sides of trunk and face.
3. Pruritus frequently accompanies the dryness.

STRATEGIES FOR SKIN CARE

1. Teach the client to:
   a. Avoid use of sun lamps and tanning salons.
   b. Sunbathe in the early morning or late afternoon rather than midday.
   c. Apply a sunscreen (oil, cream, gel, or lotion that absorbs or scatters ultraviolet light) to all skin areas not covered by clothing. A sun protection factor (SPF) of 8 to 15 provides extra to maximal protection. The sunscreen should be applied ½ hour before sun exposure and reapplied after swimming or perspiring.
   d. Protect the face and neck from drying effects of wind with hats or scarves.
   e. Prevent drying and thermal injury of hands by wearing rubber gloves when washing dishes and when using cleaning agents or other chemicals.
   f. Use tepid water for bathing, and avoid exposure to hot water.
   g. Avoid use of drying soaps, strong washing detergents, and fabric softeners. Use mild, creamy soaps.
   h. Lubricate skin after bathing with preferred emollient moisturizers containing petrolatum, lanolin, or light mineral oil, which form occlusive and semiocclusive films to reduce evaporation from the skin surface and make rough, dry skin appear smooth.
   i. Avoid adding oil to bath water, as it makes the tub slippery and difficult to clean.
   j. Wear soft, loose-fitting clothing (preferably cotton).
   k. Use humidifiers, water pans on radiators, plants, and hanging laundry to add moisture to the air.
   l. Prevent loss of moist air from a room by closing and caulking cracks in windows.
   m. Check skin daily for minimal trauma, as early diagnosis and treatment of a skin erosion or superficial ulcer may prevent severe damage.
   n. Avoid exposure to excessive heat, as reduced ability to produce sweat increases susceptibility to hyperthermia.
   o. Dress adequately to prevent hypothermia associated with reduced subcutaneous fat.
   p. Avoid prolonged pressure on areas such as the sacrum, where pressure pads are reduced.

    q. Report extensive spontaneous bruising or persistent itching to the health care provider.

    r. Have blemishes and warts evaluated for premalignant or malignant neoplasms.

    s. See a dermatologist yearly if he or she is older than 65 years of age with a history of skin cancer.

    t. Provide daily foot care.

      (1) Inspect skin of feet daily.

      (2) Check feet, particularly toenails, for external lesions.

      (3) Cut toenails straight across and not too near the nail base.

      (4) Trim nails frequently enough to prevent curling, thickening, and development of self-inflicted wounds on feet.

      (5) Wash feet daily in warm water. Dry feet well, particularly between toes; apply a moisturizing lotion; and wear clean dry stockings.

      (6) Wear properly fitting shoes with smooth linings that allow the foot to "breathe." Vinyl shoes are not advisable.

      (7) Avoid walking barefoot, and protect feet from injury.

2. Advise the older woman about the use of cosmetics.

    a. The use of proper cosmetics cleanses the skin, relieves skin problems, covers imperfections, and beautifies.

    b. A mild soap and tepid water should be used to cleanse facial skin rather than cold cream or an oil, which may clog the pores.

    c. By penetrating and filling the crevices caused by wrinkles, moisturizers may mask superficial lines and make the skin smooth and silky to touch.

    d. Facial creams applied sparingly neutralize drying effects of soap and provide a matte finish to the complexion.

    e. As skin tone and hair color change, makeup and hair-coloring shades used in the past may be too rich or strong and may result in a garish effect.

    f. A good source of light and a magnifying mirror are essential for appropriate application of cosmetics when visual acuity is reduced.

    g. Makeup should be applied sparingly to avoid a garish effect.

    h. Planning cosmetic use with a consultant trained in the use of beauty products, such as a beautician or a hairdresser, helps achieve best results.

    i. The expertise of cosmetic consultants and salespersons in stores can be helpful in choosing and applying cosmetics.

    j. Use of unscented and allergy-tested products is best.

    k. The use of hormonal creams and cosmetics should be discontinued for a trial period if pruritus occurs. For persistent dry skin and pruritus, a dermatologist specializing in geriatric skin should be consulted.

The Hair

PRIMARY AGING CHANGES

1. Hair grows more slowly.
2. Hair is finer, as atrophy of follicles results in decreased diameter of the hair shaft.
3. Thinning of hair occurs over scalp, axillae, pubic area, and extremities. Coarse hair is replaced by extremely thin, light-colored hair.
4. Men experience decreased body and facial hair. Women have increased facial hair.
5. Graying usually begins in the third decade. Body hair usually remains pigmented longer.
6. Coarse hair grows in certain areas of the skin, such as in external ear canals.

STRATEGIES FOR GROOMING HAIR

1. Teach the client to:
    a. Brush and comb hair at least twice daily to stimulate circulation and distribute natural oils.
    b. Shampoo hair weekly with mild shampoo containing conditioners.
    c. Use styling mousse, gel, glaze, or hair spray with conditioners to give body and to style hair after shampooing. Only pump hair sprays (not aerosol) should be used, with eyes and nose covered, in a well-ventilated room.
    d. Trim hair about every 8 weeks to maintain hair style and remove split ends.
    e. Consider changing hair style or using a hairpiece or a wig as hair thins over the scalp.
    f. Avoid using hair-coloring products that are hazardous.
    g. Trim coarse hair growing out of ear canals with blunt-tipped scissors.
    h. Protect the scalp from the sun with a cap or sunscreen.
2. Advise the older man about the following:
    a. Daily shaving and regular trimming of mustache, beard, and sideburns enhance appearance.
    b. Lathering creams protect the face against sharp razors.

c. If he is unsteady or has a tremor, an electric razor is advisable.

d. After-shave lotions or moisturizers protect facial skin.

e. Use of alcohol on the skin is contraindicated after shaving.

3. Advise the older woman about the following:

a. Facial hair may be removed by tweezing, waxing, or electrolysis.

b. Facial hair may be bleached with dilute solutions of hydrogen peroxide or lemon juice. Commercial bleaches are available for use on facial hair.

The Nails

PRIMARY AGING CHANGES

1. Nail growth slows down to 0.5 mm (0.125 inch) per week.
2. Brittleness and longitudinal ridging may occur.
3. Nails may fragment at the proximal end.
4. Cuticles increase in thickness and width.
5. Toenails are more likely to thicken and become dull and opaque with longitudinal ridging.

STRATEGIES FOR NAIL CARE

1. Teach the client to:

a. Avoid excessive immersion of hands in water.

b. Wear rubber gloves when washing dishes or doing other chores with cleaning solutions.

c. Use cotton gloves when gardening or working in the yard.

d. Carry out daily nail and cuticle care, including moisturizing, filing, and buffing.

e. Avoid use of nail polish or nail polish remover if nails fragment.

f. Manicure nails weekly to achieve optimum condition.

g. Keep brittle nails short, and avoid use of nail polish and nail polish remover.

CONSTIPATION

1. The elderly tend to have an increased concern with bowel function and believe that each person must have regular bowel movements.
2. Theoretically bowel function is considered normal when there are at least two bowel movements a week. Even one a week may be normal for an individual.

3. The person experiencing constipation complains of less than three bowel movements per week, difficulty in defecating, feelings of incomplete evacuation, and infrequent small or hard stools.
4. Constipation is a functional colonic motor disorder, the etiology of which is multifactorial.

Predisposing Factors

1. Poor toilet habits.
   a. Not allowing for enough time to empty the bowel.
   b. Ignoring the natural urge to defecate.
2. Diet lacking bulk and fluids.
   a. Decreased fiber and fluids lead to decreased stooling.
   b. A shift away from high-fiber foods (vegetables, fruits, and whole grains) to foods high in animal fats and refined sugars (rich desserts and other sweets) and low in fiber occurs.
   c. Lack of interest in eating or difficulty in shopping, preparation, or storage may lead to use of convenience foods, which usually are low in fiber.
3. Cutting back on liquids.
   a. Insufficient water intake may lead to concretion of stool in the lower bowel (fecaloma).
   b. Impaction and ulcers of the colon may result.
4. Lack of exercise.
5. Prolonged bed rest.
6. Laxative and enema misuse (abuse).
   a. About $250 million dollars a year are spent on over-the-counter (OTC) laxatives.
   b. Laxatives and enemas are habit forming and dull sensation for bowel elimination.
   c. Natural emptying mechanisms fail to work as body becomes dependent on laxatives and enemas.
7. Underlying illness (rarely).
   a. Irritable bowel syndrome occurs mostly in the young with periods of constipation alternating with normal or diarrheal stools.
   b. Diverticulitis, producing constipation by intestinal muscle spasm or stricture formation.
   c. Structural tumors, strictures, or volvulus.
   d. Anal stenosis and hemorrhoids, leading to spasm.
   e. Metabolic states such as hypokalemia and hypocalcemia.
   f. Endocrine malfunction such as hypothyroidism.
   g. Diabetes with diabetic autonomic neuropathy.
8. Side effects caused by prescription or OTC drugs used to treat other

conditions. Such drugs include analgesics, opiates, anticholinergics, antidepressants, antacids with aluminum or calcium, antiparkinsonism drugs, and diuretics.

Assessment Guidelines

1. Review general history, physical assessment, and laboratory findings.
2. Data of history for constipation should include the following:
   a. Age of onset.
   b. Description of bowel function: frequency, consistency, size, color, and amount of stool.
3. Assess for precipitating factors.
   a. Toilet habits.
   b. Diet and fluid intake.
   c. Activity and exercise restrictions.
   d. Laxative and enema use.
   e. Illness.
   f. Drug usage for other conditions.

Strategies to Prevent and Relieve Constipation

Teach the client to:
1. Avoid laxatives, follow the recommended regimen, and be patient.
2. Recognize normal bowel function.
3. Use good toilet habits.
   a. Provide a regular time for elimination.
   b. Try toileting after breakfast or dinner for at least 10 minutes.
   c. Try rocking the trunk from side to side or back and forth to stimulate bowel function when toileting.
4. Increase physical activity.
5. Increase daily dietary fiber intake.
   a. Include cooked fruits and vegetables, whole-grain breads, and cereals.
   b. Relieve constipation gradually by adding to food about two to four tablespoons (10 to 20 gm) a day of unprocessed wheat (miller's) bran. Some clients may require eight to ten tablespoons per day.
   c. Make bran (which looks and tastes like sawdust) more palatable by sprinkling it on cereals, mixing it with juice, or adding it to foods.
   d. Start with one tablespoon and then gradually increase intake to minimize initial gastrointestinal distress. The use of bran may

initially cause bloating, gas, and cramps, but these symptoms usually subside in a few weeks.
  e. Maintain fluid intake at eight to ten glasses of water a day.
  f. Bran is not helpful for atonic constipation, as it may add to the problem by increasing bulk in a distended colon.
  g. Cooked cereals of refined wheat, corn, rice, or oatmeal are not helpful in relieving constipation, as they tend to harden stools.
6. Limit the use of laxatives.
  a. Avoid laxative abuse.
  b. Avoid the use of mineral oil because it interferes with absorption of fat-soluble vitamins, may precipitate hydrocarbon pneumonitis if aspirated, and may cause fecal soiling.
  c. Avoid straining.
  d. Bulk laxatives or surfactant laxatives may be employed.
  e. A high-bulk laxative such as psyllium (e.g., Metamucil), a fiber supplement, may be mixed with juice or water by those who cannot tolerate the bran program.
  f. Avoid irritant laxatives, such as cascara, bisacodyl, and castor oil.
7. Limit the intake of antacids (particularly those with aluminum, which inhibit smooth muscle contraction).
8. Consult with a health practitioner if persistent constipation is not relieved by the above regimen, as impaction may result.

THERMAL REGULATION

1. The elderly are more at risk for accidental hypothermia and hyperthermia, as primary aging changes (particularly in those over 70 years of age) reduce the efficiency of physiologic mechanisms for heat conservation and heat reduction.
2. How the elderly adapt to thermal stress is further affected by health, socioeconomic, and environmental factors.
3. Prevention or early treatment of errors in thermoregulation is vital to reducing mortality in the elderly.

Physiology of Thermoregulation

1. A balance between heat production and heat loss results from physiologic and behavioral responses to thermal discomfort.
2. Heat conservation and dissipation are controlled by the autonomic nervous system, which responds to thermal discomfort by dilating or constricting cutaneous blood vessels; stimulating perspiration;

and stimulating increased muscular activity, such as shivering, to generate heat.

3. The central control of physiologic responses in the thermoregulatory center of the hypothalamus responds to stimuli from the following:

    a. Superficial thermoreceptors in the skin that respond to changes in the skin surface temperature.

    b. Deep thermoreceptors in or near the hypothalamus that respond to changes in the temperature of blood flowing through this area.

Accidental Hypothermia

1. Accidental hypothermia occurs when there is an unintentional drop in body temperature to 35° C (95° F) or below.

2. Two and one-half million Americans over age 65 are estimated at risk for hypothermia in their homes in the winter.

3. About 540,000 elderly are thought to enter hospitals yearly with occult hypothermia, i.e., temperatures on admission indicating hypothermia, even though the original reason for admission was not hypothermia.

4. High-risk clients for hypothermia are thin, debilitated elders of low socioeconomic status living in poor housing.

5. Lowered sensitivity to environmental temperature renders the elderly person less likely to take appropriate action to conserve heat or produce more heat even if he is capable.

6. Diagnosis of hypothermia may be missed, as thermometers are rarely shaken down below 35° C (95° F) and digital thermometers rarely measure temperatures below this level.

7. Early diagnosis of hypothermia is vital to reducing mortality, which ranges from 20 to 85%, depending on the following:

    a. Severity of the hypothermia when diagnosed.

    b. Existing disease processes.

    c. Degree of hypotension when admitted.

    d. Length of hypothermia prior to treatment.

    e. Development of complications.

8. The precipitating environmental temperature may be at 18° C (65° F) but is usually below 15° C (60° F).

9. Body temperature that falls below 35° C (95° F) usually continues to fall and results in death if treatment is not initiated.

10. Once an episode of accidental hypothermia is experienced, there is greater likelihood of the condition recurring.

11. Recovery, when core temperature reached normal, in many cases

has been reported even after prolonged asystole that necessitated cardiopulmonary resuscitation.

PREDISPOSING FACTORS

1. Reduced heat production related to:
   a. Decline in basal resting heat production (metabolic rate) with age.
   b. Chronic lower body heat that allows for less loss of body heat before reaching hypothermic levels.
   c. Voluntary or forced inactivity, resulting from illness or falls.
   d. Lack of awareness of cold and absence of shivering because cutaneous sensitivity is reduced.
   e. Diminished physiologic responses to cold stress, such as shivering, extremity vasoconstriction, and increase in metabolic rate.
2. Inability to conserve heat related to:
   a. Poor body insulation, as subcutaneous fat is reduced.
   b. Inability to take normal steps to keep warm by way of clothing or making other adjustments to a cool environment.
   c. Chronic diseases associated with decreased muscular activity, such as Parkinson's disease, rheumatoid arthritis, and cerebrovascular accidents.
   d. Malnutrition and dehydration.
   e. Acute illness, such as infection, heart or renal failure, endocrine dysfunction, and neurologic disorders.
   f. Inflammatory skin disease.
   g. Vasodilation induced by alcohol.
   h. Exposure to an environment below 18° C (65° F).
3. Impaired central thermoregulation related to:
   a. A variety of direct anatomic insults to the brain, such as stroke, subarachnoid hemorrhage, brain tumor, and subdural hematoma.
   b. Acid base imbalance.
   c. Drugs, such as antidepressants, antipyretics, phenothiazines, and sedatives.
   d. Combining drugs such as barbiturates and sedative hypnotics with alcohol.
   e. Defects in the autonomic nervous system that are more common in aging.
4. Psychosocial problems related to:
   a. Lack of finances for or availability of adequate food, clothing, shelter, and fuel.
   b. Living alone.

  c. Lack of knowledge or ability for self-care.
  d. Depression.

ASSESSMENT GUIDELINES

1. Thermometers should be shaken down below 35° C (95° F) for assessing the temperature of the elderly.
2. A thermometer registering from 24° C (75.2° F) should be available to assess clients suspected of having accidental hypothermia.
3. A temperature of less than 35° C (95° F) in a sample of freshly voided urine is a criterion for establishing hypothermia.
4. The following signs and symptoms are suggestive of accidental hypothermia:*
   a. Bloated face; waxy or pink skin.
   b. Irregular, slow heart beat.
   c. Thick voice and slurred speech.
   d. Shallow, very slow breathing (may be barely noticeable).
   e. Weak pulse and low blood pressure.
   f. Confusion, disorientation, or drowsiness.
   g. Uncontrollable shivering.
   h. Trembling of just one side of the body but not shivering.
   i. Stiff muscles; difficulty moving.

5. As the hypothermia worsens, all systems become depressed.
   a. Abdomen, perineum, and back are cold.
   b. The skin has a cadaveric appearance and is covered by purpuric or bullous patches.
   c. Subcutaneous tissues become firm as edema develops.
   d. Pupils dilate.
   e. The electroencephalogram (EEG) becomes flat.

STRATEGIES TO PREVENT ACCIDENTAL HYPOTHERMIA

1. Be alert to presence of risk factors and to symptoms of hypothermia.
2. Shake the thermometer down to 34.4° C (94° F) when assessing the temperature or use a digital thermometer that registers temperatures below 34.4° C (94° F).
3. Use objective measurements when assessing for hypothermia, as subjective thermal sensitivity in the elderly may be reduced by pri-

---

*Adapted from Accidental Hypothermia, NIH Publication No. 86-1464.

mary or secondary aging changes or by the actual onset of hypothermia.

4. Teach the elderly and their families (particularly those with known risk factors) to:

a. Maintain ambient temperature.

   (1) Residential temperature should be maintained at least at 18° C (65° F).

   (2) A thermometer separate from the thermostat should be checked at least daily to evaluate the temperature of the home.

   (3) Fuel-assistance programs may provide funds for fuel.

   (4) Inadequate heat in a rented apartment should be reported to the appropriate regulatory agency.

   (5) Insulation should be checked for adequacy, and sources of drafts should be eliminated. An energy audit may be requested to identify ways to prevent heat loss from the home. Local electric companies may provide audits as a free service.

   (6) If a fireplace is used in extremely cold weather, the dampers should be closed immediately after the fire is extinguished to reduce heat loss.

   (7) A quartz heating unit is safer and less expensive to operate than oil or kerosene space heaters when additional heating is needed.

b. Keep warm and dry with appropriate clothing.

   (1) Additional indoor clothing, particularly covering exposed areas of the hands, feet, and head, is desirable.

   (2) Wearing a hat or head covering indoors and a bedcap at night prevents heat loss, as two thirds of body heat is lost through the head.

   (3) Layered clothing adds insulation.

   (4) Exposure to wind and cold temperatures when outdoors can be avoided by adequate clothing and limiting the time spent outside. Errands are best done during warmer parts of the day.

c. Exercise to improve circulation and heat production.

   (1) Frequent periods of even mild exercise in a chair are beneficial.

   (2) Periodically shifting position avoids immobility.

d. Maintain adequate nutrition and fluid intake.

   (1) Alcohol should not be used for warming, as it causes gastric and peripheral dilatation with subsequent heat loss.

e. Review the medication regimen periodically to avert untoward drug effects on thermoregulation, and take appropriate preventive action.

5. Check isolated elderly persons daily, particularly for falls, as hypothermia may result from immobilization and exposure.

STRATEGIES TO PREVENT FURTHER DROP IN CORE TEMPERATURE

1. If the client's temperature is 35° C (96° F) or below, contact a physician or call an ambulance to take the patient for emergency help.
2. While awaiting help, keep the client warm and dry.
   a. Remove wet clothing.
   b. Wrap the client in a warm dry blanket.
   c. Lie close to the client to provide additional heat.
   d. Do not rub the client's limbs because this may cause vasodilation and result in further heat loss.
   e. Handle the unconscious client gently to minimize cardiac arrhythmias.
   f. If the client is conscious, offer warm drinks.
   g. Do not provide alcohol, as it causes vasodilation and increases heat loss.
   h. If the client is able to move, encourage isometric exercises.

TREATMENT FOR MODERATE TO SEVERE ACCIDENTAL HYPOTHERMIA

1. Client usually hospitalized.
2. Active external rewarming.
3. Core rewarming.
4. Treatment of cardiovascular, renal, and endocrine disease.
5. Supportive care.

Heat-Related Illnesses

1. Interference with normal loss of heat can result in serious changes in organ function and temperature regulation.
2. The frail elderly over age 70 and the obese elderly with excessive subcutaneous insulation are most vulnerable to environmental conditions because their ability to lose heat by sweat evaporation is reduced.
3. Heat stroke occurs in response to a disturbance in the body's heat-regulating mechanism and to prolonged exposure to intense heat.
4. The incidence and mortality rate of heat stroke in individuals over

age 50 have been found to be three to eight times greater than in younger people.
5. Heat exhaustion develops over a relatively long time as the body is exposed to excessive heat and is depleted of salt and fluids.
6. Distinguishing between *heat stroke* and *heat exhaustion* is most important, as the former is much more serious and is treated differently.

PREDISPOSING FACTORS

1. Reduced efficiency in heat reduction related to:
   a. Inability to compensate hemodynamically with tachycardia to perfuse skin for needed heat loss.
   b. Reduced ability to acclimatize by sweating. Sweating takes longer to initiate, as the elderly have fewer active sweat glands, and a longer time is required to activate those remaining.
   c. Electrolyte disturbances from reduced salt or fluid intake.
   d. Illness, such as circulatory disease (heart and stroke) or diabetes.
   e. Obesity.
   f. Poor preconditioning for sports.
2. Environmental conditions.
   a. Several days of high humidity and temperature.
   b. Low air flow.
   c. Use of belladonna-like drugs.

STRATEGIES TO PREVENT HEAT-RELATED ILLNESSES IN HOT, HUMID WEATHER

1. Teach the client to:
   a. Avoid direct exposure to the sun.
   b. Avoid excessive physical activity.
   c. Take more frequent rest periods.
   d. Wear light-colored airy clothing made of natural fibers to facilitate sweating. Vinyl shoes should not be worn.
   e. Eat a high-carbohydrate, low-protein diet, with added fluids and salt.
   f. Use air conditioners and fans when possible or air-conditioned community shelters.
   g. Apply to government-funded programs for assistance in paying for emergency repairs to a cooling system or in paying high energy bills.

Assessment Guidelines for Heat Stroke

1. Signs and symptoms of heat stroke include the following:
   a. Initially: headache, dizziness, weakness, and nausea.
   b. Rapid pulse.
   c. Flushed skin.
   d. Increased restlessness and irritability.
   e. Reduced interest in activity.
2. Critical state suddenly appears.
   a. Flushed face becomes ashen.
   b. Rectal temperature rises to 40° C (104° F) or higher.
   c. Skin is hot and dry with absence of perspiration.
   d. Breathing is labored.
3. If the client is not cooled promptly, collapse, coma, and convulsions ensue.

Strategies for Heat Stroke

1. Lower the client's temperature.
   a. Remove all clothing except for underclothes.
   b. Wet the client with cool water.
   c. Direct air flow from fans over the client.
   d. Apply packs of crushed ice to the head and back of the neck.
   e. Provide iced drinks by mouth.
   f. Administer cold-water enemas.
2. After temperature returns to normal, bed rest is indicated for a few days in a cool, well-ventilated room.

Assessment Guidelines for Heat Exhaustion*

1. Signs and symptoms of heat exhaustion include the following:
   a. An insidious or sudden appearance with severe weakness, nausea, giddiness, gastrointestinal upset, dizziness, and faintness.
   b. Thirst, oliguria, dysphagia, and dry mucous membranes are better guidelines to use in assessing for hydration.
2. Temperature may be normal or below normal.
3. Heat cramps—painful tonic spasms of skeletal muscle—may occur abruptly.
4. If heat exhaustion remains untreated, collapse with central nervous system depression may occur.

---

*Anhidrotic with or without salt or water depletion.

STRATEGIES FOR TREATING HEAT EXHAUSTION

1. Have the client rest in bed away from heat.
2. Provide cool liquids for drinking.
3. Arrange to provide cool sponge baths.

SLEEP DISTURBANCES

1. Complaints about sleep increase with age and have been found to be in 25 to 40% of individuals over 65 years of age.
2. Although routine use of sedative hypnotic medications is contraindicated for sleep disorders, their use increases in the elderly.
3. Sleep disorders that are most common in the elderly are:
   a. Disorders of initiating and maintaining sleep.
   b. Disorders of the sleep-wake schedule.
   c. Disorders of excessive somnolence.

Physiology and Function of Sleep

1. Theoretically, sleep is attributed to reduced activity of the reticuloactivating system resulting from neuronal fatigue or inhibition by other brain centers.
2. Sleep is essential as a restorative process.
   a. Tissue repair and renewal of epithelial and specialized cells, such as brain tissue, take place.
   b. Review and organization of the day's activities occur.
   c. During rapid eye movement (REM) sleep, important information is stored and trivial data are discarded.
   d. Problems are sometimes solved, and new insights are gained.
   e. Sorting of emotions and a clearing of the mind during dreaming prepare the mind for fresh input of the next day.
3. Extended wakefulness is frequently associated with progressive malfunction of the mind and of behavioral activities of the central nervous system.
4. The circadian cycle of wakefulness and sleep improves the somatic function of the body.
   a. During wakefulness, there is enhanced sympathetic activity with increased numbers of impulses to the skeletal musculature that increase muscle tone.
   b. During sleep, sympathetic activity decreases while parasympathetic activity increases. Arterial blood pressure falls, pulse rate decreases, skin vessels dilate, muscles relax, and gastrointestinal

activity may increase. The overall basal metabolic rate of the body falls 10 to 20%.

5. Each stage of the sleep cycle is thought to be essential to health.

Stages of the Sleep Cycle

Non–Rapid Eye Movement (NREM) Sleep

1. Alpha state
    a. As the threshold of the sleeper goes down, the sleeper enters the alpha state.
    b. Alpha rhythm brain waves begin.
    c. After the alpha state is reached, many people experience a sudden jerking (myoclonic jerk) that wakens them. This signals neural changes and a sudden burst of activity in the brain. Usually the sleeper jerks half awake and then enters stage 1.
2. Stage 1
    a. Muscles relax and the pulse slows. If the sleeper should awaken, he is likely to feel that he has not slept.
    b. Unawakened, the sleeper enters stage 2.
3. Stage 2
    a. The EEG tracings show a burst of activity as the brain waves grow larger.
    b. In transitional sleep, the sleeper's eyes roll from side to side.
    c. If eyes are open, they do not see.
    d. After about 20 minutes, stage 3 is reached.
4. Stage 3
    a. Brain waves are large and slow.
    b. Muscles are relaxed.
    c. Breathing is even.
    d. The sleeper enters stage 4, or delta sleep.
5. Stage 4
    a. Delta sleep is deepest and lasts longer in the first part of the night.
    b. After about 20 minutes of delta sleep, the sleeper ascends near waking, then goes into REM sleep.

Rapid Eye Movement (REM) Sleep

1. The sleeper dreams during the first 85% pf REM sleep.
2. The heart beat is irregular, blood pressure fluctuates, and brain waves resemble those of a waking person.

3. The first REM sleep lasts 10 minutes; then the cycle begins again, with the sleeper entering stage 2, and repeats about every 30 minutes.
4. Toward morning there is less NREM sleep and more REM sleep.
5. A person deprived of REM sleep becomes hostile, irritable, and anxious.

Alterations in Sleep

1. The initial cycle of stages 1, 2, 3, and 4 remains similar throughout life.
   a. Stage 4, delta sleep (restorative sleep) is reduced.
      (1) Decreased slow-wave sleep is associated with increased complaints of sleep disturbance with aging.
      (2) A person deprived of delta sleep seems depressed, apathetic, and lethargic.
   b. The amount of REM sleep remains fairly constant throughout life.
      (1) A decrease in REM sleep is associated with reduced intellectual functioning, as in organic mental disorder, or with reduced cerebral blood flow.
      (2) The dreams of older people during REM sleep reflect concerns about losses and death.
2. Sleep time stays the same or is reduced in the elderly.
   a. Sleep time averages 6½ to 7 hours, partially at night and partially distributed during day naps.
   b. The anxious elder has difficulty falling asleep, but total sleep time is not diminished.
   c. Women tend to take naps only when they are not fully employed.
   d. Men tend to increase the number of daily naps whether or not they are employed.
   e. Napping is more common in the elderly with chronic physical illness that disrupts normal sleep.
3. The sleep efficiency ratio of total sleep time to time spent in bed is reduced.
4. The time from the decision to sleep to onset of sleep (latency period) is increased to 20 minutes or more.
5. There is difficulty maintaining sleep with increased likelihood of waking three to four times, especially during latter part of the night. Women have more difficulty maintaining sleep at night.
6. Factors that may alter the quality of sleep include the following:
   a. Change in the sleeping environment and noise.
   b. Ruminative insomnia experienced by some elderly as they are

kept awake at night trying to solve problems not perceived with anxiety during waking.
   c. Fear of
      (1) Not getting to sleep.
      (2) What may happen during sleep.
      (3) Loss of consciousness.
      (4) Death during sleep.
      (5) Nightmares.

Sleep Disorders in the Elderly (Insomnias)

1. *Insomnia* is the subjective experience of lack of sleep associated with complaints of difficulty in falling asleep, maintaining sleep, or early awakening.
   a. Some elderly feel they have not slept because periods of light sleeping and wakefulness have fused.
   b. Others have difficulty in judging time at night and overestimate wake time.
   c. Women tend to be more insomnious than men, possibly owing to hormonal factors.
2. *Transient insomnia* is precipitated by acute short-term stress, such as hospitalization for elective surgery or air travel to a different time zone.
   a. Insomnia lasts only 3 to 5 days.
   b. Optimally, the reasons for sleep loss are explored to identify the problems and to relieve the stress.
   c. Sleep loss may be tolerated or reduced by using good sleep hygiene.
   d. At most, drug therapy should be used for only 1 to 3 nights.
3. *Short-term insomnia* is precipitated by a situational stress, such as acute personal loss often related to work, family, or illness.
   a. Insomnia lasts up to 3 weeks.
   b. Good sleep hygiene, relaxation techniques, and sleep-promoting medications may be helpful.
4. *Chronic or long-term insomnia* may be caused by pain, dyspnea, pruritus, nocturia, anxiety, depression, or mania. All are symptoms of underlying medical or psychiatric illnesses that interfere with sleep.
   a. A thorough physical and psychosocial assessment is warranted to identify the cause to ensure appropriate treatment (e.g., insomnia from dementia occurs as a result of reduced REM and stage 4 sleep, decreased total sleep time, and increased time spent awake at night).

    b. Hypnotics would be contraindicated for controlling dementia-induced insomnia, as they would further deprive the client of REM sleep.

5. *Persistent psychophysiologic insomnia* not related to an identifiable stress is experienced by some elders.
    a. High levels of anxiety and tension are experienced without classic psychologic conflicts.
    b. Nondrug strategies are considered the most appropriate approach to psychophysiologic insomnia.
    c. A short trial period (1 month) may be instituted with sleep-promoting medication.
    d. Referral to a sleep clinic for further evaluation is appropriate for patients free of major medical or psychiatric problems and for whom behavioral treatments and a short trial of sleep-promoting medication have not met with success.

6. *Rebound insomnia* occurs when tolerance to hypnotic sedatives leads to increased drug usage with a cycle of higher doses and successive periods of insomnia.
    a. Sudden termination of the drug leads to a withdrawal syndrome with anxiety-provoking dreams and rebound insomnia. Gradual withdrawal of hypnotics over a 7- to 10-day period to prevent withdrawal syndrome is indicated.
    b. Rebound insomnia may also accompany the use of alcohol, an ineffective hypnotic.
        (1) A mild withdrawal period occurs 3 to 4 hours after sleep starts.
        (2) Progressive disintegration of sleep patterns with persistent sleep interruptions and fragmented and reduced REM sleep characterizes drinking periods.

7. *Disorders of the sleep-wake schedule* occur with an irregular sleep-wake pattern or a delayed or advanced sleep phase syndrome.
    a. Improved sleep patterns have been achieved with chronotherapy, which involves helping the individual better synchronize circadian rhythms and achieve an appropriate sleep pattern.

Dysfunctions Associated with Sleep

The nurse should be alert to sleep dysfunctions, as often the client may be unaware that he is experiencing them.

1. *Sleep apnea* is an abnormal event with marked reduction or cessation of air flow during sleep.
    a. The cause may be an anatomic obstruction within the upper

airway, a central mechanism that stops diaphragmatic movement (central apnea sleep syndrome), or both.

  b. Sleep apnea has been found in as many as 28% of elderly persons in one study.

  c. The condition ranges from mild to severe and may be fatal.

  d. With the onset of REM sleep, breathing may stop for 10 seconds to 2 minutes. Sleep lightens, and the individual usually takes a breath or wakens.

  e. Excessive sleepiness, depression, and irritability are usually associated with upper airway obstruction.

  f. Insomnia is usually the complaint associated with central apnea sleep syndrome.

  g. Sleep apnea is more common in obese elderly males.

  h. Sleep partners may complain of loud excessive snoring or may note an absence of breathing during sleep.

  i. The report of the sleep partner may be the only means of making the diagnosis.

  j. Numerous treatments for obstructive apnea include permanent tracheostomy, uvulopalatopharyngoplasty, mandibular lengthening operations, a tongue-retaining device designed to hold the tongue slightly forward while sleeping, nocturnal oxygen, weight loss, and nonintervention.

2. *Nocturnal myoclonus*, or intense muscle jerks, occurs primarily in the legs (every 20 seconds).

  a. This sign is unnoticed by the client but may be reported by the sleep partner.

  b. As a result of mini-arousals and sleep pattern disruption, the client complains of fatigue and daytime sleepiness.

  c. The condition may respond to medication such as propoxyphene.

3. *Restless legs syndrome* occurs with the complaint of an uncomfortable creeping sensation in the legs that necessitates getting up and moving around for relief.

  a. A severe insomnia results.

  b. Medical treatment with vitamin E and tryptophan has resulted in limited success.

4. *Hypersomnia* occurs with an increase in total 24-hour sleep and difficulty in arousal.

  a. This condition is less common than insomnia but more serious.

  b. Sleep apnea syndrome may be a precipitating factor.

  c. Use of central nervous system depressants, antihistamines, and antihypertensives may cause hypersomnia and impair cognitive functioning.

SUGGESTED TREATMENTS FOR SLEEP
DYSFUNCTIONS

1. Improvement of sleep hygiene.
2. Specific therapies (as mentioned above).
3. Psychotherapy.
4. Biofeedback.
5. Chronotherapy.
6. Medication.

Pharmacologic Treatment for Sleep Disturbances

1. Advantages.
   a. Client experiences subjective feeling of having slept well.
   b. Symptomatic relief of insomnia helps break a cycle and leads to increased functioning.
2. Disadvantages.
   a. All drugs cause systemic alterations in the architecture of sleep (e.g., decreased amounts of REM and delta sleep).
   b. Drugs raise the threshold for arousal from sleep.
   c. Increasing drug dosage leads to a vicious circle and severe addiction problems. Withdrawal should then be accomplished in the hospital setting.
3. Contraindications.
   a. Sleep apnea or nocturnal myoclonus.
   b. Daytime sleepiness and heavy snoring, unless it has been determined that the client does not have a primary sleep disorder.
   c. Dementia.
   d. Potentially suicidal clients outside the hospital setting.
4. Strategies to minimize untoward effects of sleeping medications.
   a. Use smaller doses for older clients.
   b. Avoid repeat doses.
   c. Consider the potential for tolerance, addiction, habituation, abuse, physical and psychologic dependence, and side effects.
   d. Restrict to short-term treatment of insomnia.
   e. Caution the client against driving, as sleeping pills may have a prolonged effect.
   f. Wean the client from sedative hypnotics gradually to prevent REM sleep rebound, nightmares, agitation, and seizures.
   g. Evaluate on the basis of the client's feeling better and functioning better against the risks.

h. Be alert to any confusional reactions and depressed cardiac and respiratory functions in the client.

i. Check that the client has no more than 2 weeks' supply, as drugs do not seem to work longer than a 2-week period. Drugs may be withdrawn and then reinstituted at the same dosage.

Assessment Guide for Sleep Disturbances

1. General history, physical assessment, and review of laboratory findings.
2. Data of sleep history, including a review of the client's usual sleeping habits:
   a. Bedtime routines.
   b. Waking schedule.
   c. A specific description of the sleep complaint: difficulty falling asleep, frequent wakening, early morning arousals.
   d. Presence of pain, dyspnea, pruritus, or nocturia.
   e. Existence of psychosocial problems, such as role loss, bereavement, grief, retirement, isolation, boredom, anxiety, loneliness, sexual deprivation, and depression.
   f. Use of prescription and nonprescription drugs, cigarettes, and alcohol.
   g. Description of the client's sleep from family or sleep partner.

Strategies for Promoting Sleep

Help the client improve sleeping, eating, drinking, exercise, and relaxation habits.

SLEEP

1. Advise the client to establish regular sleep habits, as a regular arousal time and bedtime are important in establishing circadian rhythms.
   a. Acquire an accurate assessment of daily sleep needs. Include time spent napping as part of total sleep in a 24-hour period.
   b. Do not allow time in bed to become substantially greater than total sleep time.
   c. Limit daytime naps. Avoid naps in the early afternoon or evening.
   d. Occupy oneself with some restful activity, such as reading or watching television, rather than fighting wakefulness.
2. Advise the client to maintain an environment conducive to sleep.
   a. Avoid the bedroom except at night.
   b. Keep the bedroom cool rather than warm.

   c. Use an electric blanket if extra covers are required. An electric blanket often feels lighter in weight.

   d. Keep bedclothes clean and neat.

   e. Use an adequate number of pillows to prevent dyspnea and arousal.

   f. Use a mattress that is not so soft that it may contribute to orthopedic problems but not so hard that it leads to more body movements during sleep and more frequent wakenings.

   g. Avoid noise and frequent changes in the environment.

EATING AND DRINKING

Advise the client to:

1. Avoid heavy dinner meals.
2. Eat a high-protein dinner, as deprivation of amino acids has been associated with a drop in REM sleep.
3. Eat a light snack at bedtime. A glass of milk is recommended, as milk contains tryptophan, which may promote sleep.
4. Avoid tea, coffee, cocoa, and carbonated drinks that contain caffeine. Caffeine-stimulation peak occurs 2 to 4 hours after ingestion.
5. Avoid alcohol at bedtime; although one drink may help induce sleep, mild withdrawal 3 to 4 hours later may cause a wakening.

EXERCISE AND RELAXATION

Advise the client to:

1. Exercise regularly to release energy and mental tensions but not to exercise too strenuously at bedtime.
2. Use relaxation techniques, such as relaxing deep muscles, tensing and relaxing muscles, practicing Hatha Yoga, and meditating.
3. Take a warm bath before bedtime.

ADDITIONAL STRATEGIES

Advise the client to:

1. Discuss fears related to sleeping with a support person.
2. Take an analgesic at bedtime if arthritic pain interrupts sleep.
3. Take an antiparkinsonian drug at bedtime that may prevent rigidity of Parkinson's disease, which interrupts sleep.
4. Avoid regular use of sedative hypnotics because rebound insomnia may occur.
5. Refer insomniacs with persistent sleep disorders for physical and

psychosocial assessment to rule out pathology. Following assessments, referral to a sleep clinic may be appropriate.

6. Refer for behavioral therapy those who associate sleeplessness with the bedroom and bring their anxieties with them to bed. Behavioral therapy is helpful in reconditioning individuals to associate the bedroom with sleep and not with worry.

References

Coping with Skin, Hair, and Nail Changes

Cornell RC: Aging and the skin. Geriatric Medicine Today 5:26–37, 1986.
Dotz W, Berman B: The facts about treatment of dry skin. Geriatrics 38(9):92–100, 1983.
Palmer MH: Assisting the older woman with cosmetics. Journal of Gerontological Nursing 8:340–342, 1982.
Tonnesen MG, Weston WL: Aging of skin. In Schrier RW, ed: Clinical Internal Medicine in the Aged. Philadelphia: WB Saunders Co, 1982.

Constipation

Jahnigen DW, La Force FM: Little things. In Schrier RW, ed: Clinical Internal Medicine in the Aged. Philadelphia: WB Saunders Co, 1982.
Sklar M: Gastrointestinal diseases. In Calkins E, Davis PJ, Ford AB, eds: The Practice of Geriatrics. Philadelphia: WB Saunders Co, 1986.

Thermal Regulation

Accidental hypothermia. In NIH Pub No. 86-1464. Washington, DC: US Government Printing Office, 1985.
Besdine RW: Accidental hypothermia: The body's energy crisis. Geriatrics December 1979, pp 51–54.
Kolanowski AM, Gunter LM: Thermal stress and the aged. Journal of Gerontological Nursing 9(1):13–15, 1983.
Navari RM, Sheey TW: Hypothermia. In Calkins E, Davis PJ, Ford AB, eds: The Practice of Geriatrics. Philadelphia: WB Saunders Co, 1986.

Sleep Disturbances

Ancoli-Israel S, Kripke DF: Sleep and aging. In Calkins E, Davis PJ, Ford AB, eds: The Practice of Geriatrics. Philadelphia: WB Saunders Co, 1986.
Blazer D: Sleep disorders in the elderly. In McCue J, Stead EA, eds: Medical Care of the Elderly. Lexington, Mass: DC Heath & Co, 1983.
Consensus Development Conference Summary, Vol 4, No. 10. Drugs and Insomnia. 621-132:3332. Washington, DC: US Government Printing Office, 1984.
Driscoll CE, Carter BL: Insomnia. In Rakel RE, ed: Conn's Current Therapy. Philadelphia: WB Saunders Co, 1986.
Lerner R: Sleep loss in the aged: Implications for nursing practice. Journal of Gerontological Nursing 8:323–326, 1982.
Pollack CP: Sleep disorders and sleep dysfunctions in the elderly. In Rossman I, ed: Clinical Geriatrics. Philadelphia: JB Lippincott, 1986.
Schirmer MS: When sleep won't come. Journal of Gerontological Nursing 9:16–21, 1983.
Willis J: On making it through the night. FDA Consumer, HHS Pub No. 80-395. Washington, DC: US Government Printing Office, 1980.

4

Meeting the Nutritional Needs of the Elderly

NUTRITIONAL GUIDELINES
FACTORS AFFECTING EATING
PROMOTING NUTRITION

1. Early identification and fulfillment of nutritional needs are essential goals for offsetting declines, stabilizing chronic conditions, and preventing disease during the aging process.
   a. The elderly in particular should be monitored for malnutrition, which develops insidiously, tends to be overlooked, and causes health problems such as anemia and osteoporosis.
   b. Early recognition of malnutrition allows for slow dietary modifications, which are associated with increased compliance.
2. In contrast to the large number of nutritional studies based on the institutionalized elderly (about 5% of the geriatric population), there are far fewer studies on the nutritional needs of the elderly in the community.
   a. Because of the paucity of studies, differing outcomes, and controversial opinions, the establishment of the specific nutrient requirements for the elderly has been delayed.
   b. There is agreement that the elderly experience a reduction in energy requirements that necessitates the ingestion of nutrient-dense food and a drastic reduction in low-density foods.
3. Dietary planning should take into account differences in individual requirements influenced by variation in age, genetic constitution, cultural habits, religious observances, and behavioral patterns.
   a. The uniqueness of the individual and his needs is demonstrated

by elders who have been known to maintain health on what appear to be markedly restricted diets.

4. Planning for nutrient intake must be geared to minimize the high risk for food-drug interactions in the elderly.
5. Increased nutrient intake is required for the elder experiencing surgery, chronic illness, or stress.
6. The nurse must be sensitive to and knowledgeable about the client's physical and psychosocial developmental status, position on the health-illness continuum, and environmental constraints as the assessment proceeds and appropriate strategies are initiated with the elderly, their families, and significant others.

NUTRITIONAL GUIDELINES

Recommended Daily Dietary Allowances

1. The recommended daily dietary allowances of the Food and Nutrition Board of the National Academy of Sciences—National Research Council indicate the essential nutrients considered adequate for meeting identified dietary needs for most healthy people in the United States (Table 4–1).
   a. Healthy individuals whose nutritional intake is somewhat above or equal to the recommended daily allowances (RDAs) are considered nutritionally sound.
   b. Individuals whose nutrient intake is below the RDAs may not be nutrient deficient but are considered at risk for nutrient defi-

Table 4–1. *Recommended Daily Dietary Allowances*†*

Age (Years)	Weight		Height		Protein (g)	Fat-soluble Vitamins			Vitamin C (mg)	Thiamin (mg)
	kg	*lb*	*cm*	*in*		*Vitamin A (μg RE)‡*	*Vitamin D (μg)§*	*Vitamin E (mg α TE)‖*		
Men 51 +	70	154	178	70	56	1000	5	10	60	1.2
Women 51 +	55	120	163	64	44	800	5	8	60	1.0

*From Food and Nutrition Board, National Research Council: Recommended Dietary Allowances. (9th ed.) Washington, DC: National Academy of Sciences, 1980.

†The allowances are intended to provide for individual variations among most normal persons as they live in the United States under usual environmental stresses. Diets should be based on a variety of common foods in order to provide other nutrients for which human requirements have been less well defined.

‡Retinol equivalents. 1 Retinol equivalent = 1 μg retinol or 6 μg β-carotene.

§As cholecalciferol, 10 μg cholecalciferol = 400 IU vitamin D.

‖α-tocopherol equivalents, 1 mg d-α-tocopherol = 1 α TE.

Table continued on following page

Table 4–1.   *Recommended Daily Dietary Allowances (Continued)*

Age (Years)	Water-soluble Vitamins					Minerals					
	Ribo-flavin (mg)	Niacin (mg NE)¶	Vitamin B₆ (mg)	Folacin (µg)	Vitamin B₁₂ (µg)	Calcium (mg)	Phos-phorus (mg)	Magne-sium (mg)	Iron (mg)	Zinc (mg)	Iodine (µg)
Men 51+	1.4	16	2.2	400	3.0	800	800	350	10	15	150
Women 51+	1.2	13	2.0	400	3.0	800	800	300	10	15	150

¶1 NE (niacin equivalent) is equal to 1 mg of niacin or 60 mg of dietary tryptophan.

ciency and associated complications if intake remains below the RDAs for a prolonged period of time.

2. The RDAs do not include the special nutritional needs of individuals with health problems, nor do they allow for the special needs of the elderly.
3. The 1980 RDAs for protein and vitamins and minerals set forth for people aged 51 and older is an extrapolation from nutrient needs of younger healthy adults and may not adequately identify the nutrients needs of the older adult.
4. Pending resolution of controversial issues in nutrient requirements, revision of the RDAs by the National Research Council Food and Nutrition Board has been delayed.

Height and Weight and Recommended Energy Intake

1. The 1980 RDAs are supplemented by a table of mean heights and weights and recommended energy intake (Table 4–2).
2. Particular needs of the elderly are acknowledged by the division of adults into two groups: those 51 to 75 years of age and those 76 years of age and older. A reduction in energy intake is recommended for each group of older adults.
3. In addition to age and sex, the extent of physical activity should be considered in determining energy requirements for each individual.
4. Desirable weights for heights are shown in Table 4–3. Approximate ideal body weight may also be calculated as follows:
   a. Ideal body weight for men equals 106 pounds for first 5 feet of height plus 6 pounds for every inch over 5 feet (±10%).

Table 4–2.   *Mean Heights and Weights and Recommended Energy Intake**

Category	Age (Years)	Weight (Pounds)	Height (Inches)	Energy Needs (with Range) (Calories)	
Men	51–75	154	70	2400	(2000–2800)
	76+	154	70	2050	(1650–2450)
Women	51–75	120	64	1800	(1400–2200)
	76+	120	64	1600	(1200–2000)

*Adapted from Food and Nutrition Board, National Research Council: Recommended Dietary Allowances, 9th ed. Washington, D.C.: National Academy of Sciences, 1980.

Table 4–3. *Suggested Desirable Weights for Heights and Ranges for Adults**

Height† (Inches)	Weight‡ (Pounds)			
	Men		*Women*	
58			102	(92–119)
60			107	(96–125)
62	123	(112–141)	113	(102–131)
64	130	(118–148)	120	(108–138)
66	136	(124–156)	128	(114–146)
68	145	(132–166)	136	(122–154)
70	154	(140–174)	144	(130–163)
72	162	(148–184)	152	(138–173)
74	171	(156–194)		
76	181	(164–204)		

*From Food and Nutrition Board, National Research Council: Recommended Dietary Allowances, 9th ed. Washington, DC: National Academy of Sciences, 1980.
†Without shoes.
‡Without clothes. Average weight ranges in parentheses.

   b. Ideal weight for women equals 100 pounds for first 5 feet plus 5 pounds for every inch over 5 feet ($\pm 10\%$).

5. Longevity seems to be better predicted by a body weight greater than 10 to 25% considered ideal in the past. This suggests that thinner people may be less healthy, as they limit essential nutrients in their diet to maintain low weight.

6. As reported by The National Health and Nutrition Examination Survey, the weight peak for men is between ages 45 to 55 and for women it is between ages 55 to 65. Weight then falls, but the fall is more gradual in women. After peaking in the early forties, height is reduced about 1 cm (0.4 inch) per decade, accelerating in women.

Daily Food Guide

1. Nutritionists and home economists have translated the RDAs into specifications of the kinds and amounts of foods needed for daily consumption to meet nutritional needs.
   a. The leader nutrients have been identified as protein, carbohydrates, fats, vitamin A, vitamin C, thiamin, riboflavin, niacin, calcium, and iron.
   b. When the proper amount of the ten leader nutrients is consumed in the daily diet, the approximately 40 other nutrients needed are usually obtained as part of the identified nutrient food groups.
   c. Adherence to this daily dietary pattern by a healthy individual ensures an adequate intake of nutrients and trace elements (89.7 to 99.9% of the leader nutrients in 64.4% of the calories).

2. The following daily dietary pattern is advocated in guiding daily food intake to ensure an adequate intake of essential nutrients for a healthy individual:

milk and milk products	at least two servings
fruits and vegetables	four servings
meat and meat equivalents	two servings
grain and grain products	four servings
others*	

Nutritional Recommendations

In accordance with the U.S. Senate Select Committee on Nutrition and Human Needs, Dietary Goals, of 1977 and the results of research in the field of geriatric nutrition, the following recommendations have been made and are considered pending the next revision of the RDAs.

CALORIES

1. Ideal body weight should be maintained on a diet of 30 calories per kilogram of body weight with consideration for variation in body build and level of activity. This recommendation takes into consideration the 2% decrease in basal (resting) metabolic rate per decade and a reduction of activity of 200 kcal/day for men and women between 51 to 75 years of age and a reduction of 500 kcal/day for men over 75 years and 400 kcal/day for women over 75 years of age.
2. The customary range of daily energy output is 1800 to 2400 kcal (Food and Nutrition Board, 1980).

PROTEIN

1. Intake of protein should be at 0.8 mg/kg to 1 mg/kg representing 12 to 12.7% of total daily caloric intake.
2. In a diet of 1800 to 2400 kcal, there should be 50 to 70 g/day of protein.
3. Protein needs are increased with surgery, chronicity, or skin ulcerations.
4. Excessive protein intake may lead to glomerular sclerosis and inordinate urinary losses of calcium.

---

*Carbohydrates and fats complement the diet but are low-density nutrients that should be limited by caloric need.

5. Too little protein intake results in negative nitrogen balance with associated muscle wasting.
6. Animal protein should be decreased and plant protein increased as part of the effort to reduce saturated fats prevalent in animal protein (particularly red meats).
7. The following foods are good sources of protein:

Animal Proteins
- Meat
- Poultry
- Fish
- Milk
- Cheese

Plant Proteins
- Dried beans
- Dried peas
- Lentils
- Nuts
- Peanut butter

*Complementary Proteins**
- Cereal and milk
- Macaroni and cheese
- Beans and rice
- Peanut butter sandwich
- Cheese sandwich
- Textured vegetable protein†

FATS

1. Total fat intake should be reduced to about 30 to 35% to control weight, reduce cholesterol, and subsequently decrease atherosclerosis with the associated risk of coronary heart disease.
2. The calories derived from fats should be no more than 10% from saturated fats and the remainder from polyunsaturated and monounsaturated fats.
3. Cholesterol intake should be restricted to about 300 mg/day.
   a. The goal is to reduce serum cholesterol and low-density lipoproteins (LDL), which contribute to atherosclerosis.
   b. The percentage of polyunsaturated fats and high-density lipo-

*Combinations provide complete protein
†Made from soy beans, may be used as a meat extender.

proteins (HDL), which tend to lower serum cholesterol, should be raised.
c. Monounsaturated fats do not seem to have any effect on serum cholesterol.
d. Diet, exercise, and ideal weight help bring down cholesterol levels or improve cholesterol : HDL ratios.
e. Alcohol in moderation raises HDL.

4. The following lists identify fat sources and differentiate saturated and unsaturated fats:

Saturated Fats
- Animal fats in beef, pork, duck
- Lard
- Butter
- Cream
- Coconut oil
- Palm oil

Unsaturated Fats*
- Safflower oil
- Sunflower oil
- Corn oil
- Soy bean oil
- Cottonseed oil
- Olive oil†
- Peanut oil†

CARBOHYDRATES AND FIBER

1. Complex carbohydrates (starch) and fiber should be increased, as they tend to lower blood pressure and total blood cholesterol, moisten the stool, and move the stool faster through the bowel.
2. Simple refined carbohydrates (sugar) should be restricted, as they are characterized by low-nutrient density and tend to increase cholesterol levels and glucose intolerance.
3. The following foods are sources of simple, complex, and high-fiber carbohydrates:

Simple Carbohydrates
- Sugar (granulated)
- Syrups
- Flavored sodas

---

*Arranged with the highest degree of polyunsaturated fat in ascending order.
†High in monounsaturated fats.

- Fruit drinks
- Yucca
- Candy

Complex Carbohydrates
- Bread
- Cereal
- Pasta
- Starchy vegetables (corn, yams, potatoes)

High-Fiber Carbohydrates
- Whole-grain breads and cereals
- Legumes (dried beans, peas, green beans, snow peas, peanuts with skins)
- Root vegetables (beets, carrots, sweet potatoes, turnips)
- Nuts
- Popcorn
- Seeds
- Fruits and vegetables with edible skins

CALCIUM

1. There is increasing consensus for raising the calcium intake to 1000 to 1500 mg/day for the elderly to maintain calcium balance and prevent osteoporosis.
2. Long-term insufficient calcium intake, low vitamin D availability, reduced ability for metabolic calcium conversion, ingestion of a high-protein diet, and reduced intestinal absorption lead to bone loss.
3. Postmenopausal white women with small bone frames are at greatest risk for reduction in bone mass.
4. If supplementation is indicated, calcium carbonate (40% elemental calcium) is most convenient because fewer pills are required for the same amount to be absorbed.
5. The following foods contain high sources of calcium:

- Skim milk
- Dry nonfat milk
- Buttermilk
- Low-fat yogurt
- Cheese*
- Sardines and salmon with bones

---

*Harder cheeses are higher in calcium.

- Collard greens, kale, mustard, turnip greens
- Tofu (soybean cake or curd)

VITAMIN D

1. Ingestion of at least 400 to 800 IU/day of vitamin D is recommended for the elderly to improve calcium and phosphorus intestinal absorption and to prevent malabsorption of calcium by the bones.
2. Sufficient amounts of vitamin D may be synthesized by exposure to the sun for 15 minutes twice a week.
   a. With exposure to sunlight, the skin of whites synthesizes 250 IU of vitamin D daily.
   b. Heavily pigmented skin screens out about 95% of ultraviolet rays and synthesizes far less vitamin D.
3. Supplementary sources of vitamin D are often needed because of the following:
   a. Exposure to the sun is not possible.
   b. Lactose intolerance is experienced.
   c. Limitations are set on consumption of egg yolk because of their high cholesterol content.
4. When supplementing vitamin D, keep in mind the following:
   a. A multivitamin containing 400 IU/day of vitamin D is recommended as the cheapest, most practical form of supplementation.
   b. Commercially available tablets should be avoided, as they often contain excessive amounts of vitamin D (50,000 IU).
   c. Calcium supplements with vitamin D may be used if the total amount of vitamin D daily does not exceed 800 IU.
5. The following are good sources of vitamin D:

- Vitamin D–fortified dairy products
- Fish oils
- Egg yolk

WATER

1. Intake of at least 1500 ml of water a day is recommended.

SODIUM

1. Restriction of sodium intake to 2 to 3 g/day is optimal.
2. Salt may be used in cooking but should not be added at the table.
3. Fast foods should be avoided, as they are very high in sodium content.

4. Salt substitutes should not be used unless the physician agrees because many substitutes contain large amounts of potassium chloride, which may be detrimental to electrolyte balance.
5. The use of herbs as substitute for salt is recommended for seasoning (Table 4–4).
6. The following foods are high in sodium and should be avoided:

- Canned and dehydrated soups
- Canned vegetables
- Meat tenderizer (monosodium glutamate, e.g., Accent)
- Fast foods
- Canned tomato juice and sauces
- American processed cheese
- Spice salts
- Sauces: soy, steak, chili, and Worcestershire
- Prepared mustard, ketchup, pickles, relish, and olives
- Baking powder, baking soda
- Pretzels, potato chips, and salted popcorn
- Anchovies, herring, sardines
- Smoked or cured meats and fish

POTASSIUM

1. Elders medicated with non–potassium-sparing diuretics should include foods high in potassium in their diet.
2. The following foods are good sources of potassium:

- Citrus fruit and juice (orange and grapefruit)
- Bananas

Table 4–4. *Herb Blends to Replace Salt*†*

Saltless surprise:	2 teaspoons garlic powder and 1 teaspoon each of basil, oregano, and powdered lemon rind (or dehydrated lemon juice). Put ingredients into a blender and mix well. Store in glass container, label well, and add rice to prevent caking.
Pungent salt substitute:	3 teaspoons basil; 2 teaspoons each of savory (summer savory is best), celery seed, ground cumin seed, sage, and marjoram; and 1 teaspoon lemon thyme. Mix well, then powder with a mortar and pestle.
Spicy saltless seasoning:	1 teaspoon each of cloves, pepper, and coriander seed (crushed); 2 teaspoons paprika; and 1 tablespoon rosemary. Mix ingredients in a blender. Store in airtight container.

*From the FDA Consumer HHS Pub. No. 84-2192. Washington, DC: US Government Printing Office, 1984.
†The herb blends can be placed in shakers and used instead of salt.

- Dried prunes
- Apricots
- Raisins
- Potatoes
- Carrots (raw)
- Broccoli

IRON, FOLATE, AND VITAMIN B$_{12}$

1. Healthy elders who meet the recommendations of the daily food guide and are not subject to drug and food interactions usually have adequate amounts of iron, folic acid, and vitamin B$_{12}$.
2. Those elders eating a nutritious diet and demonstrating iron deficiency should be assessed for bleeding, as it is unusual for elders to be anemic when their dietary requirements are being met.
3. The following foods are good sources of iron:

    - Liver
    - Red meat
    - Soybeans
    - Fortified breads and cereals

4. The following foods are good sources of folate:
    - Liver
    - Legumes
    - Green leafy vegetables

5. Vitamin B$_{12}$ is available in most foods. Supplementation for healthy persons is not recommended.

FLUORIDE

1. Drinking water with high natural concentrations of fluoride may promote good bone and dental health.
2. Since the effects of low-dose supplementation have not been adequately studied, fluoride needs of the elderly have not been determined and pharmacologic doses for treatment of osteoporosis have not been approved by the Food and Drug Administration (FDA).

ZINC

1. Sufficient amounts of zinc are normally ingested with red meat, liver, fish, and dark poultry.
2. Supplementation is not recommended for healthy elders.

3. High-dose supplementation may impair dietary absorption of copper and cause diarrhea and nausea.
4. Prior to initiation of therapy with zinc for chronically ill patients with serious infection, leg or decubitus ulcers, or other conditions known to be zinc responsive, zinc status should be assessed to avoid excessive supplementation.

VITAMIN A

1. The elderly person should not exceed the RDA of 5000 IU except when vitamin A deficiency has been demonstrated.
2. The nurse should check all of the client's over-the-counter (OTC) vitamin preparations to determine whether any contain toxic amounts of vitamin A and should advise the client accordingly.
3. When excessive amounts of fat-soluble vitamins stored in adipose tissue (as a result of high supplementation) are released, toxicity may result.

CHOLINE

1. Many elderly erroneously believe that choline (lecithin) will improve memory or prevent senility.
2. Dietary requirements for choline have not as yet been established by the FDA.

SUMMARY

1. Maintain ideal weight
2. Fats
   a. Decrease fat and cholesterol.
   b. Decrease percentage of saturated animal fat.
   c. Increase percentage of polyunsaturated fat.
3. Protein
   a. Decrease animal protein.
   b. Increase plant protein.
4. Carbohydrates and fiber
   a. Decrease simple carbohydrates (sugar).
   b. Increase complex carbohydrates and fiber.
5. Increase calcium and vitamin D.
6. Maintain a water intake at of least 1500 ml per day.

7. Avoid excessive salt intake.
8. Avoid high doses of supplementary vitamins.

FACTORS AFFECTING EATING

1. Eating in late life is affected by the biologic status of the individual and physical and social environment.
2. Often what appears to others as rigid, depressed, or cantankerous behaviors are the attempts of the elderly to cope with primary and secondary aging changes that affect them in the physical and psychosocial dimensions. The elderly rightly feel that few understand the impact of these changes.
3. At times even the elderly themselves do not fully understand the character of the changes and lack the energy to explain changes motivating their preferences and habits.
4. Consideration of the effects of primary changes and the physical and social environment will assist nurses in planning with the elderly for satisfying, nutritional eating experiences.

Physiologic Factors

1. Reduction in body mass and decreased metabolism reduce caloric needs.
   a. A gradual loss of weight after age 60 is desirable, as it reflects a loss of excess adipose tissue.
   b. In accordance with reduced needs, appetite is reduced in the elderly.
   c. Smaller amounts of food at more frequent intervals are often satisfying.
   d. Nutrient-dense foods are essential; low-density foods should be kept to a minimum.
2. Hearing losses as a result of advancing age (presbycusis) may influence the choice of the eating environment.
   a. Hearing losses that cause difficulty in understanding speech and in discriminating conversation in a noisy environment cause many elderly to be unwilling to eat in public places. Although surrounded by people, elders often feel isolated because they cannot enjoy the conversation of people with whom they are eating. This problem is usually not alleviated by a hearing aid, which tends to pick up background noise.
   b. For the elderly who have difficulty in understanding speech in a noisy environment, it may be less frustrating to have meals in

a quieter atmosphere rather than at a nutrition center or a restaurant.

c. Motivations of the elderly for choosing an eating environment should be assessed.

3. Presbyopia, cataracts, and slowed accommodation to darkness require older people to need brighter light than younger people.

a. The objection of some elderly to a romantic atmosphere with dim lights and flickering candles is fostered by their inability to see under these conditions.

b. Provision of a well-lighted eating area is more desirable for the elderly.

4. Taste is affected by primary aging changes.

a. As the taste buds that detect salt and sweet sensations deteriorate and the taste buds for bitter and sour sensations remain intact longer, the elderly tend to report that everything tastes bitter or sour. The elderly should be cautioned against excessive use of salt or sweeteners in their attempt to regain these tastes.

b. Decrease in taste acuity may be further reduced by upper dentures covering secondary taste sites. Temporary removal of upper dentures may provide the elder with opportunities for more gustatory pleasure in eating and drinking.

5. Smell is greatly reduced as the olfactory bulbs atrophy.

a. Research indicates that a threshold concentration of at least 11 times that needed by a young person may be necessary for an elderly person to perceive the odor of a substance.

(1) The elderly should be cautioned not to rely on taste or smell when checking for food spoilage but rather to base their evaluation more on color and consistency. When in doubt, food should be discarded.

(2) The elderly should be cautioned to check that gas appliances are turned off properly and that pilot lights are lit to avoid suffocation. A large number of accidental gas-related deaths have occurred among the elderly.

b. The lack of olfactory stimulus may reduce salivation. In turn, the lack of salivary gland secretion reduces the solubilization of flavoring agents, delays the digestion of starches, reduces liquid available for moistening the oral mucosa, and hinders swallowing and softening foods ingested.

6. Loss of all teeth occurs in about 66% of the elderly by 75 years of age. Future cohorts may not present with as widespread a problem as a result of improvements in preventive action, dental care, and nutrition.

a. The elderly should be referred for appropriate dental care.

    b. Poorly fitting dentures are a problem for many and cause avoidance of hard and sticky foods.

    c. Easily chewed foods, rather than only puréed foods that ignore the individual's preferences and habits, should be available for edentulous people.

7. Gastrointestinal functioning is affected by several primary changes.

    a. Reduction in secretion by digestive glands and reduction in absorption of food affect nutritional status.

    b. For many elderly, unpredictable changes in the peristalsis of the esophagus occur with delayed emptying, a common distressing problem.

    c. Chronic atrophic gastritis and a decrease in gastric motility causes delayed emptying and maldigestion.

    d. Smaller, more frequent meals help avoid discomfort related to delayed emptying of the esophagus and stomach. The elderly should not be burdened by others' expectations for them to eat large meals. Several small meals a day may be preferable.

    e. Identifying and eliminating foods from the diet that cause gastric distress and flatulence are recommended.

8. Slowed intestinal peristalsis often results in constipation, which is associated with laxative abuse.

    a. With aging, there is a general increase in concern with bowel function and a belief that each person should have regular bowel movements.

    b. Fluids and fiber in the diet should be encouraged.

    c. Laxative-induced "constipation" should be avoided. (The bowel is so thoroughly cleaned out that no bowel movement is possible for 2 to 3 days, and the elder attributes the absence of bowel movements to constipation and uses another laxative.)

Psychosocial Factors

1. Age-related changes, increase in social and personal losses, and a decline in social opportunities that are a source for maintaining self-esteem precipitate an increase in hypochondriacal reactions (anxious preoccupation with bodily functions).

    a. Increased concern with bodily function usually occurs between 60 and 70 years of age. During this period, food preferences are influenced by real or imaginary connections between the choice of food and drink and the bodily response.

    b. The elderly should be assisted in developing better coping mechanisms that will free them from hypochondriacal preoccupation and dietary restrictions. Elders with hypochondriasis often ex-

perience spontaneous remission as stressful factors decline and better coping mechanisms are acquired.
   c. The elderly should be assisted in meeting their food and drink preferences.
2. The elderly may revert to food choices associated with pleasant experiences earlier in life.
   a. When there are increased problems with maintaining self-esteem, foods that remind the elderly of rewarding experiences earlier in life have positive symbolic value as these individuals once more experience the pleasures associated with the food.
   b. The elderly should be encouraged to make or obtain foods associated with pleasant past life experiences. The very act of baking or cooking special foods may reinforce their self-esteem.
3. The environment, timing, preparation, and presentation of food significantly influence the quality, enjoyment, and nutritional value of mealtimes. The following arrangements facilitate eating:
   a. Provision of easily chewed foods rather than puréed food for edentulous people is important because the texture and consistency of food adds to its enjoyment.
   b. Cutting meat, buttering bread, or arranging food conveniently increases nutrient intake for the aged with weak, unsteady hands.
   c. Provision of appropriate utensils for food preparation and eating is essential for assisting the elderly with handicapping conditions. Local surgical supply stores will provide catalogues of daily living aids. (See Table 11–1.)
   d. Providing the opportunity for people to eat at their own pace and the opportunity for conversation after meals promotes positive eating habits.

Ethnic and Religious Food Patterns

1. In these latter years of the 20th century, there are millions of seniors in the United States who represent widely diverse ethnic and religious backgrounds.
2. The symbolic meaning of food, religious tenets, regional preferences, and childhood experiences influence acceptance and compliance with a diet.
3. The health care provider alert to the nutritional problems in ethnic and religious dietary patterns may help the client to improve nutrient intake with acceptable dietary adjustments (Table 4–5).

Table 4–5.   *Ethnic and Religious Groups: Nutritional Concerns and Dietary Recommendations*

Nutritional Concerns	Dietary Recommendations
Black	
Low milk intake (related to lactose intolerance)	Use milk treated for lactose intolerance (available in stores) and use hard cheeses
Excessive use of pork (high in saturated fats)	Use polyunsaturated fats for frying
Use of salty meats (ham, bacon, sausage)	Instead of frying, broil or stew
Vegetables cooked for a long time in a large amount of water (pot liquor) that is later eaten with corn bread	Reduce water when cooking vegetables
	Use grccn leafy vegetables
Use of gravies	Reduce use of fatty, salty meats
Deep fat frying with lard (saturated fat)	Reduce snack foods with empty calories
Excessive use of soft and fruit drinks	
Chinese	
Excessive sodium in sauces (e.g., hoisin and soy sauce)	Reduce use of salty sauces
Excessive sodium intake from monosodium glutamate, smoked and dried meat, and dried fish	Use polyunsaturated fats for stir-frying (safflower, sunflower, corn, or soybean oil)
Monosaturated oil (peanut oil) used for stir-frying	Instead of deep frying, boil, steam, or lightly stir fry
Low in dairy products (related to lactose intolerance)	Increase use of tofu (soy bean curd) and soy beans to increase protein and calcium intake
Tend to be low in meat group	Use milk treated for lactose intolerance (available in stores)
Deep frying used for some dishes	Supplement with vitamins A and D if necessary
Greek	
Excessive salt from anchovies, feta cheese, and olives	Limit use of anchovies, feta cheese, and olives
Italian	
Excessive use of bread and pasta	Use less salty cheeses, such as ricotta and mozzarella, rather than Parmesan and other hard cheeses
Low milk intake	
Excessive use of salt in tomato sauce, anchovies, olives, and processed meats	Reduce use of salty and starchy foods
Japanese	
Excessive sodium in sauces and in dried and pickled foods	Reduce use of salty sauces and dried and pickled foods
Low in dairy products (related to lactose intolerance)	Use milk treated for lactose intolerance (available in stores)
	Increase use of tofu (bean curd) and soy-beans to increase calcium and protein intake
	Supplement with vitamins A and D if necessary
Mexican-American	
Low in dairy products	Discontinue use of lard
Low in meat	Use polyunsaturated oils in cooking

Table 4–5. *Ethnic and Religious Groups: Nutritional Concerns and Dietary Recommendations* Continued

Nutritional Concerns	Dietary Recommendations
Use of lard in cooking	Fry less; steam tortillas instead of frying
Excessive use of coffee	Increase use of green leafy vegetables for folacin
	Increase use of lean meats
	Increase use of dark green and yellow vegetables and fruits
	Continue use of corn tortillas (high in calcium as a result of soaking corn in limewater)
Puerto Rican	
Use of salt cod	Decrease use of salt pork
Use of lard	Soak salt cod very well and rinse well before using
Use of salt pork	Substitute polyunsaturated oil for lard in cooking
High-caloric diet	Increase green and yellow vegetables
Lack of yellow and green vegetables	Use more milk and cheese
	Add meat to rice and beans
	Use margarine instead of butter
Scandinavian	
Excessive use of milk, cream, butter, and cheese	Reduce intake of high-cholesterol dairy products
Central European	
Overcook vegetables, resulting in loss of vitamins	Reduce water and cooking time for vegetables
Jewish	
High in saturated fats and cholesterol	Reduce use of high-cholesterol dairy foods
	Substitute polyunsaturated fat for butter in cooking
	Reduce use of meats, especially organ meats high in cholesterol, such as liver and tongue
Catholic	
Possible excessive restriction of nutrients during Lenten season	Maintain a balanced diet and use acceptable nutritious substitutes
Seventh Day Adventist	
Exclusion of meat and fish from diet	Maintain sufficient intake of protein from dairy products and combinations of foods (see under "Protein" in text)
	Use meat analogs (e.g., textured vegetable protein made from soybeans may be used as a meat extender)

Risk Factors Predisposing to Malnutrition

1. Physiologic Risk Factors
    a. Alterations in respiratory and cardiovascular function: fatigue, weakness, and shortness of breath.
    b. Alterations in gastrointestinal function: heartburn, gas, and constipation.
    c. Alterations in genitourinary function: incontinence.
    d. Alterations in musculoskeletal function: deficits in strength, mobility, and dexterity.
    e. Alterations in neurologic status: dysphagia and deficits in hearing, vision, taste, and smell.
    f. Polypharmacy (multiple-drug medication regimen).
2. Psychosocial Risk Factors
    a. Depression (working toward intentional or subintentional suicide).
    b. Grief, recent loss of spouse or significant other.
    c. Loneliness, isolation.
    d. Denial of need for a special diet.
    e. Alcohol or drug abuse.
    f. Low income.
    g. Lack of motivation.
    h. Incorrect or lack of nutrition knowledge.
    i. Susceptibility to quackery or fad diets.
    j. Inability to meet cultural, religious, or personal preferences.

PROMOTING NUTRITION

1. Data are limited on the consequence of age-related physiologic and psychosocial changes on the nutrient needs of the elderly.
2. Since anthropometric, chemical, and clinical norms traditionally used for assessing nutritional status have not been standardized for the elderly, their use in geriatric nutrition is of limited value.
3. Overt signs and symptoms of nutritional deficiency are rarely observed in the elderly even though the client's intake and biochemical analysis suggest that the individual is at high risk for malnutrition associated with dietary imbalance.

Guide for Nutritional Assessment

1. Present an interested, accepting manner when obtaining a food history.

2. Assess the client's ability to recognize and accept his health status and his knowledge of required care.
3. Compute weight for height (see under "Height and Weight and Recommended Energy Intake" previously) and compare with ideal weight for height.
4. Review the physical and psychosocial assessments of the client for the risk factors predisposing the elderly to malnutrition.
5. Assess for malnutrition (Table 4–6).
6. Assess for environmental constraints.
   a. Inaccessible shopping area.
   b. Lack of space or equipment to store or cook food.
7. Assess for smoking, alcohol consumption, work, exercise, recreation, and socialization.
8. Obtain a diet history. A casual conversational approach at a time when the client is willing and able to talk about his diet is most productive. Several methods are available for developing a nutritional assessment.
   a. *Diet recall*: Ask the client to list all foods eaten in the last 24 to 48 hours. This method is inappropriate for elders with short-term memory deficit or a problem with writing.
   b. *Food use list*: Using a list of commonly used foods, ask the client how frequently each food is used.
   c. *Activity-associated general day's food pattern*: Ask the client to associate his eating with actitivies during the day. This gives structure to the interview (a beginning, a middle, and an end) and jogs the patient's memory, enabling him to elaborate on his eating habits.
9. Compare the assessment data with the daily food guide and nutritional recommendations (see previous sections) to evaluate how the elder is meeting nutrient needs.
10. Having completed the nutritional assessment with the elderly client, family, and significant other (friend, neighbor, or caretaker), analyze the data and with the client identify nutritional problems and physiologic or psychosocial barriers to meeting nutritional needs. Strategies are then developed to help meet these nutrient needs.

Strategies for Promoting Nutrition

Be alert to physiologic and psychosocial risk factors that may predispose the client to malnutrition and develop with the client adaptive coping mechanisms that will minimize nutritional impact. Discuss risk factors identified with the health team.

Table 4–6.   *Physical Signs of Malnutrition**

Body Area	Normal Appearance	Signs Associated with Malnutrition
Hair	Shiny; firm; not easily plucked	Lack of natural shine; hair dull and dry; thin and sparse; hair fine, silky and straight, color changes (flag sign); can be easily plucked
Face	Skin color uniform; smooth, pink, healthy appearance; not swollen	Skin color loss (depigmentation); skin dark over cheeks and under eyes (malar and supraorbital pigmentation); lumpiness or flakiness of skin of nose and mouth; swollen face; enlarged parotid glands; scaling of skin around nostrils (nasolabial seborrhea)
Eyes	Bright, clear, shiny; no sores at corners of eyelids; membranes healthy, pink, and moist; no prominent blood vessels or mound of tissue on sclera	Eye membranes are pale (pale conjunctivae); redness of membranes (conjunctival injection); Bitot's spots; redness and fissuring of eyelid corners (angular palpebritis); dryness of eye membranes (conjunctival xerosis); cornea has dull appearance (corneal xerosis); cornea is soft (keratomalacia); scar on cornea; ring of fine blood vessels around corner (circumcorneal injection)
Lips	Smooth, not chapped or swollen	Redness and swelling of mouth or lips (cheilosis); especially at corners of mouth (angular fissures and scars)
Tongue	Deep red in appearance; not swollen or smooth	Swelling; scarlet and raw tongue; magenta (purplish color) of tongue; smooth tongue; swollen sores; hyperemic and hypertrophic papillae; atrophic papillae
Teeth	No cavities; no pain; bright	May be missing or erupting abnormally; gray or black spots (fluorosis); cavities (caries)
Gums	Healthy; red; do not bleed; not swollen	"Spongy" and bleed easily; recession of gums
Glands	Face not swollen	Thyroid enlargement (front of neck); parotid enlargement (cheeks become swollen)

Table 4–6. *Physical Signs of Malnutrition** Continued

Body Area	Normal Appearance	Signs Associated with Malnutrition
Skin	No signs of rashes, swellings, dark or light spots	Dryness of skin (xerosis); sandpaper feel of skin (follicular hyperkeratosis); flakiness of skin; skin swollen and dark; red swollen pigmentation of exposed areas (pellagrous dermatosis); excessive lightness or darkness of skin (dyspigmentation); black and blue marks due to skin bleeding (petechiae); lack of fat under skin
Nails	Firm, pink	Nails are spoon-shaped (koilonychia); brittle, ridged nails
Muscular and skeletal systems	Good muscle tone; some fat under skin; can walk or run without pain	Muscles have "wasted" appearance; baby's skull bones are thin and soft (craniotabes); round swelling of front and side of head (frontal and parietal bossing); swelling of ends of bones (epiphyseal enlargement); small bumps on both sides of chest wall (on ribs)—beading of ribs; baby's soft spot on head does not harden at proper time (persistently open anterior fontanelle); knock-knees or bowlegs; bleeding into muscle (musculoskeletal hemorrhages); person cannot get up or walk properly
Internal systems:		
Cardiovascular	Normal heart rate and rhythm; no murmurs or abnormal rhythms; normal blood pressure for age	Rapid heart rate (above 100 tachycardia); enlarged heart; abnormal rhythm; elevated blood pressure
Gastrointestinal	No palpable organs or masses (in children, however, liver edge may be palpable)	Liver enlargement; enlargement of spleen (usually indicates other associated diseases)
Nervous	Psychologic stability; normal reflexes	Mental irritability and confusion; burning and tingling of hands and feet (paresthesia); loss of position and vibratory sense; weakness and tenderness of muscles (may result in inability to walk); decrease and loss of ankle and knee reflexes

*From Nutrition assessment in health programs. Part I. Methodology, clinical assessment of nutrition status. Am J Publ Health, 63(Supplement):18, 1973.

STRATEGIES FOR ENVIRONMENTAL CONSTRAINTS

1. Assist the client in contacting the following places or services for transportation assistance to inaccessible shopping areas:
   a. The local area Agency on Aging, listed among the community service numbers in the front pages of the telephone book or in the local directory of services for the aged or for the disabled.
   b. Senior Citizen Center in the area, which may provide transportation for shopping or to a nutrition center for meals.
   c. Supermarkets, which may supply bus service for seniors.
   d. Taxi services, which may provide transportation at reduced fees.
   e. Welfare services, which may provide extra funds for transportation.
   f. Senior citizen housing, which often provides busing for meal programs or shopping.
2. Assist in arranging for a neighborhood store to deliver food if the client is unable to shop.
3. Evaluate the possibility of family or friends doing the food shopping for the client.
4. Plan with the client to optimize the use of available equipment for food storage and preparation.
5. Review safe storage, refrigeration, and cooking practices.
6. Check on the availability of gas and electricity. Payment for utilities and fuel may be arranged under the Home Energy Assistance Program (HEAP).
7. Make adjustments in placement or use of equipment that will provide accessibility and maximize safe usage.
8. Arrange for the use of adaptive equipment that enables the disabled senior to store, cook, and eat food.
9. Suggest and help obtain necessary equipment, such as an electric hot plate, hot pot, food heater, electric food processor, or broiler. Older clients may be unaware of equipment with which they may reasonably and safely prepare food.
10. Inform the client that the following foods may be stored and prepared when a stove or refrigerator is unavailable. These foods may supplement meals obtained from Meals-On-Wheels or in a nutrition center:

    • Nonfat dry milk (may be reconstituted with water)
    • Cocoa mixes (may be reconstituted with hot tap water)
    • Peanut butter
    • Whole-grain cereals
    • Dried fruits
    • Whole-grain crackers

- Fresh fruits (1 to 2 days)
- Canned vegetables (small cans to be used for one meal)

STRATEGIES FOR FINANCIAL NEED

1. Help the client to review his existing budget or to develop a budget.
2. If there appears to be financial need, refer the client to local agencies for financial aid or services.
3. If there is a need for provision of meals, refer to the local Area Agency on Aging for meal programs funded by private organizations or supported by the government under the Title VII Nutrition Program for the Elderly in the Older Americans Act.
    a. Meals are planned to meet one third of the RDAs for people over age 51.
    b. Individuals are not expected to pay, but some seniors prefer to pay a token amount rather than accept the meals without payment.
    c. Meals are provided at project centers, such as schools, church buildings, or senior citizen centers. Meals-On-Wheels delivers food to the home of those seniors unable to attend the centers.
    d. Often a light evening meal that does not require refrigeration accompanies the larger noontime meal. Alternative arrangements usually must be made for weekend meals.
4. When total income including Social Security payments is insufficient for meeting nutritional needs, refer the senior to the local Department of Social Services to apply for Emergency Assistance and Supplemental Social Security.
5. Arrange payment for adaptive equipment for eating through Medicaid if the client is eligible.
6. Apply to a food stamp center (see food stamps information under community service numbers in local telephone directory) for food stamps that may be used to buy food in stores, home-delivered meals, and meals in centers at reduced cost. There is no gross limit on income if at least one member of the household is age 60 or older. An assets limit and a net income limit apply.
7. Suggest shopping at local stores that offer discounts to senior citizens.
8. Encourage the use of manufacturers' discount coupons.
9. See under "Nutrition Services," Chapter 17.

STRATEGIES FOR ASSESSED INCORRECT OR LACK OF NUTRITION KNOWLEDGE

1. Review with client appropriate materials on nutrition and plan with client for improved nutrition.

2. Refer client for nutrition services at local health department or hospital when appropriate.

Resources

Consumer Information Center-D
P.O. Box 100
Pueblo, CO 81002
  The Consumer
  Diet and the Elderly
  The Gender Gap at the Dinner Table
  What about Nutrients in Fast Foods?

General Mills Inc.
Nutrition Department
Department 45, P.O. Box 1112
Minneapolis, MN 55440
  Meal Planning for the Golden years (Charge $0.45)
  For Professionals: Contemporary Nutrition Order Form

National Institute on Aging/Food
Building 31, Room 5C35
Bethesda, MD 20205
  Age Pages
  Dietary Supplements: More Is Not Always Better
  Nutrition: A Lifelong Concern
  Hints for Shopping, Cooking, and Enjoying Meals
  Be Sensible About Salt

References

Abraham S, Johnson CL, Najar MF: Weight by height and age for adults 18–74 years of age: United States—1971–74. DHEW Publication No.(PHS) 79–1656 (Vital and health statistics; series 2; No. 208). Hyattsville, Md: National Center for Health Statistics, 1979.

Bailey LB, Cerda JJ: Diagnosis and treatment of nutritional disorders in older patients. Geriatrics 39(8):67–72, 1984.

Burr ML, Sweetnam PM, Barasi ME: Dietary fibre, blood pressure and plasma cholesterol. Nutrition Research 5:465–470, 1985.

Busse E: Eating in later life: Physiologic and psychologic factors. Contemporary Nutrition (General Mills Nutrition Dept.) 4(11), 1979.

Crapo P: Nutrition in the aged. In Schrier R, ed: Clinical Internal Medicine. Philadelphia: WB Saunders Co, 1982.

Dietary Goals for the United States. (2nd ed.) Select Committee on Nutrition and Human Needs, US Senate, Stock No. 051-070-04367-8. Washington, DC: US Government Printing Office, 1977.

Dietary Guidelines for Americans. US Department of Agriculture and US Dept of Health and Human Services. Washington, DC: US Government Printing Office, 1980.

Fehiley AM, Burr ML, Phillips KM, Deadman NM: The effect of fish on plasma lipid and lipoprotein concentrations. Journal of Clinical Nutrition 38(9):349–351, 1983.

Freedman ML, Ahrenheim JC: Nutritional needs of the elderly: Debate and recommendations. Geriatrics 40(8):45–62, 1985.

Howard RB, Herbold NH: Nutrition in Clinical Care. New York: McGraw-Hill, 1978, pp 268–285.

Hui Y: Human Nutrition and Diet Therapy. Monterey, Calif: Wadsworth Health Sciences, 1983.

Kohrs MB: New perspectives on nutritional counseling for the elderly. Contemporary Nutrition (General Mills Nutrition Dept.) 8(3), 1983.

Mannenberg D: Nutrition. In Ernst N, Glazer-Waldman H, eds: The Aged Patient. Chicago: Year Book Medical Publishers, Inc, 1983.

Miller RW: On being too rich, too thin, too cholesterol laden. FDA Consumer HHS Pub. No. 81-1087. Washington, DC: US Government Printing Office, 1983.

Millis RM, Bowen PE: Process guides for nutrition care in community health. Journal of the American Dietetic Association 85(1):73–76, 1985.

National Research Council, Food and Nutrition Board: Recommended Dietary Allowances. (9th ed.) Washington, DC: National Academy of Sciences, 1980.

Natow A, Heslin J: Geriatric Nutrition. Boston: CBI Publishing, 1980.

Nelder K: Nutrition, aging, and the skin. Geriatrics 39(2):69–87, 1984.

Nelson RA: Clinical nutrition in the elderly: Its time has come. Geriatrics 39(8):15, 1985.

O'Hara-Devereaux M, Andrus L, Scott C, eds: Eldercare: A Practical Guide to Clinical Geriatrics. New York: Grune & Stratton, 1981.

Schulz TD, Leklem JE: Dietary status of 7th Day Adventists. Journal of the American Dietetic Association 83(1):27–33, 1983.

Williams SR: Essentials of Nutrition and Diet Therapy. St. Louis: CV Mosby, 1978.

Drugs and the Elderly

RISK FACTORS IN DRUG THERAPY
ADVERSE DRUG REACTIONS
DRUG INTERACTIONS
FOOD-DRUG INTERACTIONS
DRUG MISUSE AND ABUSE

In an effort to maintain health and combat acute and chronic disease processes, the elderly use far more drugs than does the younger population. Although the elderly compose only 11% of the population of the United States, they use about 25% of drugs prescribed. The elderly are at greater risk for adverse drug reactions, drug-drug interactions, food-drug interactions, noncompliance, and potential abuse.

RISK FACTORS IN DRUG THERAPY

1. Primary and secondary changes alter pharmacokinetics (how a drug acts in the body) and pharmacodynamics (how a drug acts at receptor sites).
2. Interaction of primary and secondary changes causes unpredictable responses.
3. Complex drug regimens characterized by several drugs self-administered at various times of the day increase the possibility of error.
4. Self-medication with over-the-counter drugs (OTC) and use of folk medicines and quack remedies may interfere with medication regimens.
5. Many of the drugs used by the elderly are characterized by a narrow

therapeutic index that allows for only a very limited range between a therapeutic and toxic dose.
6. Conditions often experienced by the elderly, such as bed rest, dietary changes, malnutrition, dehydration, altered body temperature, stress, congestive heart failure, and thyroid disease, influence the body's reaction to drugs.

ADVERSE DRUG REACTIONS

The elderly are highly susceptible to adverse drug reactions that may occur at normal adult doses used for prophylaxis, diagnosis, or therapy.

Types

1. *Pharmacologic reactions.*
   a. Toxicity may occur with exaggerated response or extension of the desired action of the drug even at normal doses.
   b. Side effects, the undesired secondary effects of a drug, are predictable and should be kept to a minimum to prevent interference with the patient's normal functioning.
2. *Hypersensitivity (allergic) reactions.*
   a. Prior exposure to the drug must have occurred and sufficient time for the production of antibodies must have elapsed before a hypersensitivity reaction may develop.
   b. After the production of antibodies, these reactions may be immediate (anaphylactic) or delayed (serum sickness).
   c. Hypersensitivity reactions range in severity from a minor skin rash to anaphylaxis and death.
3. *Idiosyncratic reactions* may occur in clients who, as a result of their genetic background, manifest an abnormal or unusual response to a drug.

Causes

ALTERATIONS IN PHARMACOKINETICS OWING TO PRIMARY CHANGES

1. Absorption of drugs by the elderly is generally not affected.
2. Distribution of a drug throughout the body is slowed.
   a. Decreased body water slows the distribution of the drug and may alter the action of water-soluble drugs. The diminished thirst

mechanism in the elderly increases the risk of dehydration and the possibility of altered drug action.

b. Large amounts of highly lipid-soluble drugs are deposited in increased body fat. The drugs remain inactive but accumulate with the potential for prolongation of drug action when they are released.

c. Decreased circulating protein (particularly albumin) in the blood reduces the availability of binding sites and increases suscepti-bility to toxicity from higher levels of freely circulating drug.

d. Decreased cardiac output, by reducing flow to the liver and kid-ney, slows the rate of drug distribution to the organs most re-sponsible for drug metabolism and excretion.

3. Metabolism (biotransformation) of a drug, usually to a water-soluble inactive metabolite, occurs mostly in the liver. As biotransformation in the liver is slowed owing to reduction in hepatic cells, microsomal enzyme activity, and blood flow, the risk of toxic accumulation of a drug is great. This is especially true for drugs associated with a high hepatic clearance.

4. Excretion of drugs occurs primarily in the kidney, with lesser amounts excreted in bile, sweat, saliva, breast milk, and expired air. The elderly are more susceptible to cumulation of a drug followed by toxicity. As excretory function of the kidney is reduced as a result of loss of nephrons, reduction in blood flow to the kidney, and decreased rate of glomerular filtration, the risk of toxic accumula-tion of a drug rises.

Alterations in Pharmacodynamics

Alterations in pharmacodynamics may occur owing to changes in end-organ responsiveness associated with primary aging changes.

Changes in Bioavailability

The amount of active ingredient available for absorption into the circulation (bioavailability) of drugs with a narrow therapeutic index may be particularly hazardous to the elderly.

1. Manfacturers' formulas often differ in the amount of active drug available.

2. Formulation (dosage form) of the drug dramatically influences the rate of absorption, serum concentration, and duration of action of the drug. The same dosage delivered in different formulations may result in undermedication or toxicity.

Strategies for Minimizing Adverse Drug Reactions

Benefit without risk in drug therapy is as yet an unachieved goal. However, the possibility of serious damage from adverse drug reactions may be minimized.

1. Review health history and assessment data. Note primary and secondary changes that may affect drug usage.
2. Obtain a careful drug history.
3. Review drug history, especially for past adverse drug reactions.
4. Check that drug dosages are maintained at conservative levels. Dosage of drugs excreted primarily via the kidney should be reduced.
5. Check that dosages are increased gradually and only as needed.
6. Monitor for adverse reactions by clinical assessment and by laboratory assessment as indicated (when norms for the elderly are established). Table 5–1 lists potentially ototoxic, nephrotoxic, and hepatotoxic drugs.
7. Teach client about drug and then evaluate the client for compliance.
8. Ascertain that drug therapy is used only as needed.
9. Encourage the client to continue using the same manufacturer's product unless the health care provider agrees to a change, because the same drug produced by different manufacturers may have differences in bioavailability.
10. Suggest changing formulations of drugs only when necessary, as changes in serum concentration may alter the pharmacokinetics of the drug. Serum concentrations are most rapidly achieved in the following dosage forms in increasing order: slow-release tablets, intact tablets, crushed tablets, and liquids.
11. Monitor closely for side effects and report their occurrence, as the side-effect profile of a drug is often more important than the pharmacokinetic profile for initiating or continuing drug therapy.

DRUG INTERACTIONS

Drug interactions occur when more than one drug is administered. As each drug is added to a therapeutic regimen, the risk increases for drug interactions.

Types

PHARMACOKINETIC INTERACTIONS

1. Interactions affecting absorption.
   a. Changes in bioavailability of a drug may be caused by another

Table 5–1. *Potentially Ototoxic, Nephrotoxic, and Hepatotoxic Drugs**

Drug	Ototoxic	Nephrotoxic	Hepatotoxic
Acetaminophen			X
Acetazolamide		X	
Acetohexamide			X
Acetylsalicylic acid	X	X	
Alcohol			X
Allopurinol			X
Amikacin	X	X	
Aminosalicylic acid			X
Amitriptyline		X	X
Amphotericin B		X	
Ampicillin	X		X
Bacitracin		XX†	
Cephaloridine		X	
Chloramphenicol	X		X
Chlordiazepoxide			X
Chlorothiazide		X	X
Chlorpromazine	X		
Chlorpropamide			X
Chlorthalidone			X
Cisplastin		XX	
Clindamycin			X
Colchicine		X	
Colistimethate sodium		X	
Colistin		XX	
Conjugated estrogenic hormones			X
Corticosteroids		X	
Dantrolene			X
Desipramine			X
Diazepam			X
Ethacrynic acid	X	X	
Erythromycin estolate			X
Fenoprofen	X	X	
Ferrous sulfate			X
Furosemide	X	X	
Gentamicin	X	XX	
Gold compounds	X	X	X
Hydralazine		X	X
Hydrochlorothiazide		X	X
Ibuprofen	X		
Imipramine	X		X
Indomethacin			X
Isoniazid			X
Kanamycin	X	XX	
Meprobamate			X
Methyldopa			X
Minocycline	X		X
Naproxen	X		X
Neomycin		XX	
Nicotinic acid		X	X
Nitrofurantoin			X
Nortriptyline	X		X
Oxyphenbutazone			X
Oxytetracycline			X
Papaverine			X

Table 5–1. Potentially Ototoxic, Nephrotoxic, and Hepatotoxic Drugs*
Continued

Drug	Ototoxic	Nephrotoxic	Hepatotoxic
Para-aminosalycilic acid (PAS)		X	
Penicillamine		XX	
Penicillin		X	X
Perphenazine			X
Phenacetin		X	X
Phenazopyridine hydrochloride			X
Phenobarbital			X
Phenylbutazone	X	X	X
Phenytoin			X
Polymyxin	X		
Polymyxin B		XX	
Probenecid			X
Procainamide hydrochloride			X
Prochlorperazine			X
Propoxyphene			X
Propranolol	X		
Quinidine	X		X
Quinine	X		
Rifampin			X
Salicylates		X	
Streptomycin	X	X	
Sulfisoxazole			X
Sulfonamides		X	X
Tetracyclines		XX	X
Thiazides		X	
Thioridazine			X
Tobramycin	X	XX	
Tolbutamide			X
Tolmetin	X		
Tripelennamine hydrochloride			X
Vancomycin	X		
Viomycin		X	
Vitamin A			X

*Adapted from Boyd JR: Therapeutic dilemmas in the elderly. In Covington TR, Walker JI, eds: Current Geriatric Therapy. Philadelphia: WB Saunders Co, 1984.
†XX indicates drugs with highest incidence of nephrotoxicity.

drug, such as when an antacid is administered concurrently. The antacid, an absorbent and a buffer, alters absorption of many drugs by altering the surface and pH of the environment.
  b. Chemical complexation of a drug may occur when a chemical such as calcium (from an antacid) combines with tetracycline and forms complexes that are not absorbable.
  c. Drugs that alter gastric emptying time, such as cholinergics, by slowing gastric motility may lead to increased absorption.
  d. Cathartics, which increase gastric motility, may reduce absorption of other drugs.
2. Interactions affecting distribution.

   a. When two drugs capable of binding to albumin are in the same drug regimen, the more strongly bound drug remains attached to the protein-binding site and the less strongly bound drug is released in the plasma with increased concentration and pharmacologic activity.

   b. The reduction in protein-binding sites in the elderly contributes to the competition between drugs for binding sites. Toxicity may occur with higher plasma levels of a drug.

   c. A high level of free circulating drug with a narrow therapeutic index may be dangerous.

3. Interactions affecting metabolism.

   a. Drug interactions that stimulate microsomal enzymes in the liver.

     (1) Biotransformation is usually faster to an inactive form with decreased activity of the drug.

     (2) Exceptions may occur, as when a drug is activated, and may produce a greater clinical response (e.g., activation of digitoxin to digoxin).

     (3) Most often the clinically significant interaction occurs when the drug causing enzyme stimulation is withdrawn. The biotransformation of the remaining drug is delayed and activity altered.

   b. Drug interactions that inhibit microsomal enzymes in the liver.

     (1) Prolonged and increased activity of a drug that is due to enzyme inhibition may lead to toxicity. An example of this is cimetidine-inhibiting enzyme systems with a reduction in metabolism, elevation of blood levels, and prolonged action of many drugs, such as propranolol, diazepam, theophylline, phenytoin, and coumarin.

     (2) The inhibition of enzymes may be used therapeutically, as, for example, when allopurinol inhibits the enzyme xanthine oxidase, needed for the metabolism of mercaptopurine and azathioprine, so that a reduction in neoplastic drugs is possible.

4. Interactions affecting excretion.

   a. In the renal tubules, competition between two or more drugs can result in a decreased rate of elimination. The use of the drug probenecid to block the excretion of penicillin is a useful application of this competitive drug interaction.

   b. Renal clearance of drugs is often enhanced or inhibited by urinary pH.

     (1) Acid drugs are eliminated more rapidly in alkaline urine, and basic drugs are eliminated more rapidly in an acidic urine, as they are ionized and cannot be reabsorbed.

(2) Reduction in excretion by acidification or alkalinization of urine by drugs may result in toxic serum levels.

(3) Speeding the elimination of potentially toxic drugs may be accomplished by administering the appropriate urinary acidifier or alkalizer.

PHARMACODYNAMIC INTERACTIONS

1. Pharmacodynamic interactions occur when drug interactions affect the receptor site where the pharmacologic action of the drug is to occur.
2. Interactions may be additive or antagonistic and may involve one or more receptors.
   a. When two drugs with the same pharmacologic action are given together, additive pharmacologic and toxic effects may occur.
      (1) Primary pharmacologic activity is obvious when the interaction is the result of primary pharmacologic activity of the drugs, such as additive central nervous system sedation from narcotics and hypnotics.
      (2) Secondary pharmacologic effects are often not noted, as when the secondary additive anticholinergic effects of antipsychotic drugs occur.
   b. Opposing pharmacologic effects may negate the action of both as the drugs act at different receptor sites. Administration of a vasoconstrictor and a vasodilator may result in no effect as they cancel action out.
   c. Antagonism at a single receptor site may be used therapeutically, as when a narcotic agonist and a narcotic antagonist compete for the same receptor sites.

Strategies for Prevention of Drug Interactions

1. Utilize a drug reference source to check for potential interactions of drugs in the medication regimen.
2. Advise the client not to take any drugs before consulting with the health care provider or pharmacist for possible interactions.
3. Monitor the client for additive and antagonistic primary and secondary actions of drugs.
4. Help the client to avoid drug reactions that affect absorption by timing administration at least 2 hours apart and sequencing administration appropriately.
5. Teach the client how to alkalize or acidify urine, if indicated, by dietary intake of the appropriate foods.

Urinary Alkalizers
- Almonds
- Baking soda and baking powder
- Carbonated beverages
- Chestnuts
- Coconuts
- Fruit (except cranberries, plums, and prunes)
- Jams, jellies
- Milk and cream
- Molasses
- Olives
- Vegetables (except corn and lentils)

Urinary Acidifiers
- Bacon
- Breads and pastries*
- Cheese
- Corn
- Cranberries
- Eggs
- Fish, shellfish
- Grains
- Lentils
- Mayonnaise
- Meat
- Nuts (Brazil nuts, peanuts, walnuts, filberts)
- Pasta, rice
- Plums
- Prunes
- Poultry

Neutral Foods
- Butter
- Coffee
- Cooking oils
- Honey
- Margarine
- Starches (corn and arrowroot)
- Sugars
- Syrups
- Tapioca
- Tea

---

*Not made with baking soda or baking powder.

FOOD-DRUG INTERACTIONS

1. The elderly are more susceptible to food-drug interactions because of primary and secondary aging changes, exposure to many drugs over an extended period of time, and susceptibility to vitamin and mineral deficiencies.
2. The physiologic and psychologic status of the elderly client may affect how the drug will act in the body.
   a. Malnutrition may reduce the therapeutic effect of the drug by altering rates of absorption and excretion.
   b. Depression may lead to reduced salivation with reduced nutritional intake that will alter the action of drugs.
3. Food may alter the pharmacokinetics of a drug. Increased or decreased therapeutic effectiveness may result. For example, toxicity may occur as a result of changes in biotransformation or delayed rate of excretion.
4. A drug may affect the way the body uses food by interfering with absorption of certain nutrients or by altering the body's ability to convert nutrients into a usable form.
   a. Vitamin and mineral deficiencies may result in the elderly who are at greater risk because of marginal diets and chronic illness.
   b. All therapeutic classes of drugs may demonstrate mechanisms that affect utilization of nutrients.

Alterations in Pharmacokinetics Caused by Food

ABSORPTION

The most common type of food-drug interaction is one in which the extent or rate of absorption of an oral drug is affected by food. A delay in the rate of absorption of the drug is usually not clinically significant unless a high serum level is required for a therapeutic response. Food may alter the absorption of drugs by:
1. Restricting by physical mass contact with the absorbing surface. Absorption is then inhibited or delayed.
2. Interacting with a drug and forming complexes that cannot be absorbed. For example, the calcium in milk will form non-absorbable complexes with tetracyclines. Enternal feedings may form gelatinous non-absorbable complexes with drugs.
3. Altering the secretion of gastric juice, digestive enzymes, and bile. Alterations in the pH of the stomach affect the degree of ionization

of weak acids or weak bases. As ionized drugs cannot pass through the lipid membranes, absorption of drugs is altered.

4. Delaying gastric emptying and increasing exposure of the drug to the environment of the stomach. For example, increased exposure of enteric-coated bisacodyl to the pH of the stomach may cause the coating to break down. The drug will then irritate the gastric mucosa. When the passage of enteric-coated aspirin to the small intestine is delayed by food, the therapeutic effect is also delayed.

5. Reducing hepatic blood flow and altering the first pass effect. As these changes reduce the rate of metabolism of a drug, circulating toxic levels of the drug may result.

METABOLISM

1. Food may cause enzyme induction, as when hydrocarbons in broiled meat increase the metabolism of phenacetin and theophylline. The therapeutic effect of the drug is then reduced.

2. Nutrients may be altered by certain drugs, as when monoamine oxidase (MAO) inhibitors suppress the monoamine oxidase enzymes that are needed to metabolize tyramine, a potent pressor contained in aged cheese, beer, broad beans, beverages containing caffeine, Chianti wine, chocolate, figs, licorice, liver, herring, cream, yogurt, and yeast extract. Failure of the enzymes to inactivate tyramine results in hypertensive crisis.

EXCRETION

1. Excessive intake of food that alters the pH of urine can affect the excretion of weakly acidic or basic drugs.

2. The type of ash, alkaline or acidic, that the food will be metabolized to is determined by the mineral content of the food and is not indicated by the taste of the food.

Strategies for Minimizing Food-drug Interactions

1. Assess the client prior to initiating drug therapy and periodically for response to drug therapy.

2. Be alert for the effects of drugs on nutrient utilization that may result in malnutrition with vitamin and mineral deficiencies. Plan for supplementation of nutrients as needed.

3. Utilize appropriate references for comprehensive information on all drugs.

4. Check that all medication dispensers are appropriately labeled with complete information for administration.
5. Help the client plan how to acidify or alkalize urine by dietary intake if indicated by drug therapy. (See foods that affect urinary pH under "Interventions for Prevention of Drug Interactions," previously.)
6. Alert the client, his family or significant other to possible food-drug interactions and advise how to minimize these. Table 5–2 shows recommended administrations for selected drugs to minimize food-drug interactions.
7. Administer drugs with a glass of water (unless contraindicated) to increase the gastric emptying rate and the exposure of the drug to the absorbing surface of the small intestine.
8. Drugs that are to be taken on an empty stomach should be administered at least 1 hour before a meal or 2 hours after a meal.

DRUG USE AND ABUSE

The elderly are at high risk for drug misuse and may also be at considerable risk for drug abuse. Some elderly may obtain illicit drugs. Some opiate addicts may reach old age and maintain some form of their habit. Most instances of inappropriate drug use in the elderly are likely to involve medications prescribed for existing physical or psychologic conditions. The extent and nature of drug abuse among the elderly is unknown, as it is often denied or unrecognized. Distinguishing between misuse and abuse is difficult. The Federal Government's Strategy Council on Drug Abuse (1979) has developed the following definition of drug misuse and drug abuse:

1. Drug misuse is the inappropriate use of drugs for therapeutic purposes. This includes inappropriate prescribing or use of drugs resulting from the following:
   a. Lack of knowledge on the part of the physician.
   b. Errors in judgment by the physician, including drugs prescribed when there is a preferable, safer alternative treatment (such alternatives may include nondrug treatment).
   c. Client use of a prescription drug not under the supervision of a physician or not in accordance with the instructions of the physician.
2. Drug abuse is the nontherapeutic use of any psychoactive substance, including alcohol, in such a manner as to adversely affect some aspect of the user's life. The use pattern may be occasional or habitual. The substance may be obtained from any number of sources, such as:

Table 5–2. *Recommended Administration for Selected Drugs to Minimize Food-Drug Interactions*

Drug	Take Without Food	Take With Food	Do Not Take With Milk or Dairy Products	Restrict Alcohol
Acetaminophen	X			
Adrenal cortical steroids		X		
Ampicillin	X			
Aspirin		X		
Barbiturates				X
Bisacodyl	X		X	
Carbamazepine		X		
Cephalosporins	X			
Chlorpropamide				X
Cimetidine		X		
Colchicine		X		
Diuretics		X		
Erythromycin stearate		X		
Estrogens		X		
Ethyl alcohol		X		
Griseofulvin		X		
Hydralazine		X		
Hydrochlorothiazide		X		
Indomethacin		X		
Iron salts			X	
Isoniazid	X			
Lincomycin	X			
Lithium		X		
Methoxsalen		X		
Metronidazole				X
Mineral oil	X			
Nitrofurantoin		X		
Penicillamine	X			
Penicillin	X			
Phenolphthalein	X			
Phenylbutazone		X		
Phenytoin		X		
Potassium chloride solutions			X	
Potassium iodide		X		
Propantheline bromide	X			
Propranolol		X		
Pyrimethamine		X		
Quinidine		X		
Riboflavin		X		
Rifampin	X			
Spironolactone		X		
Sulfadiazine	X			
Sulfasalazine		X		
Tetracyclines	X			
Thiamine		X		
Thiazide		X		
Tolbutamide				X
Triamterene		X		

a. Prescriptions.
b. Friends.
c. Over-the-counter preparations.
d. The illicit market.

Drug Misuse

1. Reasons for drug misuse.
   a. The health care provider tends to prescribe more medications (particularly tranquilizers) than needed.
   b. Tranquilizer use is widespread, especially in nursing homes, where it is particularly motivated by the desire of officials to maintain operational efficiency.
   c. The elderly misuse drugs intended for therapeutic purposes because of lack of knowledge, errors, or self-medication.
2. Strategies for reduction of drug misuse.
   a. Assume responsibility for obtaining education related to drug use, misuse, and abuse to effectively provide appropriate health supervision.
   b. Establish an empathetic relationship with the client and provide opportunity for expression of feelings related to loss of family and friends, physical changes, retirement problems, dependency, depression, and low self-esteem.
   c. Assist the elder in appropriately coping with these crises of aging rather than rendering him unable to cope by the overuse of tranquilizers.
   d. Provide comprehensive care in the community and in nursing homes.
      (1) Maintain ongoing assessment of the intellectual, emotional, social, and physical dimensions of the client.
      (2) Utilize this assessment in setting goals and planning interventions appropriate for promoting health.
   e. Develop an individual plan reflecting the unique needs of each client.
   f. Make available a variety of treatment modalities, including physical therapy; occupational therapy; recreational therapy; reminiscence groups; and socialization with children, adults, and pets.
   g. Avoid excessive use of tranquilizers that hasten decremental changes and rob elders of the opportunity to fully use their remaining faculties to adjust to the environment and live in dignity.
   h. Appropriately inform the elderly about their health status and

teach them how to adhere to the therapeutic regimen prescribed. See under "Drug Compliance" in Chapter 6.

  i. Advise the elderly to seek medical attention rather than use OTC drugs.
  j. Teach the elderly person not to share or hoard drugs by emphasizing the associated dangers.
      (1) Sharing may result in lack of appropriate treatment and adverse reactions.
      (2) Hoarding may lead to excessive accumulation of central nervous system depressants, which may be ingested accidentally or used in a suicide attempt.

Drug Abuse

CHARACTERISTICS

1. In comparison with younger age groups, the elderly probably use drugs and alcohol more as coping mechanisms for dealing with depression, losses, and problems.
2. Although some addicts "mature out" of their addiction, the majority adapt and hide their addiction by using other drugs such as hydromorphone hydrochloride (Dilaudid), by decreasing daily usage, and by substituting legally available substances such as alcohol or barbiturates.
3. Aged addicts leave the street culture, because both the subculture and new recruits have changed and no longer meet their needs for social support. The dissatisfaction (lack of social support) that motivates the older adult to drop out of the street culture may be used as the basis for programs to rehabilitate them.
4. In contrast to the stereotype of drug addicts is a group of elderly Chinese who became addicted early in the century after emigrating from China. Burdened with the necessity of meeting their opiate needs, these Chinese—in contrast to most other addicts—have been hard-working, productive, and otherwise law-abiding citizens all their lives.

STRATEGIES FOR REDUCTION OF DRUG ABUSE

1. Encourage use of methadone maintenance clinics, which provide a legal free means of meeting addiction needs and opportunities for counseling and social network support.
2. Develop outreach programs in cities to reach older drug-dependent persons.

3. Create public education campaigns.
4. Work toward re-educating health professionals as needed.
5. Develop strategies to convince nursing homes to accept methadone-maintained patients.

Alcoholism

CHARACTERISTICS

1. Alcoholism is more prevalent among the elderly than previously recognized and is a significant problem.
2. Whereas the alcohol problems of some older persons are an extension of a lifelong behavior pattern, some elders (about one third) experience alcohol problems as a reaction to loss of family and friends, physical changes, retirement problems, dependency, depression, and low self-esteem.
3. Late-onset alcoholics do not seem to have the deep-seated psychologic problems of the early-onset alcoholics.
4. Frequency of alcoholic consumption appears the same as in younger alcoholics, but the quantities of alcohol are less.
5. In the elderly, the consequences of alcohol abuse seems not to lead to as severe and obvious social or physical problems and impairments.
6. The chronic alcoholic who exhibits psychopathologic symptoms; depressive traits; and a history of employment problems, police problems, and marital instability is often known to health care providers.
7. The elderly person who in response to loss and lack of control increases his alcoholic consumption is often not recognized as having a problem. The family usually shields these individuals from public notice and in their denial may supply the elder with alcohol.

DILEMMAS ASSOCIATED WITH ALCOHOLISM

1. Alcohol and other drugs produce more pronounced behavioral and physiologic effects in the elderly.
2. Alcohol problems and aging-related pathologic conditions may be difficult to differentiate and may interact with and exacerbate each other.
3. Pathologic conditions already existing are exacerbated by excessive alcoholic consumption.
4. Diagnosis of pathologic conditions is complicated by these alcohol-induced changes.

5. Older clients are more at risk for drug interactions, as they often take many medications that, when combined with alcohol, can lead to coma and death.
6. Because the elderly metabolize alcohol differently and metabolize drugs more slowly than younger people, more time (several days) may elapse for drug interactions to occur so that there is increased risk, and interactions may be undetected or incorrectly attributed.
7. Problems associated with alcoholism are ascribed to aging (e.g., alcoholism may cause dementia that may be diagnosed as part of aging).

CONSIDERATIONS IN TREATMENT

1. Most iatrogenic side effects of alcohol are preventable or potentially reversible if recognized early.
2. There is a need for preventive programs designed specifically to develop an understanding of psychosocial factors that precipitate problem behaviors.
3. Effective programs are those working with self-concept, interpersonal relationships, and developmental change.
4. Although the objective of therapy may be an attempt to achieve complete abstinence, a reduction in the number and severity of binges may be a more realistic goal.
5. Alcoholics may fail several therapies before a certain combination is successful.

STRATEGIES FOR TREATMENT

1. Consider common treatment approaches for alcoholism (early-onset) such as behavior modification, psychotherapy, and deterrence and adversion therapies. All therapies should aim to minimize the medical, psychologic, and social problems induced by alcohol.
2. Refer alcoholics who are willing to work with a group to Alcoholics Anonymous (AA). AA has been helpful to many in achieving and maintaining abstinence.
3. Refer for individual counseling those alcoholics who prefer to work in one-to-one therapy rather than group therapy.
4. Help the families of late-onset alcoholics to recognize the needs of these elders for increased control of their lives, a social support network, and opportunity for expressive activities. Help families work toward meeting these needs of the elderly.

Recommendations for Prevention of Complications of Drug Therapy

1. The professional would best take an aggressive approach to consumer health education to minimize or eliminate the unnecessary complications of drug therapy.
2. Development and use of the following resources and activities is recommended:
   a. Consumer and professional education.
   b. Drug information hotline.
   c. Medication counseling.
   d. Crisis intervention.
   e. Health referral and follow-up.
3. The National Institute on Drug Abuse (1980) recommends the following prevention activities along a continuum:
   a. Information modalities: production and distribution of materials.
   b. Education modalities: activities that focus on skill building to encourage personal growth and development.
   c. Alternative modalities: activities that focus on reduction, elimination, or delay of drug use, drug use–related dysfunctional behavior, and other problem behaviors prior to onset of serious chronic, debilitative behaviors.

References

Boyd JR: Therapeutic dilemmas in the elderly. In Covington TR, Walker JI, eds: Current Geriatric Therapy. Philadelphia: WB Saunders Co, 1984.

Fielo S, Rizzolo, MA: The effects of age on pharmacokinetics. Geriatric Nursing November-December, 6:328–331, 1985.

Gerber JG: Drug abuse in the elderly. In Schrier RW, ed: Clinical Internal Medicine in the Aged. Philadelphia: WB Saunders Co, 1982.

Glantz MD: Alcohol use and abuse. In Glantz M, Petersen DM, Whittington FJ, eds: Drugs and the Elderly Client. DHHS No. 83-1269. Washington, DC: US Government Printing Office, 1983.

Glantz MD: Drugs in the elderly. In Glantz M, Petersen DM, Whittington FJ, eds: Drugs and the Elderly Client. DHHS No. 83-1269. Washington, DC: US Government Printing Office, 1983.

Hayes JE: Normal changes in aging and nursing implications of drug therapy. Nursing Clinics of North America 17(2):253–262, 1982.

Kastarup EK, ed: Facts and Comparisons. St. Louis: Facts and Comparisons, Inc, 1981.

Lamy PP: Modifying drug dosage in elderly patients. In Covington TR, Walker JI, eds: Current Geriatric Therapy. Philadelphia: WB Saunders Co, 1984.

Lamy PP: Pharmacology and therapeutics. In Glantz M, Petersen DM, Whittington FJ, eds: Drugs and the Elderly Client. DHHS No. 83-1269. Washington, DC: US Government Printing Office, 1983.

Lamy PP: Physician drug abuse of the elderly. In McCue JD, ed: Medical Care of the Elderly. Lexington, Mass: DC Heath & Co, 1983.

Lehmann P: Food and drug interactions. HHS No. 84-3070. Washington, DC: US Government Printing Office, 1984.

Loebl S, Spratto G, Heckheimer E: The Nurses' Drug Handbook. New York: John Wiley & Sons, 1983.

Malseed RT: Pharmacology: Drug Therapy and Nursing Considerations. Philadelphia: JB Lippincott, 1982.

Mayer SE, Melmon KL, Gilman G: Introduction: The dynamics of drug absorption, distribution, and elimination. In Gilman AG, Goodman LS, Gilman A, eds: Goodman and Gilman's The Pharmacological Basis of Therapeutics. New York: Macmillan, 1980.

Mullen E, Granholm M: Drugs and the elderly patient. Journal of Gerontological Nursing 7(2):108–113, 1981.

Oppeneer JE, Vervoren, TM: Gerontological Pharmacology. St. Louis: CV Mosby, 1983.

Peterson DM: Epidemiology of drug use. In Glantz M, Petersen DM, Whittington FJ, eds: Drugs and the Elderly Client. DHHS No. 83-1269. Washington, DC: US Government Printing Office, 1983.

Peterson DM: Illegal drug use, older addicts, and the maturing-out hypothesis. In Glantz M, Petersen DM, Whittington FJ, eds: Drugs and the Elderly Client. DHHS No. 83-1269. Washington, DC: US Government Printing Office, 1983.

Roe DA: Therapeutic effects of drug-nutrient interactions in the elderly. Journal of the American Dietetic Association 2:174–178, 1985.

Smith CH, Bidlack WR: Dietary concerns associated with the use of medications. Journal of the American Dietetic Association 84:901–914, 1984.

Vicary JR: Prevention and treatment programs. In Glantz M, Petersen DM, Whittington FJ, eds: Drugs and the Elderly Client. DHHS No. 83-1269. Washington, DC: US Government Printing Office, 1983.

Wiener MB, Pepper GA, Kuhn-Weisman G, Romano, JA: Clinical Pharmacology and Therapeutics in Nursing. New York: McGraw-Hill, 1979.

Whittington FJ: Consequence of drug use, abuse, misuse, and abuse. In Glantz M, Petersen DM, Whittington FJ, eds: Drugs and the Elderly Client. DHHS No. 83-1269. Washington, DC: US Government Printing Office, 1983.

Whittington, FJ: Misuse of legal drugs and compliance with prescription directions. In Glantz M, Petersen DM, Whittington FJ, eds: Drugs and the Elderly Client. DHHS No. 83-1269. Washington, DC: US Government Printing Office, 1983.

Drug Therapy and Compliance

ALTERATIONS IN ACTION AND RECOMMENDATIONS FOR
   DRUG THERAPY WITH FREQUENTLY USED DRUG CLASSES
   AND DRUGS
STRATEGIES FOR SUCCESSFUL DRUG THERAPY
DRUG COMPLIANCE

ALTERATIONS IN ACTION AND RECOMMENDATIONS FOR THERAPY WITH FREQUENTLY USED DRUG CLASSES AND DRUGS

1. Drug therapy for the elderly, whether with medically prescribed or over-the-counter (OTC) preparations, consists of a large number of drugs taken over a long period of time to ameliorate chronic conditions.
2. The drugs most used are analgesics, cardiovascular agents, laxatives, vitamins, antacids, and antianxiety agents.
3. A basic knowledge of the classification, pharmacokinetics, pharmacodynamics, indications, contraindications, side effects, dosage, administration, and storage is essential for assisting the elderly client in complying with a drug regimen. This information is available in a comprehensive drug reference book.

Analgesics

1. Analgesics are among the most frequently purchased OTC drugs.
2. The choice of drug is influenced by advertising, recommendations by friends, past experience, and cost.
3. More professional guidance in the selection and use of OTC analgesics is needed to reduce the incidence of adverse reactions in the elderly.

ACETAMINOPHEN (APAP [TYLENOL, DATRIL])

1. Acetaminophen is the preferred analgesic for noninflammatory pain.
2. Chronic oral intake of more than 4 to 5 g/day may cause liver damage.

ACETYLSALICYLIC ACID (ASA, ASPIRIN)

1. The cheapest analgesic is aspirin.
2. For inflammatory pain, aspirin is better than acetaminophen.
3. Aspirin is as effective as propoxyphene and codeine.
4. An adverse effect of aspirin is gastrointestinal bleeding in 75% of users. Concomitant administration of a liquid antacid may be used to minimize bleeding.
5. The antiplatelet effect of aspirin is employed to prevent recurrent myocardial infarction and transient ischemic attacks.
6. Aspirin may have greater potential for adverse effects in the elderly.

PHENACETIN

1. Phenacetin, used chronically alone or in combination analgesics, is known to lead to nephropathy.
2. Chronic use is contraindicated.

PROPOXYPHENE AND PROPOXYPHENE COMBINATIONS (DARVOCET-N 100 AND DARVON COMPOUNDS)

1. Propoxyphene alone is not as effective as ASA or APAP.
2. Propoxyphene combinations are as effective as ASA or APAP.

3. In the elderly, confusional reactions are increased.
4. Long-term full-dose use is contraindicated.

NARCOTIC ANALGESICS

Doses should be lowered by one third to two thirds, or longer dosage intervals should be used.
1. *Codeine* alone is as potent as ASA and APAP, and combinations with APAP are more effective.
   a. Adverse reactions, nausea, vomiting, and constipation, occur more in the elderly than in other groups.
2. *Pentazocine hydrochloride* (Talwin) is not as effective as aspirin.
   a. Talwin may be addictive.
   b. Talwin may cause confusional reactions.
3. *Meperidine hydrochloride* (Demerol), *morphine,* and *hydromorphone* (Dilaudid) all are more potent in the elderly and should be reduced in dosage.

Antacids

1. Antacids are frequently used by the elderly to relieve heartburn or as part of a medication regimen.
2. Commercial antacids vary in neutralizing ability, depending on the amount of antacid included and the formulation.
3. Antacids should be used cautiously because they may contain significant amounts of sodium, may affect electrolyte balance, and may interfere with the absorption of other drugs.
4. In order to minimize alterations in absorption of other drugs, a person should not take any oral medication within 2 hours of taking antacids.
5. *Magnesium-containing antacids* produce a laxative effect and may cause diarrhea.
   a. Magnesium-containing antacids must be given cautiously to patients with impaired renal function, as high levels may precipitate central nervous system depression.
6. *Aluminum-containing* and *calcium-containing* antacids may cause constipation.
7. Mixtures of aluminum-containing and magnesium-containing antacids are used to avoid adverse effects upon bowel function.

Antibiotics

1. Dosages of antibiotics excreted by the kidney should be reduced, as half-life is usually extended in the elderly.
2. *Penicillin* may cause increased central nervous system toxicity, with seizures caused by the reduced rate of renal excretion of the drug.
3. The low therapeutic index of *aminoglycosides,* associated with the potential for causing ototoxicity and nephrotoxicity, requires that elderly clients receiving these antibiotics be closely clinically monitored.
4. *Tetracyclines* are best administered with at least 120 ml of water to prevent gastrointestinal irritation. They are not to be administered with dairy products or iron salts, with which they form insoluble complexes.
5. *Clinadamycin* has caused an increased incidence of diarrhea and pseudomembranous colitis in the elderly.
6. *Methenamine mandelate* (Mandelamine) has no therapeutic value for patients with an indwelling catheter, as the drug is active only in bladder urine.
7. *Sulfonamides* may cause hematologic toxicity in elderly clients on diuretic therapy.
   a. The client should be encouraged to drink large amounts of liquid to avoid crystalluria when receiving therapy with soluble sulfonamides.
   b. Sulfonamides increase the risk of a hypoglycemic reaction, especially if a client is using a oral hypoglycemic.
8. *Isoniazid* is associated with increased susceptibility to hepatotoxicity in the elderly, with anorexia and vomiting. The use of alcohol potentiates hepatotoxicity caused by isoniazid.

Anticoagulants

1. Elderly clients on anticoagulant therapy are more at risk for bleeding. They should be alerted to signs of bleeding and cautioned about activities that may cause bleeding, such as vigorous toothbrushing.
2. Hemorrhage is more likely to occur in the elderly as a result of decreased plasma binding, reduction in vitamin K intake, and alteration in liver function.
3. The use of aspirin is contraindicated with anticoagulants, as bleeding may occur as a result of drug interaction. One possible exception to this is the use of aspirin with anticoagulants for a client with a heart valve prosthesis.

Anticonvulsants

1. Diphenylhydantoin (Dilantin) is the drug of choice for seizure disorders in the elderly.
   a. Toxicity with diphenylhydantoin is more likely to occur in the elderly, as toxic serum levels of the drug occur quickly owing to reduced serum albumin available for binding and reduced renal clearance rate.
   b. The probability of a drug-drug interaction is increased when the elderly have several drugs in their regimen in addition to diphenylhydantoin.

Antidiabetic Oral Agents

1. The majority of maturity-onset diabetics may best be controlled by weight reduction and dietary changes.
2. For some diabetics with a blood glucose level of 200 to 300 mg/dl, oral drugs such as *tolbutamide* (Orinase), *chlorpropamide* (Diabinese), and *acetohexamide* (Dymelor) are used to prevent diabetic complications.
3. In the elderly, there is increased risk of overtreatment with antidiabetic drugs, such as chlorpropamide and acetohexamide, that have extended half-lives. These drugs cause periodic mild episodes of hypoglycemia that may, over a period of a few weeks, do permanent damage to the brain.
4. Hypoglycemic signs in the elderly are bizarre behavior, slurred speech, disorientation, and confusion. The classic signs of hypoglycemia, such as tremor, sweating, and tachycardia, are not as visible in the elderly.
5. Increased photosensitivity and cardiovascular morbidity are associated with the use of oral antidiabetic agents in the elderly.

Antihypertensives

1. The elderly taking antihypertensives must be carefully monitored, as the drugs often make clients lethargic, depressed, and subject to giddiness and postural hypotension.
2. Titrating antihypertensives accurately is complicated by the inability to obtain accurate blood pressure levels. Increased rigidity of the arterial wall affects blood pressure readings obtained with a manometer and cuff. These readings are not as reliable as previously believed. Intra-arterial transducers have revealed diastolic pressures 20 to 25 mm Hg lower than sphygmomanometer readings.

3. There is further reduction in baroreceptor response and peripheral venous tone by antihypertensive drugs that alter sympathetic nerve response. Severe hypotension that may result may be catastrophic, as the blood and oxygen supply to the brain and heart is already compromised by cerebral and coronary arteriosclerosis. Orthostatic hypotension may occur and predispose the elderly client to falling.
4. In the elderly, blood pressure maintained below 120/70 mm Hg may precipitate orthostatic hypotension, impaired sexual function, and drowsiness or sedation.
5. *Clonidine hydrochloride* (Catapres) is not recommended for use with poorly compliant clients or for those with renal problems.
6. *Hydralazine hydrochloride* (Apresoline) may aggravate angina, but this effect may be blocked by propranolol.
7. *Methyldopa* (Aldomet) may be used with a diuretic to prevent sodium retention. One bedtime dose may improve compliance and may have a sedative effect as well as lower blood pressure.
8. *Prazosin hydrochloride* (Minipress) lowers blood pressure profoundly with the first dose. Clients should be alerted to the rapidity of effect.
9. Clients taking *propranolol* (Inderal) do not require a diuretic to prevent sodium retention. See "Beta-adrenergic Blockers" under "Cardiovascular Agents," later.
10. *Reserpine* is not recommended for use in clients experiencing depression, sinusitis, or peptic ulcer disease or in clients with a history of breast cancer.
11. *Combination drugs* (e.g., Ser-Ap-Es, Aldoril, Esimil, Salutensin, and Hydropres) with reduced diuretic, sympatholytic, or vasodilator doses minimize full-dose side effects.
    a. Use of diuretics is preferable to the use of combinations when treating elderly hypertensive patients.

Anti-Inflammatory Analgesics

PHENYLBUTAZONE AND OXYPHENBUTAZONE

1. Phenylbutazone and oxyphenbutazone have longer half-lives, greater incidence of gastrointestinal side effects, increased oral anticoagulant effects, and severe toxic reactions in the elderly.
2. Fluid retention and blood dyscrasias may occur in adverse reactions.

3. Administration with meals or a liquid antacid is necessary to reduce gastrointestinal side effects.
4. Full dosage is not recommended for longer than 14 days.

INDOMETHACIN

1. Indomethacin (Indocin) frequently causes lightheadedness and headaches.
2. Gastrointestinal effects are more insidious than with phenylbutazone.
3. Full dosage is not recommended for longer than 14 days.

OTHERS

Tolmetin sodium (Tolectin), *fenoprofen calcium* (Nalfon), *sulindac* (Clinoril), *ibuprofen* (Motrin), and *naproxen* (Naprosyn) are less effective than ASA in inflammatory disease, but gastrointestinal side effects occur less often. All are more expensive than aspirin.

Antiparkinsonian Agents

1. Therapy should start with small doses that are gradually increased as needed.
2. *Trihexyphenidyl* (Artane), *procyclidine hydrochloride* (Kemadrin), and *benztropine mesylate* (Cogentin) are antiparkinsonian drugs that are generally not recommended for prophylaxis against the appearance of side effects of antipsychotic agents.
   a. If extrapyramidal symptoms appear as a result of use of antipsychotic drugs, the antiparkinsonian drugs may be administered for 1 to 3 months with beneficial effects.
3. *Anticholinergic blocking agents* such as benztropine mesylate have limited use because they tend to exacerbate side effects (dry mouth, constipation, tachycardia, and urinary retention).
4. *Diphenhydramine hydrochloride* (Benadryl) is utilized for treatment of extrapyramidal symptoms in geriatric clients unable to tolerate more potent drugs.
5. The elderly client taking *levodopa* (L-Dopa) should be advised not to use vitamin supplements containing 10 to 25 mg of vitamin B_6, as that reverses the antiparkinsonian effect of levodopa.

Cardiovascular Agents

ANTIARRHYTHMICS

1. Declines in organ function, changes in tissue sensitivity, drug-drug interaction, stress, and other age-related changes are considered in selecting a particular antiarrhythmic and dose for treatment of the elderly.
2. Generally, the loading dose is reduced.
3. Dosage of antiarrhythmics such as quinidine, procainamide hydrochloride (Pronestyl), and disopyramide phosphate (Norpace) is reduced by as much as 50% for the elderly.
4. *Quinidine* toxicity, cinchonism (gastrointestinal effects, lightheadedness, tinnitus), occurs more frequently in elderly clients with low body weight.
5. Quinidine and *digoxin* used together maintain higher serum levels and prolonged half-life in the elderly.
6. *Pronestyl* usually must be given at 4-hour intervals to maintain therapeutic levels.

BETA-ADRENERGIC BLOCKERS

1. The elderly receiving beta-adrenergic blockers should be assessed carefully for the onset of cardiac failure because beta blockade could further depress myocardial contractility and worsen failure.
2. When beta-adrenergic blockers are to be withdrawn, they should be tapered over a 1- to 2-week period to avoid precipitating symptoms associated with coronary artery disease.

CALCIUM CHANNEL BLOCKERS

1. For management of angina in the elderly, doses should be as small as possible to prevent hypotension and syncope, which lead to falls and fractures.
2. Increase in dosage must be done very gradually.
3. Drugs should be tapered at time of withdrawal.

DIGITALIS PREPARATIONS

1. In the treatment of cardiac failure and arrhythmias, *digoxin* (Lanoxin) is preferred, as digitoxin and digitalis leaf have extended half-lives.

2. After cardiac failure has cleared and the client appears stabilized, digoxin may be discontinued.
3. The range between therapeutic effect and toxic effect is small.
4. As the mean half-life of digoxin in the elderly is lengthened with reduced urinary clearance, close monitoring is necessary.
5. The concomitant use of a diuretic makes the client susceptible to dehydration and digoxin toxicity.
6. Drug toxicity may present as delirium in the elderly. Extreme weariness; lethargy; and initial signs of gastrointestinal toxicity, anorexia, and weight loss may also occur.
7. Because noncompliance with digitalis preparations occurs in about one third to one half of clients, close monitoring for compliance is essential.

VASODILATORS

1. All vasodilators may cause orthostatic hypotension.
2. Clients should be warned against concurrent alcohol consumption, which may precipitate too low blood pressure.
3. The client should sit down prior to sublingual use to prevent falling as a result of orthostatic hypotension.
4. *Nitroglycerin ointment* should be applied on paper and not rubbed into the skin.
5. Long-acting nitrates (e.g., Isordil, Sorbitrate, and Peritrate) have variable effects on older people.
6. Central cerebrovascular and peripheral dilators (e.g., Vasodilan, nylidrin hydrochloride, Cyclospasmol, Hydergine, and niacin) may be used in a 1- to 3-month trial for senile dementia or peripheral vascular disease.

Diuretics

1. Diuretics are one of the most common drugs to cause adverse reactions in the elderly.
2. All diuretics worsen incontinence.
3. Dehydration, hypokalemia, and hypotension are easily precipitated by diuretics in the elderly. Changes in dietary intake, less effective thirst recognition, and abnormal autonomic response to hypotension by the baroreceptors predispose the elderly to these conditions.
4. Fluid intake of at least 1500 ml/day should be encouraged.
5. Fluid intake and urine output and electrolytes should be periodically monitored.

6. Foods high in potassium, such as bananas and citrus juices, should be included in the diet.
7. Potassium supplementation and salt substitutes (potassium chloride) should be used cautiously to avoid life-threatening hyperkalemia, especially with potassium-sparing diuretics.
8. Dosage should be reviewed if blood pressure is less than 120/70 mm Hg.
9. Administration of too high a dose may result in mild dehydration, lethargy, and dizziness on standing.
10. Dehydration and hypokalemia associated with diuretic therapy may potentiate the toxicity of cardiac glycosides.
11. Diuretics may not be an essential part of maintenance therapy after congestive heart failure. After the client is stabilized and the edema has cleared, the dosage of the diuretic may be reduced.

THIAZIDES

1. Therapy using chlorothiazide (Diuril) or hydrochlorothiazide (HYDROdiuril) should by started with the lowest possible dose.
2. Thiazides are ineffective if creatinine clearance is less than 30 to 40 ml/min.

FUROSEMIDE

1. Furosemide (Lasix) is effective with creatinine clearance less than 30 ml/min.
2. Furosemide may cause electrolyte imbalance, as it promotes sodium, potassium, calcium, and chloride excretion.
3. If the client is susceptible to precipitancy of micturition, a slower-acting diuretic (one of the thiazides) rather than furosemide may be preferable to avoid incontinence.

SPIRONOLACTONE

1. Spironolactone (Aldactone) is a potassium-sparing diuretic.
2. Spironolactone is used often in combination with thiazide (Aldactazide).
3. Use of supplemental potassium and salt substitutes, which may lead to fatal hyperkalemia, should be limited.

TRIAMTERENE

1. Triamterene (Dyrenium) is a potassium-sparing diuretic.
2. Triamterene is most often used in combination with thiazide (Dyazide).
3. Use of supplemental potassium and salt substitutes, which may lead to fatal hyperkalemia, should be limited.

Hormones

1. *Prednisone, dexamethasone* (Decadron), and *methylprednisolone* (Medrol) are used primarily for crippling inflammatory diseases (rheumatoid arthritis) or disabling allergic disease (asthma).
   a. When treatment is discontinued, dosage is to be tapered.
   b. With long-term use, there is a greatly increased risk of gastrointestinal bleeding, loss of diabetic control, osteoporosis, myopathy, cataracts, psychic disturbances, and fluid retention.
2. *Thyroid* replacement should be started with low doses and gradually increased to avoid increased risk of cardiovascular and cerebrovascular morbidity.

Laxatives

Excessive laxative usage by the elderly may precipitate problems. After the bowel is cleaned out by a laxative, the patient will not have a bowel movement for a day or two. During this period "imaginary constipation" occurs; the client is convinced that he is constipated because he has not had a bowel movement for a day or two, and so he takes another laxative. Teaching the client about a normal stool pattern may be helpful in reducing laxative use.

1. *Mineral oil* may be aspirated and may lead to pneumonitis and even pneumonia.
   a. This laxative should not be taken with food, as it interferes with the absorption of vitamins A, D, E, and K and the mineral calcium in the gut.
2. *Irritant cathartics* (e.g., Dulcolax, Ex-Lax, Modane) or saline cathartics (e.g., milk of magnesia, Epsom) should be discouraged, as they tend to foster more constipation.
3. *Stool softeners* (e.g., Colace, Surfak) and bulk laxatives (e.g., Metamucil, Effersyllium, or Konsyl) produce the most normal type of stool. (See under "Constipation, in Chapter 3.)

Potassium Chloride Supplements

1. Liquid potassium chloride (KCl) must be used with sufficient water to prevent osmotic diarrhea.
2. Salt substitutes (e.g., Neocurtasal, Co-Salt) must be measured carefully, as each tablespoonful contains about 65 mEq KCl.
3. Efferevescent KCl (K-lyte) is expensive but tastes better than liquid KCl.
4. Solid KCl (Slow K, Kaon-Cl) is expensive but well tolerated except in delayed gastrointestinal transit time or esophageal or pyloric obstruction.

Psychotropic Agents

1. Informing the elderly that psychotropic drugs affect libido and potency in varying degrees will be helpful to them in distinguishing side effects from primary aging changes. The physician should be aware of these problems, as reduction in libido and potency caused by side effects may be relieved by dosage reduction or change to another drug.
2. Simple drug intoxication may be demonstrated by lethargy, confusion, and disorientation.
3. Secondary effects, such as postural hypotension and disinhibition reactions, such as restlessness, agitation, paranoia, and aggression, may occur.
4. It may be not advisable to administer psychotropic drugs at bedtime to the elderly client who voids at night, as he may fall as a result of orthostatic hypotension precipitated by the drug.

ANTIDEPRESSANTS

1. Depression occurs in many elderly as they experience bereavement and relocation. Therapeutic counseling, socialization, and exercise all play a valuable part in assisting the elderly to cope with depression.
2. Care should be taken not to suppress the expression of grief by drugs. Antidepressant drug therapy should be used judiciously, as it may worsen feelings of anxiety and depression and initiate or contribute to acute and chronic brain syndromes.
3. *Monoamine oxidase inhibitors* are contraindicated in the treatment of depression because side effects such as orthostatic hypotension, inhibition of ejaculation, weakness, and hypertensive crisis are more

likely to occur in association with polypharmacy and lack of necessary diet compliance by the elderly.

4. *Tricyclic antidepressants* include imipramine hydrochloride (Tofranil) and amitriptyline hydrochloride (Elavil).
   a. Adverse reactions most likely to occur in the elderly are dry mouth, constipation, dizziness, tachycardia, palpitations, blurred vision, urinary retention, orthostatic hypotension, and cardiac arrhythmia.
   b. Tricyclics are to be used cautiously in a client with narrow-angle glaucoma or increased ocular pressure.
   c. Once the client has been stabilized on a dose, one nightly administration is preferable because it has a sedative effect and yet prevents the client from experiencing the worst side effects, such as dry mouth. Also, the client is less likely to forget to take the drug at bedtime.
   d. Because tricyclics tend to worsen already existing conditions, such as glaucoma, confusion, cardiac arrhythmias, and urinary retention, careful evaluation of benefit versus risk must be done on an individual basis.
5. *Methylphenidate hydrochloride* (Ritalin) may be used for the treatment of mild depression, but caution must be used because the drug may exacerbate anxiety and tension and worsen glaucoma.
6. *Lithium carbonate* (Eskalith, Lithane, and Lithonate) is used effectively in much lower doses in the elderly for preventing recurrence of manic attacks and for modifying mood swings associated with bipolar depression.
   a. Clients over age 60 are more susceptible to lithium toxicity, demonstrated by diarrhea, vomiting, tremor, mild ataxia, drowsiness, thirst, polyuria, muscular weakness, slurred speech, and confusion.
   b. Normal amounts of sodium must be available to prevent lithium retention and toxicity. Therapy with lithium for a client on diuretic therapy may be inadvisable, as low levels of sodium would predispose the client to lithium retention and toxicity.

MINOR TRANQUILIZERS (BENZODIAZEPINES)

1. Benzodiazepines, including *chlordiazepoxide hydrochloride* (Librium) and *diazepam* (Valium), are used for relief of tension and anxiety, but they have debilitating effects, particularly in the elderly.
   a. Benzodiazepines are seldom life threatening but are more likely to cause confusion, drowsiness, fatigue, lethargy, nystagmus, ataxia, dysarthria, and muscle weakness in the elderly.

b. Since these features are characteristic of illness, the benzodiazepines may in this way confuse the clinical picture and debilitate the patient.

c. As the medicated lethargic patient may not eat or drink, mild dehydration may develop that further intensifies the adverse effects of the drug.

d. Muscle weakness and nightmares with self-destructive features have been associated with use of the benzodiazepines.

e. Librium and Valium have greatly extended half-lives with the potential for accumulation in the elderly. *Oxazepam* (Serax) is the preferred drug of the group, as it is safer by virtue of its shorter half-life (3 to 21 hours).

f. Use of benzodiazepines for the elderly is questionable, with no greater benefit demonstrated by these agents than by other drugs that are less hazardous and debilitating.

Major Tranquilizers and Antipsychotics

1. The *phenothiazines* (chlorpromazine hydrochloride [Thorazine] and thioridazine hydrochloride [Mellaril]) and *butyrophenone* (haloperidol [Haldol]) are administered to tranquilize or sedate and for antipsychotic effect, or a normalizing of mood, thought, and behavior. They are used to control anxiety and restlessness displayed in schizophrenic and other psychiatric disorders.

2. Close monitoring for the elderly on phenothiazine therapy is essential, as elders are more susceptible to hypotension, oversedation, dryness of mouth, blurred vision, photosensitivity, altered libido and potency, hypothermia, urinary retention, and constipation.

3. Decreased thirst owing to central nervous system inhibition has been know to precipitate dehydration, hemoconcentration, reduced pulmonary ventilation, and pneumonia.

4. Clients must be cautioned not to drink alcohol or use other sedatives that will potentiate the tranquilizer.

5. Driving a car or operating other machinery is contraindicated.

6. Extrapyramidal pseudoparkinsonism symptoms demonstrated by muscle tremors, rigidity, muscle spasms, extreme restlessness, and involuntary movements may occur.

7. Tardive dyskinesia (involuntary and repetitive movements, including tongue protrusion, licking of the lips, smacking and sucking lip movements, chewing, puffing of cheeks, facial grimacing, grunting, and other strange sounds, wrinkling of the forehead, and blinking of the eyes, may occur).

a. Tardive dyskinesia is more likely to occur with high-dose therapy in the elderly. There is a higher incidence in elderly women and in the elderly who have a previous history of brain damage.

   b. There is no effective treatment for tardive dyskinesia, and for some patients the symptoms are irreversible.

   c. If these symptoms appear, all antipsychotic medication should be stopped.

   d. An early sign of impending tardive dyskinesia is vermicular (wormlike) movements of the tongue.

   e. If medication is stopped when the early signs appear, tardive dyskinesia may not develop.

8. Close monitoring of the elderly on therapy with antipsychotics and major tranquilizers is essential to maximize the effect of the drug, minimize side effects, and support the client during untoward reactions.

9. Clients must be carefully evaluated for adherence to the drug regimen, as lack of compliance has been associated with the attempt to reduce untoward reactions and with hoarding pills for attempts at suicide.

10. The use of a liquid formulation rather than pills may be more reliable in ensuring compliance.

11. After a steady level of drugs in the body has been achieved, one dose administered at bedtime with a warm drink may have both a sedative and antipsychotic effect with reduction in the side effects of dry mouth and hypotension.

12. The aim of therapy is to achieve a steady level of the drug that will help the patient maintain a more rational attitude.

SEDATIVES

1. Preferable to the use of sedatives for complaints of insomnia is identification of the stressor causing insomnia. Emotional support and encouragement to read or drink warm milk often are helpful (see under "Insomnia," Chapter 3).

2. Use of barbiturates (e.g., phenobarbital, Nembutal, Seconal, Amytal) is contraindicated in the elderly, as barbiturates tend to accumulate in the body and cause a syndrome that resembles dementia with intellectual impairment and slowing of speech and gait.

3. Barbiturates in the elderly may cause paradoxical excitement, the reverse of the desired effect.

4. *Chloral hydrate* is used for nighttime sedation for the elderly because it is quickly excreted from the body and causes mild gastrointestinal upset only in a few clients.

5. *Flurazepam hydrochloride* (Dalmane) or *oxazepam* is also administered

for insomnia. Flurazepam should not be taken more than 5 nights a week, in order to prevent toxic accumulation.

6. *Diphenhydramine hydrochloride* (e.g., Benadryl) may be utilized for sedation in the elderly who cannot tolerate more potent sedation.

7. *Meprobamate* (Equanil, Miltown) is no more effective than a placebo. Continual use is not recommended, as it has a narrow therapeutic index.

Theophylline

1. Dosages of theophylline should be reduced by an average of 30% in the elderly.
2. Congestive heart disease, cirrhosis, influenza vaccine, and viral upper respiratory infection reduce hepatic clearance.
3. Smoking increases metabolism of theophylline and influences dosage requirements.

Vitamin and Mineral Supplements

1. Vitamin and mineral supplements may be indicated when diets are marginal.
2. *Calcium* supplementation is frequently necessary, as the requirement rises to 1000 to 1500 mg/day to prevent osteoporosis.
3. The elderly should be cautioned against oversupplementation with vitamins or minerals, which may lead to imbalance or toxicity.
4. The anemic elderly should always be assessed for bleeding or systemic diseases before hemapoietic therapy is started.

STRATEGIES FOR SUCCESSFUL DRUG THERAPY

1. Encourage the use of one pharmacy, as it is most helpful for the client to establish rapport with a pharmacist who will develop a drug profile (record of all drugs prescribed for client).
2. Assist the client in developing a medication card listing all medications and amount and frequency of dosage. Teach the client to carry this card with him at all times. Advise the client to enroll in a Medic Alert System (Fig. 6–1).
3. Inform seniors that they may request regular bottle caps rather than child-proof bottle caps. Regular caps are usually easier for the elderly to open.
4. Encourage the use of generic drugs at the onset of therapy (if ap-

1. Your emblem, bearing the internationally recognized medical symbol, triggers Medic Alert®, the world's only comprehensive emergency medical information system.

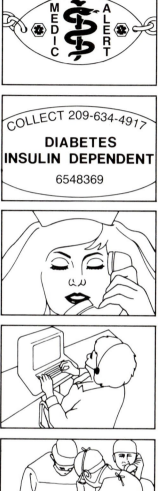

2. The emblem is engraved with your primary medical conditions, personal identification number, and Medic Alert's 24-hour hotline phone number.

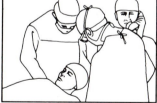

3. A hotline call from a medical professional starts the information retrieval process.

4. Within seconds, Medic Alert's emergency operator responds with your computerized information.

5. Your vital data relayed back to emergency room staff help medical personnel provide appropriate diagnosis and care, and could save your life.

As a back-up to the Medic Alert System, you are provided with an annually updated wallet card.

Figure 6–1. *How the Medic Alert® System works. Medic Alert is an international emergency medical system. A person pays a fee to enroll in the system and receives a bracelet or neck chain to wear at all times. If the person is found unconscious or unable to communicate, the health care worker telephones the Medic Alert number and receives information about the patient's health problem. (From Medic Alert Foundation International.)*

proved by prescriber of medication) to avoid changes in bioequivalence after the client has been stabilized on another drug.

5. See Chapter 7 for adaptive equipment for the client who experiences vision loss and Chapter 11 for assistive devices for the client who experiences loss of dexterity.

6. Suggest to the physician the use of a formulation most easily swallowed by the elderly client (e.g., liquids or caplets instead of large tablets or capsules). Changes in bioequivalence of formulations must be considered.

7. Evaluate the elderly client who appears to be deteriorating in all dimensions for possible adverse drug reactions.

8. Be alert to the client presenting signs of acute brain syndrome that may be due to adverse drug reactions.

9. Be alert to signs of dehydration that will affect drug action. Assess tongue for furrows indicating dehydration. The tongue is the best indicator of state of hydration in the elderly.

10. Provide enough fluids to promote easy swallowing of the medication and to help it move through the gastrointestinal tract. The elderly should be assisted into a position that prevents aspiration and promotes swallowing.

11. Ensure that medication has not adhered to dry mucous membranes and that it has been swallowed.

12. Discourage drug-induced immobility that leads to perceptual changes, dehydration, and decubitus.

13. Plan for a longer period of time for absorption of rectal suppositories, as the elderly have reduced body temperature.

14. Monitor injection sites, as reduced cutaneous sensation may mask pain, infection, intravasation, or other trauma.

15. Include a family member or significant other and the pharmacist as part of the support system for achieving compliance.

16. Refer to a community health agency as needed.

DRUG COMPLIANCE

1. Noncompliance with a prescribed medication regimen is estimated in 25 to 50% of the elderly population.

2. The elderly require assistance to improve compliance, as they experience changes in all dimensions that add to the problems of adhering to a medication regimen.

3. The results of noncompliance may be:
   a. A poor therapeutic response.
   b. Toxicity associated with improved compliance after dosage increases.

Table 6–1. *Factors That Promote or Interfere with Compliance**

Factors	Compliance	Noncompliance
Disease Factors		
Mental or emotional problems		X
Client's perception of diagnosis as life-threatening	X	
Severe symptoms and degree of disability	X	
Prolonged illness		X
Good response to therapy		X
Characteristics of Therapy		
Prolonged duration of treatment		X
Complex drug regimen		X
Increased frequency of dosing		X
Increased side effects		X
Increased cost		X
Client Factors		
Increased age		X
High satisfaction with provider	X	
Low educational level		X
Low socioeconomic status		X
Low income		X
Ability to contact pharmacy	X	
Understanding of the diagnosis, need, and benefit of drug	X	
Lack of desire to regain health		X
Ability to make judgments	X	
Cultural or religious conflicts		X

*Adapted from Boyd JR: Therapeutic dilemmas in the elderly. In Covington, TR, Walker, JI, eds: Current Geriatric Therapy. Philadelphia; WB Saunders Co, 1984.

    c. Unnecessary therapy with agents that produce more adverse effects.
    d. Increases in morbidity and mortality.
  4. Factors that promote or interfere with compliance are indicated in Table 6–1.
  5. Problems involving medication errors that result in noncompliance and strategies to promote compliance are listed in Table 6–2.

Table 6–2. *Problems Involving Medication Errors That Result in Noncompliance and Strategies to Promote Compliance*

Problems	Strategies
Failure to Fill the Prescription	*Strategies to Promote Obtaining the Medication*
Lack of finances and expense of the medication	Arrange for financial assistance if client is unable to afford medication or equipment (see Financial Assistance, Chapter 17).
Inaccessibility of pharmacy	Assist client in selecting a pharmacist with whom communication can be established by phone or mail.
Lack of understanding of diagnosis, need, and benefit of drug	Explain diagnosis, need, and benefit of each drug. Provide client with appropriate educational materials.

Table continued on following page

Table 6–2. *Problems Involving Medication Errors That Result in Noncompliance and Strategies to Promote Compliance* Continued

Problems	Strategies
Failure to Fill the Prescription	*Strategies to Promote Obtaining the Medication*
Conflict with cultural or religious beliefs	Explore cultural or religious beliefs regarding illness and treatment. Identify conflicts and assist client in resolution that will permit compliance. Find appropriate references and individuals who may clarify beliefs and suggest alternatives that will promote compliance.
Lack of desire to regain health	Assess whether lack of desire to regain health is due to cognitive impairment, secondary gains, or desire to end life. Develop with client or family or significant other interventions that will better meet his needs and involve him in society. The cognitively impaired individual requires family or significant other to assume responsibility for compliance.
Incorrect Administration of Medication	*Strategies to Promote Correct Administration of Medication*
Complexity of regimen	Reduce complexity of medication regimen by minimizing number and frequency of medications.
Medication to be taken at different times throughout the day	Check with physician for possibility of using timed-release capsules, especially for patients with failing memory.
Dosage errors	Identify type of error and reasons for incorrect administration.
Errors in frequency (taking too many or too few), errors in timing (taking before or after meals)	
Lack of knowledge of purpose of medication	Provide cards with name of drug, reasons for use, benefit expected, route of administration, possible adverse reactions, and interactions and interventions to minimize adverse reactions.
Unclear directions on container (printing too small on label); vague directions on label (e.g., p.r.n. [as necessary] requires judgment)	Check that each container is labeled clearly with name of drug, frequency, and route of administration.
Failing memory	Develop calendar indicating day of the week and time medication is to be taken. Instruct client to associate taking medication with daily events, such as before or after meals or at bedtime. Associating taking medication with a program that the client watches daily on television may be helpful. Promote compliance by clients on a regimen of several medications a day to be dosed at various times. 1. Encourage client to obtain a medication container (or to use an egg carton) and number compartments. 2. Teach client to stock compartments of container with appropriate medications for the day. 3. Client should then check container for medication to be taken at agreed upon intervals. This process is especially helpful for clients with poor memory.

Table 6–2. *Problems Involving Medication Errors That Result in Noncompliance and Strategies to Promote Compliance* Continued

Problems	Strategies
Failure to Fill the Prescription	*Strategies to Promote Obtaining the Medication*
	4. Commercially made containers are available with seven small containers, one for each day of the week.
	5. Assist client in stocking the receptacles for each day of the week.
	This is convenient for client with difficulty organizing, remembering, and handling medication. This method also is helpful in alerting client in time to reorder medication.
Inability to open containers or use equipment because of sensory or motor changes	Help client to obtain equipment for administration that is easily purchased, meets his needs, is adaptable to home use, and can be replaced as needed.
Self-administration by wrong route or using wrong technique (e.g., failing to unwrap a suppository before insertion)	Teach client, family, or significant other technique for proper administration of medication, and observe return demonstrations at appropriate intervals.
Lack of assistance or supervision	Refer for home health care services as needed. As a check for compliance, record number of tablets or capsules or amount of solution that client receives from pharmacist. Record amount used and count or measure remaining medication periodically.
Premature Discontinuation of a Medication	*Strategies to Prevent Premature Discontinuation of Medication*
Feeling better as signs and symptoms of illness fade	Stress health benefits of maintaining drug compliance. Provide appropriate recognition for client's drug compliance.
Adverse effects	Advise client to check with physician if he experiences untoward effects from drug(s) rather than discontinuing the drug himself. Teach appropriate intervention for minimizing side effects when physician is aware of side effects and believes the benefit is worth the discomfort or risk.
Inability to refill prescription because of lack of accessibility to a pharmacy	Periodically evaluate client's motivation, intention, and ability to refill prescription. Assist with arranging for refill.
Lack of finances to pay for refilling prescription	Refer for financial assistance. Encourage use of generic drugs if physician agrees.
Misunderstanding directions; lack of education about benefit expected, how to minimize adverse reactions, and consequences of premature discontinuation.	Periodically evaluate client's knowledge of medication information as to name, use, frequency, dosage, anticipated side effects, mode of administration, and consequences of premature discontinuation. Correct misconceptions and reteach as needed.
Difficulty making judgments	Review with client those areas in medication regimen that require judgment, as when a medication is ordered 3 to 4 hours p.r.n. Many seniors require specific guidelines to assist them in making judgments.

Table continued on following page

Table 6–2. *Problems Involving Medication Errors That Result in Noncompliance and Strategies to Promote Compliance* Continued

Problems	Strategies
Failure to Fill the Prescription	*Strategies to Promote Obtaining the Medication*
Fear of dependency on drugs	Assist client in resolving fears of drug dependency by developing with him an acceptable regimen that will best meet his emotional and physical needs. Stress benefit to be derived by drug.
Use of Inappropriate Medication	*Strategies to Prevent Use of Inappropriate Medication*
Failure by doctor or pharmacist to limit refills	Check that client does not exceed number of refills authorized by health care provider before returning for reevaluation.

Failure to discard discontinued medication; hoarding unused pills; using outdated pills	Emphasize to client importance of discarding and replacing outdated pills (e.g., nitroglycerin sublingual tablets lose potency after 6 months and should be replaced).
	Urge client to discard discontinued pills.
	  1. Their use may lead to unfortunate side effects and toxicity.
	  2. Unused tablets lose their potency over time and should not be used even if reordered at a later date.

Sharing pills with relatives and friends	Discuss with client the detriments of sharing drugs with relatives and friends.
Self-treatment with OTC (over-the-counter) drugs	Emphasize need for health supervision and individual medication regimens. Explain need to consult with health care provider if use of OTC drugs is contemplated, as symptoms may be masked and drug interactions may occur.
Failure to report self-medication or medication ordered by another health care provider	Emphasize the necessity of reporting to health care provider self-medication or use of medication ordered by another physician.

References

Boyd JR: Therapeutic dilemmas in the elderly. In Covington TR, Walker JI, eds: Current Geriatric Therapy. Philadelphia: WB Saunders Co, 1984.

Butler RN, Lewis MI: Aging and Mental Health. St. Louis: CV Mosby, 1982.

Cape R: Aging: Its Complex Management. New York: Harper & Row, 1983.

Cooper JW: Pharmacology: Drug related problems of the elderly. In Ohara-Devereaux MO, Andrus LH, Scott CD, eds: Eldercare: A Practical Guide to Clinical Geriatrics. New York: Grune & Stratton, 1981.

Gerber JG: Drug usage in the elderly. In Schrier RW, ed: Clinical Internal Medicine in the Aged. Philadelphia: WB Saunders Co, 1982.

Kastrup EK, ed: Fact & Comparisons. St. Louis: Facts & Comparisons, Inc, 1981.

Lamy PP: Modifying drug dosage in elderly patients. In Covington TR, Walker JI, eds: Current Geriatric Therapy. Philadelphia: WB Saunders Co, 1984.

Loebl S, Spratto G, Heckheimer E: The Nurse's Drug Handbook. New York: John Wiley & Sons, 1983.

Mullen E, Granholm M: Drugs and the elderly patient. Journal of Gerontological Nursing 7(2):108–113, 1981.

Oppeneer JE, Vervoren TM: Gerontological Pharmacology. St. Louis: CV Mosby, 1983.

Wiener MB, Pepper GA, Kuhn-Weismann G, Romano JA: Clinical Pharmacology and Therapeutics in Nursing. New York: McGraw-Hill, 1979.

7

Vision and Aging

CHANGES IN VISUAL FUNCTION ASSOCIATED
  WITH PRIMARY AGING
PROBLEMS OF THE EYE THAT MAY
  IMPAIR VISION
STRATEGIES FOR PROMOTING VISION
STRATEGIES FOR ASSISTING THE VISION-IMPAIRED

1. About 5 million elderly people in the United States (20% of those over age 65) report difficulty in seeing.
2. There are currently about 990,000 elderly who are severely visually impaired. This number is expected to almost double by the year 2000.
3. Primary aging changes within the eye and secondary aging changes are largely responsible for increased visual impairment in the elderly.
4. The leading causes of legal blindness for those age 65 and over are glaucoma, macular degeneration, optic nerve atrophy, senile cataracts, and diabetic retinopathy.
5. After heart disease and arthritis, visual impairment is the greatest handicap among the aged.
6. Visual impairment may range from low vision to total blindness.
   a. *Legal blindness* exists when after correction with lenses visual acuity in the good eye is 20/200 or less or when the visual field is restricted to 20 degrees or less. (The higher number is the distance from the chart, and the lower number refers to the line on the chart. The higher the lower number, the larger the letters on the line.)
   (1) A full visual field is 180 degrees.

      (2) The vision loss may be central, peripheral, or both.

      (3) *Total blindness* occurs when there is no light perception. See Figure 7–1.

  b. *Low vision* refers to the relationship between normal field of vision and visual acuity and visual function.

      (1) An individual is identified as having low vision when distance and near vision cannot be corrected to within the normal range of 20/20 with conventional eyeglasses or contact lenses. This person requires low vision aids to see. Corrected vision may range from 20/60 to 5/200.

      (2) There are two major low vision problems.

         (a) A central field defect interferes with reading ability or any task that requires vision for detail.

         (b) Reduced peripheral vision interferes with mobility and orientation to surroundings.

      (3) An individual classified as legally blind may not necessarily be totally blind and may benefit from low vision aids.

7. Although early recognition of eye problems followed by prompt treatment may prevent 50% of cases of blindness, the availability and utilization of care are limited for the following reasons:

  a. Lack of coverage for routine eye examinations and glasses by insurance policies, Medicare, and Medicaid discourages the financially pressed elderly from seeking appropriate care and purchasing prescribed glasses.

  b. Some elderly believe that failing eyesight is normal and that nothing can be done to maintain vision.

  c. Some elderly, fearing that visual problems may interfere with independence, deny the problem.

  d. The rate of decline in function is so gradual that the elder is not aware of the magnitude of loss and does not seek care.

  e. Some aged incorrectly believe that they should resist the effects of aging and that wearing glasses will hasten the aging process.

  f. Care providers may not recognize the problem or may consider it unimportant.

8. The need for education of the public to the importance of eye care and the need for coverage of services are evidenced by the consequences of inadequacy of service and poor utilization of existing services. These consequences include:

  a. Accidents and falls.

  b. Fewer work and leisure activities.

  c. Diminished feelings of status and emotional security.

  d. Higher cost of living.

  e. Reduced ability to function and maintain a desired lifestyle.

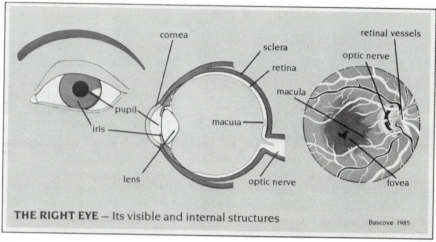

A

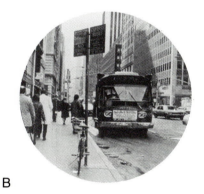

B

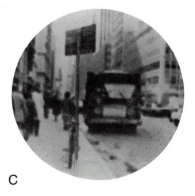

C

Normal Vision. A person with normal vision or vision corrected to 20/20 with glasses sees this street scene. (The area of the photographs is the field of vision for the right eye.)

Cataract. An opacity of the lens results in diminished acuity but does not affect the field of vision. There is no scotoma, but the person's vision is hazy overall, particularly in glaring light.

Figure 7–1. A, *Structures of the eye. B–M, A photographic essay on partial sight. (From The Lighthouse Low Vision Service.* © *1988 Lighthouse Low Vision Service. The New York Association for the Blind. Reprinted by permission.)*

Illustration continued on following page

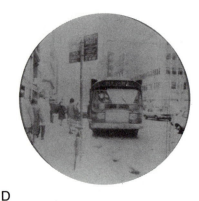

D

Corneal Pathology. An injury or damage to the cells of the cornea results in a distorted or clouded image and increased glare sensitivity. Clear detail is no longer discernible, but the field of vision is normal.

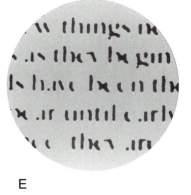

E

With cataracts and corneal disease, print appears hazy or lacking in contrast.

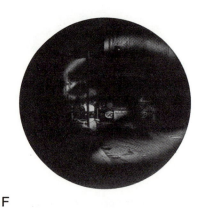

F

Glaucoma. Chronic elevated eye pressure in susceptible individuals may cause optic nerve atrophy and loss of peripheral vision. Early detection and close medical monitoring can help reduce complications.

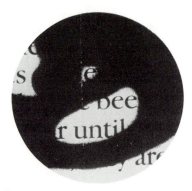

G

In advanced glaucoma, print may appear faded and words may be difficult to read.

Figure 7–1. Continued

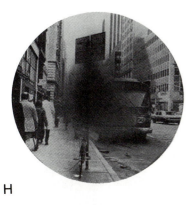

H

Macular Degeneration. The deterioration of the macula, the central area of the retina, is the most prevalent eye disease. This picture shows the area of decreased central vision called a central scotoma. The peripheral or side vision remains unaffected so mobility need not be impaired.

I

With macular degeneration, print appears distorted and segments of words may be missing.

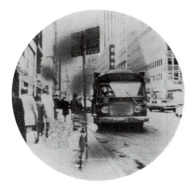

J

K

Diabetic Retinopathy. The leaking of retinal blood vessels may occur in advanced or long-term diabetes and affect the macula or the entire retina and vitreous. Not all diabetics develop retinal changes, but the likelihood of retinopathy and cataracts increases with the length of time a person has diabetes.

In diabetic retinopathy, reading vision is variable and print may be distorted or blurred. If cataracts are also present, print is hazy as well as distorted.

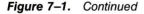

Figure 7–1. *Continued*

Illustration continued on following page

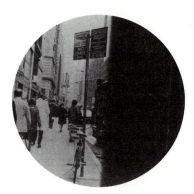

L

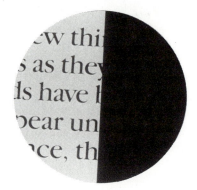

M

Hemianopia. A defect in the optic pathways in the brain can result in vision loss in half of the field. The most common defect, right homonymous hemianopia, occurs in corresponding halves of the right field of vision, causing reading impairment.

It can also occur in corresponding halves of the left field of vision, in the upper half of the field (superior hemianopia), the lower half (inferior hemianopia), or both outer halves of the field (bitemporal hemianopia). In hemianopia, half of the reading field is blanked out.

Figure 7–1. *Continued*

f. Restriction of daily activities.
g. Information deficits.
h. Social isolation.
i. Intellectual inertia.
j. Sensory deprivation.
k. Sense of isolation and hopelessness.
l. Predisposition toward fear, paranoia, and even hallucinations.
m. Depression triggered by the visual loss.

CHANGES IN VISUAL FUNCTION ASSOCIATED WITH PRIMARY AGING (TABLE 7–1)

1. Decreased acuity (acuteness or sharpness of vision).
2. Decreased ability to discriminate color, especially blues, blue-green, and violet.
3. Decreased depth perception.
4. Decreased peripheral vision.
5. Decreased adaptation to light change.
6. Decreased tolerance for glare.
7. Decreased accommodation (ability of the eye to adjust for various distances by changing the curvature of the lens so as to focus the image of an object on the retina).
8. Decreased convergence (ability to focus both eyes together on an object).
9. Decreased ability to look up.

Assessment for Visual Impairment

1. A client history of familial or personal eye problems, allergies, disease, or trauma is taken.
2. A medical eye examination should include:
    a. A visual acuity test with and without glasses with the Snellen Eye Chart or the Rosenbaum Pocket Screener.
    b. A visual field test for central and peripheral vision.
    c. Inspection of the external eye for the condition and function of lids and extraocular muscles.
    d. Funduscopy examination for the clarity of the media; the shape of the anterior chamber; and the condition of the cornea, lens, and retina.
    e. Tonometry for intraocular pressure.

Table 7–1. *Primary Aging Changes of the Outer and Inner Eye and Their Implications*

Tissues	Change	Implications
Structures supporting the eye	Decreased subcutaneous fat	Eyes appear sunken
	Decreased elastic tissue	Lids wrinkle
	Decreased muscle tone	Decreased ability to look up
		Increased difficulty focusing
	Laxity of lid	Increased susceptibility to ptosis (drooping of lid), entropion (turning-in of the lower lid), and ectropion (turning-out of the lower lid)
Lacrimal gland	Atrophy of glandular tissue	Decreased tears, dry eyes
Conjunctiva	Thin and friable	Pinguecula and pterygium (benign degenerative growths) appear more frequently
Cornea	Endothelial cells degenerate	Decreased transparency
		Light scatters, causing glare
	Deposits of fat from arcus senilis	
	Deposits of pigment from the iris	
	Flattens	Asymmetry results in astigmatism (light rays do not focus at the same point on the retina)
Sclera	Thins with loss of water	
	Yellowish tinge due to fatty deposits	
	Decreased opacity	Stray light enters the eye
Iris	Decreased pigment	Decreased color
Pupils	Decreased size	Limits amount of light entering eye
		Increased illumination required
	Decreased reactivity to light changes	Increased time to adjust to light changes
		Decreased night vision
Lens	Decreased elasticity	Decreased accommodation, decreased visual acuity, and increased glare experienced
	Increased opacity	Cataracts further filter light
	Increased density	Decrease in light reaching retina
	Yellowing	Decreased sensitivity to light spectrum
		Difficulty discriminating blue-green and violet
	Enlarges	May cause acute-angle glaucoma (by occluding the outflow of aqueous humor)

Table 7–1. *Primary Aging Changes of the Outer and Inner Eye and Their Implications* Continued

Tissues	Change	Implications
Fundus	Blood vessels narrow	Interference with blood supply to optic nerve can result in atrophy of the nerve and blindness in the affected eye
	Decrease in brightness of macular and foveal light reflex	Decreased visual acuity due to macular or retinal degeneration
	Blood vessels of choroid change	Increased susceptibility to macular degeneration
	Increase in drusen	Spots of pigment and waste materials that appear as small yellow round spots in the macular area; may indicate a tendency to develop senile macular degeneration
	Decrease in speed of cones to recover from adaptation to darkness	Decreased accommodation to light change
	Decrease in blood and oxygen to rod dense area	Decreased visual field. Increased time for adaptation to dark
Vitreous	Gelatinous substance shrinks and becomes more liquid	Floaters form owing to vitreous condensing. "Lightning flashes" occur as the vitreous body shrinks and causes traction on retina at points of attachment; traction may lead to retinal detachment
	Opacities develop	Light scatters and glare is experienced

3. Observation of how an elder manages the activities of daily living, socialization, communication, diversional activities, and transportation is preferable to asking the client how he sees. Evaluating function may reveal visual problems that the client is denying in fear of loss of vision and independence.

PROBLEMS OF THE EYE THAT MAY IMPAIR VISION

The Outer Eye

ENTROPION (TURNING-IN OF THE LOWER LID)

1. As a result of laxity of lid structures, the margin of the lower lids

turns in. The lashes irritate the cornea and cause tearing and a gritty feeling.

2. Persistent irritation may lead to inflammation of the conjunctiva and the cornea (keratitis).
3. Temporary relief may be obtained by using adhesive strips to evert the lid.
4. For correction, surgery is the treatment of choice.

ECTROPION (TURNING-OUT OF THE LOWER LID)

1. As a result of laxity of supporting lid structures, the lower lid turns outward, exposing the conjunctiva. The incidence of chronic infection is increased.
2. Wiping tears in an upward, inward motion and use of artificial tears (methylcellulose) may promote comfort.
3. For correction, surgery is the treatment of choice.

TUMORS OF THE LID

1. Benign tumors (senile keratosis, pedunculated papillomas, horns, and keratin cysts) of the lid that are annoying may be surgically removed.
2. Malignant tumors, usually basal cell carcinomas of the lower lid, are best removed by surgery or cryotherapy.

INFLAMMATION OF THE GLANDS OF THE LID

1. *Blepharitis* (inflammation involving hair follicles and glands) occurs more frequently in the elderly than in younger individuals.
2. Squamous blepharitis (chronic inflammation with scaling) appears to be associated with seborrheic dermatitis, which is treated with a cleansing shampoo, selenium sulfide (e.g., Selsun). The lid margins are cleansed twice daily. An antibiotic ointment is used to treat squamous blepharitis in the inner angle of the lids.

PTOSIS

1. Drooping of the upper lid may occur as a result of laxity of the skin of the lid, weakness of the levator muscle, and herniation of orbital fat into subcutaneous lid tissue.

2. The lowered lid may obscure the superior aspect of the pupil and thereby cause loss of the superior portion of the visual field.
3. Surgery may be necessary to prevent loss of vision.

DERMATOCHALASIS

1. The skin of the upper lid may hang as a fold over the lid margin as a result of loss of elasticity of the upper lid.
2. The sagging lid impinges on normal vision. The client may complain of tiring when reading or of inability to read for a normal length of time.
3. Surgical excision of excess tissue is indicated if the visual field is compromised by the overhanging tissue.

DRY EYES AND TEARING

1. Reduction in tearing is due to atrophy of glandular tissue.
2. The eyes feel dry, burn, and have a constant foreign body sensation.
3. Instillation of methylcellulose eye drops is a palliative treatment for dry eyes.
4. A normal amount of tears may appear present because of ectropion or stenosis of the outlet of the lacrimal duct. Diagnosis is made by the Schirmer test, in which filter paper is placed over the lower lid and the moistening is measured. A wet distance of 5 mm is considered positive for tearing.
5. Treatment of tearing is geared toward the cause of tear overproduction.

BENIGN DEGENERATIVE LESIONS OF THE CONJUNCTIVA

1. *Pinguecula,* a whitish yellow oval mass on either side of the cornea on the conjunctiva, occurs frequently in the aged.
2. *Pterygium,* a whitish pink raised fold of conjunctiva that overlaps the cornea on the nasal side, occurs frequently in the aged.
3. Surgical removal is indicated if lesions limit vision or cause significant discomfort.

CONJUNCTIVITIS (RED EYE)

1. Red eye may be due to viral, bacterial, or allergic conditions; glaucoma; iridocyclitis; or a systemic disease.
2. Medical treatment is determined by causation.

Problems of the Inner Eye

ERRORS OF REFRACTION

1. Refraction is concerned with the bending of light as it passes through the cornea, the aqueous humor, the lens, and the vitreous body so that the rays ultimately focus on the retina. Two errors of refraction seen in the elderly as a result of primary aging changes are presbyopia and astigmatism.
2. *Presbyopia* generally occurs in people over age 40 with a decrease in efficiency of accommodation of near vision as the lens becomes less elastic and light rays cannot be focused on the retina. Near objects appear blurred, and visual fatigue is experienced when doing "close work." Presbyopia may be corrected with lenses. Accommodation is reduced and continues to decrease until age 65 to 70 and then changes very little.
3. *Astigmatism* occurs most often as the curvature of the cornea becomes asymmetric or the lens changes so that light rays do not focus at the same point and vision is distorted. Astigmatism may be corrected with lenses.

CATARACTS

1. Ninety-five per cent of persons over age 65 demonstrate some lens opacity as the lens increases in density (nuclear sclerosis) and size and loses water content and elasticity.
2. Senile cataracts are caused by physical and chemical changes in the lens that produce progressive clouding of the lens.
3. As the cataract grows, it becomes noticeable as a milky or yellowish spot on the normally black pupil.
4. The rate of growth of cataracts varies from slow development over a period of years to rapid development over a few months.
5. When the clouding is small and not in the center of the lens, there may be little interference with vision. If the cataract begins in the center of the lens or grows rapidly, the person will experience a decrease in accommodation, depth perception, and glare tolerance (see Fig. 7–1).

6. As the cataract interferes with activities of daily living, the client complains of blurred vision, double vision, spots, ghost images, and the impression of a film over the eyes.
7. More light is needed on the work area, but less light is needed near the eyes.
8. Surgery may be initiated earlier than in the past, as new techniques reduce the risk of removing a cataract before it is "ripe" (mature).
9. Indications for surgery include:
   a. Reduced vision that interferes with what the client considers necessary activity to maintain his lifestyle.
   b. An enlarged lens that may precipitate a secondary glaucoma.
   c. A cataract that begins to disintegrate and irritate the eye.
10. Cataract surgery is associated with a 95% success rate and may be scheduled for surgery in a day-care unit if there are no other medical problems. If both eyes have cataracts, surgery is performed on each eye at least 1 month apart.
    a. Intracapsular cataract extraction (ICCE) involves removal of the opaque lens of the eye with its capsule by cryoextraction. As a supercooled metal probe is applied to the lens, it adheres to the moist lens capsule. The lens is then removed by a gentle upward and then sideward pull.
    b. Extracapsular cataract extraction (ECCE) may done by phaco-emulsification (ultrasound) if the lens is soft or by irrigation and aspiration if the lens is hard.
       (1) The anterior lens capsule, which includes the cloudy lens, is removed, but the posterior lens capsule is left intact.
       (2) The posterior lens capsule can be used to provide support if an intraocular lens (IOL) is inserted.
11. Postoperative restrictions are primarily directed toward preventing an increase in intraocular pressure and providing safety for the client, who now may have a refraction problem or may lack accommodating power in the operated eye.
    a. The client usually may be assisted to the bathroom after recovering from anesthesia and may be provided with a meal before being discharged home.
    b. When lying in bed, the client may lie on his back or unoperated side.
    c. For the first 24 hours postoperatively, the client may require assistance in bathing, eating, and ambulating.
    d. Acetaminophen (Tylenol) usually relieves nominal pain. Sharp, severe pain and nausea and vomiting should be reported to the physician.
    e. Light activity and reading are usually permissible 24 hours post-

operatively. No heavy work should be done for 4 to 6 weeks after surgery.

f. Lifting heavy objects or straining during bowel movements should be avoided. The client should pick up objects by bending knees, not by bending forward.

g. Abstinence from sexual activity may be advised for up to 6 weeks after cataract and IOL implant surgery to prevent dislocation of the implanted lens because the pupils dilate during orgasm.

h. When eye drops are ordered, the appropriate method for instillation of the drops should be taught or closely reviewed with the client.

i. Use of sunglasses or an eye shield may be advisable to protect the eye from injury until healing has taken place. An eye shield will prevent the client from rubbing the eye during sleep.

12. Once the lens is removed, the client becomes aphakic (without a lens) and loses one third of focusing power of that eye. The lens may be replaced by one of the following:

a. A thick eyeglass lens that produces an image 25% larger than that produced by the normal eye. This causes distortion, double vision, and loss of peripheral vision.

b. A contact lens with an increase in image of only 8%. Elders often have difficulty tolerating or managing contacts because of problems with manual dexterity. Extended-wear, soft gas-permeable lenses may be a suitable choice for the elderly because these lens need to be removed only every 3 months either by a professional or by the client.

c. An IOL implant at the time of surgery, which allows 24-hour wear and provides full visual field, virtually no magnification of images, improved depth perception, binocular vision when one cataract has been removed, and no discomfort or inconvenience in approximately 75% of all cases.

(1) Most clients find that the IOL implants result in greatly improved vision.

(2) With intraocular lenses, the client sees well at a distance but may have to wear glasses for reading and writing.

(3) A very small number of clients experience complications following implantation of an artificial lens. These include chronic iritis, secondary glaucoma, corneal edema, endophthalmitis (inflammation of the internal structures of the eye), and displacement of the implant.

(4) With improvements in IOL surgery, there are only a few contraindications. These are axial myopia, uncontrolled glaucoma, and proliferative diabetic retinopathy.

13. Medicare pays for "reasonable charges."
    a. Spectacles are the least costly.
    b. Intraocular lenses are most expensive initially, but extended-wear contacts may be more expensive because lenses have to be replaced often and client may have to pay a professional to clean contacts.
    c. Cost of maintaining extended-wear contacts can be reduced if the client or family cleans and replaces lenses.
    d. Insurance is available for loss or damage to contact lenses.

GLAUCOMA

1. *Open-angle* and *angle-closure glaucoma* are the greatest threats to blindness in older people in the United States.
2. Early glaucoma produces no symptoms except for increased fluid pressure within the eye. Normal range of intraocular pressure is from 12 to 21 mm Hg of mercury measured by a Schiøtz tonometer.
3. The increased intraocular pressure is due to impairment in the outflow of aqueous humor at the angle of the anterior chamber through the trabecular meshwork, Schlemm's canal, and into the scleral veins that drain the eye (Fig. 7–2).
4. Increased intraocular pressure may cause optic atrophy, vision loss, and ultimately blindness.
5. Open-angle glaucoma, also referred to as wide-angle glucoma, chronic simple glaucoma, or glaucoma simplex, constitutes about 90% of primary glaucomas.
   a. The condition is familial and is due to a defect in the trabecular meshwork that interferes with the drainage of the aqueous humor.
   b. Because a person with glaucoma is often symptom-free, the condition may not be noted until the client has marked loss of peripheral vision (tunnel vision) with irreversible damage. (See Fig. 7–1.)
   c. Open-angle glaucoma is best detected by a yearly ophthalmologic evaluation that includes measurement of intraocular pressure and a funduscopic examination.
   d. Preferably, the treatment is medical with topical agents that improve aqueous outflow. Since glaucoma produces no symptoms and the side effects of the drugs include irritation or visual blurring, compliance with therapy is a problem.
      (1) Pilocarpine (miotic) drops are used alone or combined with epinephrine compounds. Pilocarpine constricts the pupil to

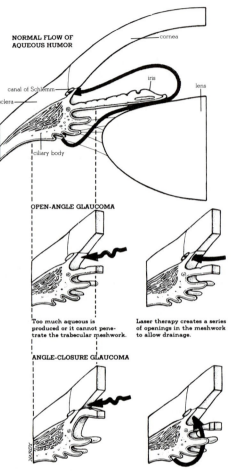

NORMAL FLOW OF AQUEOUS HUMOR

cornea

iris

lens

canal of Schlemm

sclera

ciliary body

OPEN-ANGLE GLAUCOMA

Too much aqueous is produced or it cannot penetrate the trabecular meshwork.

Laser therapy creates a series of openings in the meshwork to allow drainage.

ANGLE-CLOSURE GLAUCOMA

The iris tents up and blocks trabecular meshwork drainage to Schlemm's canal.

A hole is created in the base of the iris to permit drainage through the canal.

Figure 7–2. A, *Normal flow of aqueous humor.* B, *Open-angle glaucoma.* C, *Angle-closure glaucoma. (Illustration by Neil O. Hardy. From Resler MM, Tumulty G: Glaucoma update. American Journal of Nursing 83(5):753, 1983.)*

allow outflow of aqueous humor, but it also compounds problems of adaptation to light changes and night driving.

   (a) Compliance is improved with the "Ocusert," a capsular membrane containing pilocarpine.

   (b) The Ocusert is placed in the conjunctival sac, where it uniformly dispenses the medication.

   (c) Although the Ocusert is expensive to use, it is advantageous in that the eye drops do not have to be inserted four times a day, thus improving compliance.

  (2) Timolol maleate (a beta blocker) reduces the production of

aqueous humor and allows the pupil to dilate and respond to the environment.

   (a) The punctum should be occluded during administration to prevent a systemic effect.
   (b) Pulse rate and blood pressure should be periodically monitored for systemic side effects. A mild slowing of the pulse is most common.
   (c) Timolol maleate has precipitated status asthmaticus in clients with a prior history of asthma.
   (d) In the presence of disorientation or sensorium loss and when other beta-blocking drugs are in use, timolol maleate is contraindicated.
   (3) Oral acetazolamide (Diamox), a carbonic anhydrase inhibitor, may be used to reduce the formation of aqueous humor.
   e. If treatment with drugs fails, surgery may be performed to allow the drainage of aqueous humor.
   f. Within recent years, as an alternative to surgery, the outflow area is treated with a series of laser burns with about a 75% success rate.
      (1) Coagulation spots, 50 microns in diameter, are placed at intervals around the inner circumference of the trabecular meshwork. Following the contraction of the tissue during healing, the trabecular spaces open and drainage of aqueous humor proceeds through Schlemm's canal.
      (2) A transient postlaser pressure rise that may last for a few weeks is the major drawback. This pressure rise is offset by scheduling the treatment in two sessions of 50 burns each. If intraocular pressure drops to an acceptable level after only half the meshwork is treated, no further laser therapy may be necessary.
   g. Advantages of laser therapy over conventional surgery include the following:
      (1) It can be performed as an outpatient procedure.
      (2) The procedure takes about 15 minutes.
      (3) There is very little pain, possibly slight stinging.
      (4) Infection and severe hemorrhage can be circumvented.
      (5) Production of cataracts can be avoided.
      (6) Prophylaxis for the second eye is more easily accepted by the client.
6. Narrow-angle or angle-closure glaucoma is associated with a shallow anterior chamber and narrowing between the iris and the trabecular structure. The older client is more predisposed to angle-closure

glaucoma, as the lens increases in size and the anterior chamber decreases.

  a. Typically, an angle-closure attack is unilateral and strikes in 30 to 60 minutes after occurrence of emotional distress, dilatation of the pupil in a darkened place, or the administration of a mydriatic (pupillary dilator).

  (1) Mechanical blockage of aqueous humor moving from the posterior to the anterior chamber may cause the iris to block the outflow.

  (2) The client complains of sudden severe ocular and facial pain, nausea and vomiting, abdominal pain, decreased vision, or halo or rainbow vision; some clients may not experience any symptoms.

  (3) The cornea is edematous and cloudy, the pupil is fixed in midline, and the conjunctival vessels are congested.

  (4) An angle-closure attack must be treated as a medical emergency.

  b. The subacute form of angle-closure glaucoma is characterized by mild attacks that resolve after a short time. The client experiences mild ocular pain, headaches, halos around light, and corneal edema. The angle only partially closes and opens spontaneously in a short time.

  c. Chronic forms of narrow-angle glucoma are diagnosed on physical examination by findings of high ocular pressure. No pain is experienced. Peripheral visual field loss and optic nerve changes occur.

7. In an acute attack, the following agents are used:

  a. *Miotic drops* are administered to constrict the pupil and pull the iris out of the outflow angle.

  b. *Carbonic anhydrase inhibitors* are administered to restrict the action of the enzyme needed to produce aqueous humor.

  c. Systemic *osmotic diuretic agents* (mannitol and urea) may be administered to reduce the pressure of the aqueous humor.

  d. *Meperidine hydrochloride* (Demerol) may be administered for pain.

8. After the angle is opened and pressure is relieved, iridectomy is performed by laser beam.

  a. A minute hole is made through the iris to allow the fluid to bypass the pupil.

  b. After the fluid rushes out through the hole, the iris drops back to its normal position and the angle of outflow widens.

  c. Pieces of pigment that are loosened by the laser may clog the hole, but they are removed with the laser a week or two after treatment.

9. The results of iridectomies are permanent, but vision lost as a result of pressure that destroyed retinal cells prior to iridectomy cannot be regained.
10. Prophylactic laser surgery or surgical peripheral iridectomy is usually done on the other eye.

AGE-RELATED MACULAR DEGENERATION (AMD) OR SENILE MACULAR DEGENERATION (SMD)

1. In about 90% of clients, SMD does not lead to total blindness, although central vision is diminished. Clients are able to continue to perform their own activities of daily living and may lead productive lives.
2. SMD usually begins in persons in their sixties. Some form of macular degeneration affects nearly everyone in their seventies or eighties.
3. Causes of SMD include:
    a. Arteriosclerotic changes with aging in the capillary layers of the choroid adversely affect the macula by reducing the blood supply and nutrition.
    b. Age-related tissue atrophy occurs.
    c. Systemic disease and genetic factors may also be involved.
    d. A family history of SMD and blue or medium-pigmented eyes are the strongest indicators of possible risk.
    e. Advanced age, cardiovascular disease, and hyperopia (farsightedness) are additional risk factors.
    f. Borderline risk factors are smoking in men, occupational exposure to chemicals, and decrease in handgrip strength.
4. Usually SMD is bilateral but often presents first in one eye with the complaint of slow progressive impairment of central vision with a gray shadow in the center of the visual field (see Fig. 7– 1).
5. *Avascular* or dry SMD, a mild form, is generally asymptomatic and is characterized by the development of drusen, yellow-white specks that form under the macula. However, 10% of clients with dry SMD may experience a total loss of central vision and legal blindness. Following early diagnosis, argon laser photocoagulation can successfully treat 89% of these cases.
6. *Exudative neovascular* SMD occurs with the rapid growth of new vessel membranes into the retina from the choroid layer and destroys the macular light-sensing cells.
    a. The membranes cause blood to leak within the retina and finally scar the central vision or macular area. The new blood growth can begin near the outer edge of the macula and spread inward

toward the fovea. Within a month or two, most of the macula including the fovea may be severely damaged.

b. Speedy detection is essential to preserve central vision. The client may report sudden distortion of straight surfaces or blurring and loss of visual acuity. There is disruption of central vision as straight lines appear wavy or crooked and words blur. Untreated, a scotoma (blind spot) becomes noticeable to the client. Damage to the fovea causes irreversible loss of central vision, though peripheral vision remains intact.

c. Treatment consists of photocoagulation of subretinal or choroidal new vessel membranes with a laser beam to prevent further loss of central vision.

7. SMD that has reached the fovea cannot be treated with the laser, as the beam would destroy the sensitive tissue. Last-stage SMD is irreversible.

8. High-risk individuals should check their own vision on a regular basis with the Amsler Grid Test for visual distortion (Fig. 7–3). A home eye test for adults is available for $1.00 from:

Amsler Grid Test for Macular Degeneration

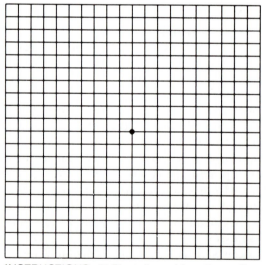

Figure 7–3. The Amsler grid. (Reproduced with permission of the National Society to Prevent Blindness, 500 East Remington Road, Schaumburg, IL 60173, a not-for-profit organization that provides sight-saving programs and services through its 267 affiliates/divisions.)

INSTRUCTIONS: 1) Place the grid on the wall at eye level. 2) View it from 12 inches. 3) If you wear glasses for reading, you should wear them for the test. 4) Test one eye at a time. 5) Look at the center dot. 6) Tell your doctor if you can't see all the lines, or if some lines appear wavy.

The National Society to Prevent Blindness
79 Madison Avenue
New York, NY 10016

9. The elderly should be encouraged periodically to look at any straight edge, such as a door frame, a telephone wire, or the intersection of a ceiling and a wall, to check whether these straight lines appear wavy. Visual distortion indicates the need for an ophthalmologic examination. Clients with complaints of mild distortion are treatable.

10. Low vision aids, such as telescopic lenses and magnifying aids, may be helpful. The client may also learn to look just to the side of the object, but relearning is difficult for many elderly.

RETINAL DETACHMENT

1. With aging, the vitreous body shrinks, becomes more liquid, and often forms vitreous condensation, or "floaters."

2. Traction is caused on the retina at points of adhesion as the vitreous body shrinks. The client experiences "lightning flashes" that may indicate retinal tears are occurring. Immediate ophthalmologic care should be sought.

3. Surgical removal of a cataract from an eye may predispose the elderly client to retinal detachment.

4. Retinal detachment causes a field vision defect, seen as a dark shadow in the peripheral field.

5. Preventive treatment is creation of a chorioretinal adhesion (a weld point) with a laser beam where retinal changes (thinning holes and tears) may lead to retinal detachment.

6. Surgery is required to reattach the retina.

DIABETIC RETINOPATHY

1. Early nonproliferative or background diabetic retinopathy appears as tiny red dots or microaneurysms in the retina of diabetics. With progression, small hemorrhages occur; blood vessels become dilated, irregular, or blocked, and retinal infarcts occur.

2. Proliferative retinopathy develops in some diabetic patients as the capillary network is lost. Ischemia results, and the hypoxic retina produces a vasoproliferative substance causing new vessel formation. Severe hemorrhage may occur in the eye. Fibrous bands of scar tissue then form on the retina, causing detachment with subsequent blindness. (See Fig. 7–1.)

3. Macular edema develops in many older diabetics as the pre-existing blood vessels in the central portion of the macula become leaky and both blood cells and plasma flow into the retina. These leaks break

down the normally impermeable blood-retinal barrier. Thickening and edema of the retina occur with many small hemorrhages and accumulation of hard fatty lipid deposits. This process leads to impairment of central vision.

4. Methods of treatment for diabetic retinopathy.
   a. Severe visual loss in patients with proliferative diabetic retinopathy is reduced by a barrage of laser burns scattered around the peripheral retina to destroy by photocoagulation existing neovascular patches and to prevent future regrowth and hemorrhage in the area.
   b. For more severely affected eyes in which blood is clouding the vitreous fluid and preventing the penetration of laser light, vitrectomy is used. The bloody vitreous gel is removed along with the fibrous bands that endanger the retina. Because these eyes are already so severely damaged, 20/20 vision rarely returns after treatment, but useful vision may be returned.
   c. Photocoagulation with a laser beam is effective in preventing vision loss from macular edema. A focal technique of coagulating only the tissue suspected of leaking fluid into the macula is used. Retinal swelling, severe visual loss, and blindness caused by abnormal development of retinal blood vessels are prevented.
5. All diabetic clients should have yearly ophthalmologic examinations for signs of retinopathy, as the effects of macular edema can be prevented and proliferative and severe proliferative diabetic retinopathy can be treated.

HEMIANOPIA

1. Hemianopia occurs in association with hemiplegia following a cerebral vascular accident as a result of a defect in the optic pathways between the eye and the brain.
2. There is interference with the client's ability to see visual cues and relearn motor skills. Susceptibility to accidents and physical hazards is increased.
3. Usually there is a loss of vision in the same half of the visual field of each eye. The client sees only one half of what a person with normal vision sees (see Fig. 7–1).
4. The most common defect occurs in the right field of vision.
5. The client cannot see past the midline toward the side opposite the lesion in the brain unless he turns his head.
6. Hemianopia can also occur in the horizontal halves of the visual field.

    a. An *inferior* hemianopia causes problems with mobility and reading.

    b. A *superior* hemianopia reduces the client's ability to see things above the midline of the eye.

7. The client experiencing hemianopia should be taught how to position his head to improve his visual field and body image.

8. In addition, the hemiplegic client may experience reduction in depth perception and visual perception in the horizontal and vertical planes.

    a. These deficits may cause problems with gait and posture.

    b. As a client may not be aware of perceptual distortion, vulnerability to accidents is increased.

    c. The client attempts to compensate for visual losses with behavior that may at times appear bizarre.

Implications for the Use of Ocular Drugs

1. The elderly are at risk for systemic side effects of ocular drugs for the following reasons:

    a. First pass effect may occur as the eye drops enter the bloodstream in therapeutic concentration and pass to target organs without prior detoxification by the liver.

    b. Eye drops are in high concentrations.

    c. The lax conjunctival sac retains higher amounts of the drug.

2. Individuals providing health supervision for the client should utilize a pharmacology reference to check on the pharmacokinetics of the drug to ensure appropriate use.

3. Clients should be taught appropriate administration of the drug, what it is used for, side effects, and when to consult with the health care provider.

4. The person administering the eye drops must apply pressure over the punctum for at least a minute after drug application to prevent the drug from entering the lacrimal duct and thereby systemic circulation.

5. Caution should be used to prevent the concomitant use of a drug that produces similar effects or similar adverse reactions.

6. Caution must be used when frequent ocular steroid applications are ordered. In one third of clients, application of topical ocular steroids leads to increased intraocular pressure that may result in permanent ocular damage.

7. Artificial tears used for dry eyes may contain thimerosal, or mercurial preservatives, which may cause a delayed allergic contact der-

matitis, conjunctivitis, or blepharitis that may be attributed to the original problem.
8. Optimum control of dosage of eye drops is provided by a bottle that provides good drop control.

STRATEGIES FOR PROMOTING VISION

1. Facilitate early diagnosis and prompt treatment for primary and secondary aging changes in the eye to prevent irreversible vision loss.
2. Refer elderly individuals to low vision services when refraction with standard lenses cannot bring vision approximately to 20/20.
3. Encourage compliance with the following recommendations of the American Academy of Ophthalmology for promoting early diagnosis and treatment of an aging or disease process in the eye.
   a. Medical eye examination including a refraction at least every 2 years for those over 65 years of age.
   b. More frequent care for the high-risk aged with diabetes or a history of eye problems.
   c. Prompt ophthalmologic care if an individual experiences the following warning signs:
      (1) Loss, distortion, or dimness of vision.
      (2) Pain in and around eyes.
      (3) Excessive tearing or discharge from the eye.
      (4) Swelling of the eyelids or protrusion of the eye.
      (5) Double vision.
      (6) Flashes of light, halos around lights, or floaters.
      (7) Sudden crossing or deviation of the eye.
      (8) A change in color of an eye.
4. Encourage participation in community programs that screen for visual acuity deficits and glaucoma. These programs provide good indications of problems that require professional care.

STRATEGIES FOR ASSISTING THE VISION-IMPAIRED

1. Recognize that each client reacts emotionally to loss of vision in a manner characteristic of his enduring personality, his attitude toward aging, and the degree of vision loss experienced. Assist the client as he grieves his vision loss.

2. Discuss with the client and family the prognosis to enable them to deal realistically with the vision loss.
3. Assist in arranging a client visit with a counselor from a low vision agency who can explain what help is available.
4. Provide support and discourage maladaptive behaviors.
5. Refer for individual or group psychotherapy as needed to help the client emotionally adjust to vision loss.
6. Promote social communication.
   a. Focus on what the client can do or may do rather than on his limitations.
   b. Do not raise your voice when speaking to the blind client.
   c. Use the words "see" or "blind" when needed rather than hedging.
   d. Be considerate and speak to the blind client when entering a room and when leaving.
   e. When an individual with low vision enters a room, guide him over to people in the room to be introduced.
   f. When guiding the client, do not grab his arm but rather offer him your arm so that he can follow your movements. Pause for curbs, steps, or other obstacles.
   g. Do not sneak up on a vision-impaired person. Walk up firmly and ask in a clear voice if help is needed.
   h. Keep the client's environment well lit.
   i. Offer to read the client's mail to him.
   j. Encourage use of the library to keep in touch with events.
   k. Suggest that the client ask the bank teller or store cashier to separate different denominations of bills so that he may fold them properly for identification.
   l. Suggest gifts for the client such as perfume or flowers to stimulate his senses or objects that will help him maintain independence.
   m. Help the client to join or form a self-help group with others with whom he shares concerns, experiences, and success in coping with vision loss.
   n. Discuss safety factors and attitudes with the client and significant others.

Low Vision Services

1. Referral to and use of low vision services are appropriate for an individual when refraction with standard lenses cannot bring his vision approximately to normal 20/20 vision.
2. The goal of low vision services is to assist the individual along the low vision continuum to maximize the use of remaining vision and to achieve his optimum function in the community.

3. Low vision services include:
   a. Evaluation of the type and extent of the eye problem by a team of professionals.
   b. An examination with special equipment for evaluating the client's remaining vision.
   c. Assessment of how the client functions in activities of daily living at home and in the community and how he wishes to function.
   d. An individual program developed with prescription of aids and devices, orientation and mobility training, and rehabilitation directed toward meeting individual needs in the home and community.
      (1) Clients are shown low vision devices that may benefit them.
      (2) The advantages and disadvantages of each device are discussed.
      (3) Instruction in the use of selected devices is provided.
      (4) Instruction is provided in proper use of lighting, essential for success with these devices.
      (5) Clients may take devices home to check which best meet individual needs and lifestyle.
   e. Evaluation of the effect of the prescribed aid on the client's function in the physical and psychosocial dimensions.
   f. Emotional support and reassurance to the client.
   g. Referral to other community services as needed. A source for a listing of low vision services is:
      American Foundation for the Blind
      15 West 16th Street
      New York, NY 10011
      (212) 620-2000
4. The degree of benefit of low vision services depends on the following:
   a. Readiness of the client to start rehabilitation.
   b. Degree and stability of remaining vision.
   c. The signs and symptoms of the secondary change causing the condition.
   d. Age of the client.
   e. State of health in the physical and psychosocial dimensions.
   f. The client's goals and how much work he is willing to do to attain them.
5. Client education and training one on one may be obtained from paraoptometric trainers (non-physician, low vision specialists) in a low vision center, clinic, or private facility.

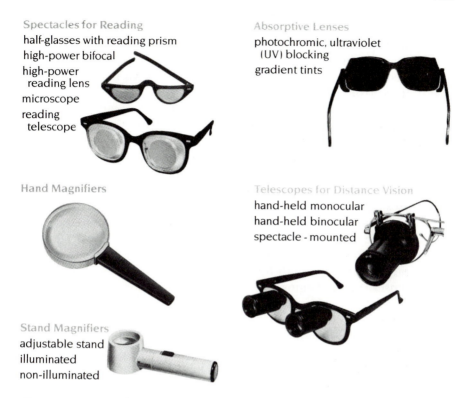

Spectacles for Reading
half-glasses with reading prism
high-power bifocal
high-power reading lens
microscope
reading telescope

Absorptive Lenses
photochromic, ultraviolet (UV) blocking
gradient tints

Hand Magnifiers

Telescopes for Distance Vision
hand-held monocular
hand-held binocular
spectacle - mounted

Stand Magnifiers
adjustable stand
illuminated
non-illuminated

Figure 7–4. *Low vision devices. (Modified with permission from The Lighthouse Low Vision Service. © 1988 Lighthouse Low Vision Service. The New York Association for the Blind.)*

Low Vision Aids (Fig. 7–4)

OPTIC SYSTEMS

1. Magnifiers
   a. The majority of magnifiers are used for improving near vision by enlargement of the visual image with convex or magnifying lenses mounted in a variety of ways.
   b. The least magnification that provides useful help is best.
      (1) Less magnification causes fewer problems with distance and lighting for the client.
      (2) The greater the magnification, the smaller the field of vision.

    c. Hand-held, neck-supported, chest-supported, and standard-mount magnification devices are useful for short tasks, such as reading directions and checking prices or labels in a store. Many people with reduced vision carry a hand-held magnifying lens away from home.

    d. Table-stand magnifiers cause less eye fatigue because a constant distance is maintained between the object and the magnifier.

    e. Magnifiers that hang around the neck are helpful for sewing or craft work.

    f. Adequate background lighting is essential if nonilluminated magnifiers are used.

2. Lenses

    a. Full-diameter *single-vision lenses* are used in conventional reading glasses.

    b. *Bifocal lenses* are divided into one strength for close magnification and another strength for more distant sight. The use of bifocal lenses usually begins after age 40 when presbyopia develops.

    c. Special *spectacles* or clip-on magnifying devices (loupes) can be used.

    d. *Microscopic lenses* may be used from distances of 13 inches away from the information source to as little as $\frac{1}{4}$ inch away. The thicker the lens, the nearer the client has to be to the material viewed.

    e. *Telescopic lenses* for reading permit the client to increase the distance from the eye to the information. However, these lenses decrease the area visible on the page and decrease the amount of light permitted to enter the eye. Because they severely reduce peripheral vision, telescopic lenses are absolutely contraindicated for driving. Proper training and lighting are essential for successful use.

    f. A *telemicroscopic lens system* combines a telescopic distance lens with a reading lens. A more convenient working distance is possible, but the visual field is reduced. Telemicroscopes may be adjusted for distance viewing, such as television, theater, or sporting events.

    g. *Telescopes* are used to attain distance vision (binocular or monocular). They are useful for stationary situations, such as viewing television, blackboards, or theater and for spotting signs and landmarks at a distance. Telescopes are most often hand-held and may be carried in a case. In a moving situation, telescopes are not of use because spatial disorientation occurs.

    h. *Prism spectacles* move images to a functioning part of the retina.

ELECTRONIC DEVICES

1. A closed-circuit television monitor adapted for reading is advantageous for clients who work in one area or who lack mobility.
   a. Reading material is magnified on a television screen to provide large-print reading. Magnification may be greater than with optical systems.
   b. A more normal field of vision at a more conventional working distance fosters increased reading speed, endurance, and reading comfort.
   c. Depending on the client's need, material may be easily switched from black on a white background or white on a black background.
2. The reading machine converts the image of a printed letter into a vibrating tactile form that is transmitted to the finger tips. The Optacon (the most widely used reading machine) may have limited value for the elderly because of their reduction in tactile sensation. More complex reading machines use a computer to convert camera input into synthetic speech.

MOBILITY AIDS

1. A long lightweight cane functions as a detector and enables the blind person to obtain information on his surroundings and to protect himself as he walks. The technique of using the cane is taught at low vision training centers.
2. A guide dog is usually not a suitable mobility aid for very old clients because many old persons do not have the physical stamina required for the strenuous program of training or to maintain the normal speed of the dog (about 3 miles per hour).

AIDS FOR INDEPENDENT LIVING

1. Aids for the 80s: What They Are and What They Do
   American Foundation for the Blind
   Consumer Products Department
   15 West 16th Street
   New York, NY 10011
   (212) 620-2000
2. Accessory aids available
   • Calculators
   • Clocks/timers
   • Communication aids

- Education aids
- Games
- Health care aids
- Household aids
- Kitchen aids
- Measuring aids
- Mobility aids
- Personal aids
- Recreation aids
- Tools
- Wrist watches
- Writing aids

BOOKS, RECORDINGS, AND LIBRARY SERVICES

1. Braille books use a code system utilizing one or more embossed raised dots in various positions within a "cell." There are 63 possible combinations of dots used for letters of the alphabet, for punctuation, for contractions, and so on.
   a. Braille is read with the fingers and is written with the aid of a metal slate or a specially constructed braille typewriter.
   b. Elderly clients may have difficulty learning the system because of slowed cognitive ability for absorbing new material and reduced sensation in their finger tips.
2. Large print books, magazines, and newspapers by commercial publishers as well as nonprofit organizations are available in public libraries.
3. Talking books (on long-playing records) and books on magnetic tape are increasing in number.
4. The National Library Service for the Blind and Physically Handicapped of the Library of Congress lends recorded books and magazines on discs and cassettes and equipment for playing cassettes and tapes to individuals with low vision. An application for these services and the address of the nearest cooperating library may be obtained from the:
   National Library Service for the Blind and Physically Handicapped
   Library of Congress
   1291 Taylor Street N.W.
   Washington, DC, 20542
   (202) 287-5100
5. *Braille Book Review* and *Talking Book Topics* are published by the American Foundation for the Blind under contract with the Library of Congress.

6. Recording for the Blind is a national, nonprofit organization that provides textbooks and other material without charge to visually and physically handicapped persons.
   Recording for the Blind, Inc.
   20 Roszel Road
   Princeton, NJ, 08540
   (800) 221-4792

Environmental Modifications that Enhance Visual Function

USE OF LIGHTING

1. Modifying light sources and reducing the number of reflective surfaces will promote visual acuity, visual function, and safety.
2. Lighting needs vary, but generally, increased illumination is needed. Twice as much illumination is needed at age 60 as at age 20.
3. Time is required for an elder's eyes to adjust when moving from one light area to a brighter or darker area.
4. For the elderly, the ability to control light in their environment with curtains, light switches, and placement of lamps is a high priority.
5. The client requires help in finding the combination of optical aid and lighting that works best for him. Lighting either may enhance vision or can make a good aid useless.
6. The area of concentration where the client's attention is directed should be brighter than the background area by a ratio of 3:1 and no greater than 10:1 for optimal visual acuity.
   a. The client should be encouraged to try different ratios of light to discover what best suits his needs.
   b. Small portable high-intensity lamps with three-way switches may be helpful in achieving the proper ratio.
7. The visual environment can be improved by use of the following:
   a. Dimmer switches instead of wall switches to control the lighting when passing from one room to another.
   b. Three-way lamps instead of a bulb with only a single brightness.
   c. Four 60-watt bulbs separately around the room instead of one 200-watt bulb.
   d. Blinds or curtains to tint or reduce bright sunlight coming through the windows.
   e. Ceiling-area lights during the day to balance strong light from windows.

  f. Fluorescent lighting for ceiling fixture if a very bright light is needed.
  g. A night light burning all night to minimize the difficulty of adjusting from darkness to light and to help locate light switches at night.
  h. A floor lamp or other light in the room that does not shine on the television screen or cause glare. (A small black-and-white television provides the clearest, sharpest picture.)
  i. Increased lighting positioned in stairwells and hallways to avoid glare or shadow that may distort vision.
  j. A gooseneck lamp for concentrated light to see and identify small objects, such as medication.
  k. A battery-lighted magnifier to make small objects more readily visible.
  l. Sunglasses, brimmed hats, and umbrellas to reduce glare from the sun.
  m. A cleaner that provides a dull finish on linoleum floors. (Wax should not be used on vinyl or linoleum floors, which reflect light and produce glare. Nonshining, nonslippery floor coverings should cover glare spots.)
  n. Covering for shiny surfaces, glass items, and polished metals. Gleaming metal bathroom fixtures may be replaced with wood or plastic if glare is a persistent problem.
  o. Flat paints, wallpaper, and paneling for walls instead of high-gloss paints.

USE OF COLOR

  1. Color contrast improves sight. (For example, dark-colored food, such as meat or green vegetables, should be served on light-colored dishes upon a dark tablecloth. Light-colored food, such as fish, cheese, or eggs, is better visualized or identified on dark dishes on a light tablecloth.)
  2. Glass dishware is inadvisable as it seems to blend into the environment and is not easily visible.
  3. Use of foods that have more intense color, such as red radishes rather than white ones or romaine rather than iceberg lettuce, makes preparation easier and the food more appealing.
  4. Use of dark surfaces for measuring light ingredients and light surfaces for measuring dark ingredients increases ease and accuracy of measuring in cooking.
  5. Use of warm colors (red or yellow) heightens the visibility of the

environment; cooler tones, such as blue, are difficult for the elderly to distinguish.

6. Contrasting handrails, floorboards, and first and last steps and brightly colored doorsills can prevent tripping.

7. A room is lightened by painting the walls a light color and having light-colored drapes.

8. Painting cupboards a bright color or covering them with bright contact paper in contrast to the door aids in seeing the doors.

9. Painting the edge of the bathtub with a stripe will help one to visualize the side of the tub.

10. Painting keys with nailpolish or sticking different colored tape around the heads of keys improves their visibility and distinguishes each key.

Use of Other Senses to Compensate for Visual Losses

1. Sensory stimulation informs the elderly more about the world, stirs their minds, and prevents or minimizes the risk of injury or accident. Wheelchair-bound individuals are particularly in need of sensory stimulation, as with deprivation come depression, confusion, and hallucination.

2. Auditory stimulation that aids orientation may be derived from socialization, radio, television, a talking clock, and talking books.

3. Touching helps a person orient himself.

   a. By skimming walls and furniture, a person may orient himself to his environment. Since a large number of objects in a room helps a person maintain orientation, furniture should be left in place unless a change is requested by the client.

   b. A cane or walker may stablize the client and provide tactile information about the environment.

   c. Holding onto both armrests of a chair before sitting down promotes a sense of security and control.

   d. Stove dials with raised dots as temperature guides are helpful in choosing appropriate cooking temperatures.

   e. Walls may be marked with Velcro strips or raised dots to aid the client in moving from room to room or in locating light switches at night.

   f. Writing guides and inexpensive cardboard forms with spaces for lines are tactile cues for letter and check writing.

4. Training sessions in which clients are asked "What do you hear?" or "What do you smell?" stimulate the use of other senses.

Strategies for the Vision-Impaired When Traveling

1. Teach the client to:
   a. Avoid leaving doors half open. When indoors, close doors.
   b. Use curtains, shades, and blinds to provide contrasting shades in the new environment.
   c. Use railings on stairs.
   d. Wear appropriate clothing and foot gear for comfort and to minimize distraction.
   e. Plan route before setting out and use landmarks to help in orientation.
   f. Hold onto the arm of a sighted person and walk about a half step behind to maintain control when being guided.
   g. Cross street at crosswalks only.
   h. Sit near the driver on buses and ask for help needed.
2. Teach the client the following strategies for night driving:
   a. Do not look at oncoming headlights.
   b. Travel on well-lit roads when possible.
   c. Travel on divided highways.
   d. Do not use yellow lenses to cut glare, as they reduce total illumination.
3. Encourage the client to:
   a. Discuss with a low-vision service the advisability of training with a cane for orientation and mobility.
   b. Check with transportation services whether there are financial concessions or other benefits available for the blind person or his traveling companion.

Financial Assistance

Legally blind individuals are eligible for a number of entitlements.
1. Supplemental Social Security.
2. Medicaid coverage for low vision services and aids.
3. Payments made to meet emergencies threatening the health, safety, and welfare of blind people, such as lost or stolen cash and losses as a result of burglary or fire.
4. Food stamps.
5. Homemaker and housekeeper services to assist with household chores, money management, and personal care.
6. Medicare coverage for clients over age 65 and disabled people under age 65 who have been entitled to Social Security Disability Benefits for 2 years or more. Does not pay for low vision services or aids.

7. Assistance for low vision services provided by state commissions for the blind and visually handicapped (funded by the state and federal government).
8. Income tax exemptions for the blind.
9. Reduction in travel charges by some companies.

Resources

The following organizations will forward detailed professional and lay information on request:

State Commission for the Blind and Visually Handicapped
Check telephone directory for addresses.

State Departments of Education and Labor.
Check telephone directory for addresses.

Office of Scientific Recording
The National Eye Institute
Building 31, Room 6A-32
Bethesda, MD 20205

American Foundation for the Blind
15 West 16th Street
New York, NY 10011
(212) 620-2000

The Lighthouse
National Center for Vision and Aging
111 East 59th Street
New York, NY 10022
(212) 355-2200

The National Society to Prevent Blindness
79 Madison Avenue
New York, NY 10016
(212) 684-3505

American Optometric Association
Communication Division
243 North Lindbergh Boulevard
St. Louis, MO 63141
(314) 991-4100

American Academy of Ophthalmology
655 Beach Street
P.O. Box 7424
San Francisco, CA 94120-7424
(415) 561-8500

Lions Club International
300 22nd Street
Oak Brook, IL 60570
(312) 986-1700

References

Aging and Vision. New York: American Foundation for the Blind & American Association of Retired Persons, 1985.

Andreasen MEK: Color vision defects in the elderly. Journal of Gerontological Nursing 6:383–384, 1980.

Bernstein C: Alerting SMD victims in time. Sightsaving 51:16–20, 1982.

Cohen S: Sensory changes in the elderly. American Journal of Nursing 81:1851–1880, 1981.

Eifrig DE, Simons KB: An overview of common geriatric ophthalmologic disorders. Geriatrics 38:55–77, 1983.

Fisher SJ, Cunningham RD: The medical profile of cataract patients. In Brindley GV, ed: Clinics in Geriatric Medicine. Philadelphia: WB Saunders Co, 1985.

Flaherty TM, Meadows MN: Specific disorders of the visual system. In Kneisl CR, Ames SW, eds: Adult Health Nursing. Reading, Mass: Addison-Wesley Publishing Co, 1986.

Frank RN: New hope in diabetic retinopathy. Sightsaving 53:2–5, 1984.

Fraunfelder FT, Meyer SM: Safe use of ocular drugs in the elderly. Geriatrics 39:97–102, 1984.

Freeman PB: Optical and nonoptical aids for patients with age-related macular degeneration. Sightsaving 54:20–23, 1985.

Greene J: The abc's of contact lenses. FDA Consumer. HHS No. 82-4021. Washington, DC: US Government Printing Office, 1982.

Hiatt RL: Blindness: The physician's role in prevention. Geriatrics 38:97–99, 1983.

Horwitz J: Laser light on glaucoma: The therapeutic burn. Sightsaving 51:12–15, 1982.

Meadows MN, Flaherty TM: Surgical approaches to visual system dysfunction. In Kneisl CR, Ames SW, eds: Adult Health Nursing. Reading, Mass: Addison-Wesley Publishing Co, 1986.

Mensher JH: Laser therapy for eye disorders. Postgraduate Medicine 76:51–56, 1984.

Randall RM: SMD: Age-related macular degeneration. Sightsaving 54:15–19, 1985.

Stern EJ: Helping the person with low vision. American Journal of Nursing 80:1788–1789, 1980.

Sullivan N: Vision in the elderly. Journal of Gerontological Nursing 9:228–235, 1983.

Taisch EA, Taisch A, Metz HS: Problems of the eyes. In O'Hara-Devereaux M, Andrus LH, Scott MI, eds: Eldercare. New York: Grune & Stratton, 1981.

Thackray P: How much does a miracle cost? Sightsaving 52:10–13, 1983.

Yurick R, Spier BE, Robb SS, Ebert NJ: The Aged Person and the Nursing Process. East Norwalk, Ct: Appleton-Century-Crofts, 1984.

Hearing Impairment in the Elderly

PHYSIOLOGY OF HEARING
TYPES OF HEARING LOSS
THE EFFECTS OF HEARING IMPAIRMENT
ASSESSMENT FOR HEARING IMPAIRMENT
COMMUNICATION AND HEARING IMPAIRMENT
AIDS FOR THE HEARING-IMPAIRED

1. It is estimated that more than 50% of the 27 million Americans over age 65 are affected by hearing impairment.
2. *Presbycusis*, associated with primary changes, is the most common cause of hearing impairment in the adult population in the United States. The degree of impairment may range from mild to severe.
3. Differences in age of onset, degree of hearing loss, and the adjustment of the individual influence the consequences of hearing impairment.
4. Changes associated with aging gradually occur in the cochlea and cause subtle hearing losses for which the elderly compensate often without realizing that hearing is impaired.
5. When auditory acuity is reduced or sounds are distorted, hearing loss has occurred.
   a. The loudness of sounds may be reduced, so that the ringing of a doorbell or the shouting of a name across a room may not be heard.
   b. Sound may be distorted. The hearing-impaired elderly person may hear the voice but cannot understand the communication.
      (1) Sounds filter through, as when a record is scratched or a broadcast produces static.

(2) The elder cannot differentiate between sounds of speech and confuses words with similar sounds, such as fit and sit.

(3) Increasing the volume may not improve the quality of sound or make words more understandable.

   c. *Recruitment,* an abnormal growth in the loudness of sound, may occur. There is a narrow range between when a sound is loud enough to hear and when it becomes too loud and thus painful.

6. The elderly hearing-impaired who have difficulty understanding speech are often regarded as senile because they may offer inappropriate responses and appear confused.

7. An older person may not admit to a hearing loss because of concern that his family may believe he is no longer capable of functioning independently and that certain freedoms and responsibilities may be taken away.

8. Aural (audiologic) rehabilitation may reduce the effects of hearing impairment through amplification of sound and speech therapy.

9. Recent innovations in assistive devices make access to various community resources possible for the hearing-impaired elderly; this enables them to continue pursuit of their interests.

10. Counseling for the elderly hearing-impaired, their family, friends, and co-workers is critical for preventing social isolation and functional dependency.

11. The increased incidence of hearing impairment in the aged, the invisibility of the hearing loss, and the reduction in quality of life substantiate the need for early diagnosis and intervention.

12. Advocacy is needed to develop public awareness to problems, rights, and privileges of the hearing-impaired.

PHYSIOLOGY OF HEARING

1. Sound passes through the external ear canal and strikes the eardrum.

2. This causes the eardrum to vibrate in tune with the sound waves striking it and transmits the vibrations to the malleus, the incus, and the stapes, the ossicles in the middle ear.

3. These bones amplify the vibrations so that the waves can pass on to the inner ear, where they cause rippling in the fluid within the cochlea.

4. The tiny hair cells in the cochlea respond to the ripples by producing

nerve impulses that travel along the auditory nerve to the brain (Fig. 8–1).
5. In the brain, these "sounds" are interpreted.

TYPES OF HEARING LOSS

Conductive Hearing Loss

1. Interference with the normal transmission of sound through the external auditory canal, tympanic membrane, or middle ear causes conductive hearing loss.
2. The most common conductive problem in the elderly is external blockage resulting from cerumen (wax) accumulation. In addition, tympanic membrane perforation, otitis media, and discontinuity or fixation of the middle ear ossicles (otosclerosis) may cause conductive hearing loss.
3. Usually, all sound frequencies are affected, but hearing losses are not severe.
4. Conductive hearing loss can usually be relieved by medical or surgical intervention. The client often benefits from the use of a hearing aid.

Sensorineural Hearing Loss

1. Damage to the inner ear, the hair cells in the inner ear, or the eighth cranial nerve results in sensorineural hearing loss.
2. A slow, progressive bilateral sensorineural degeneration of auditory function, beginning in middle to older age, is associated with cu-

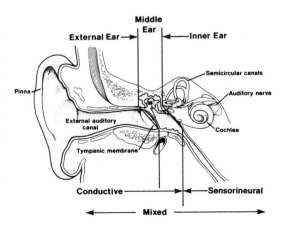

Figure 8–1. Structures of the ear and types of hearing loss. This cross section demonstrates the three regions of the ear: external, middle, and inner ears. The type of hearing loss is also classified according to the region of the ear involved. M = malleus; I = incus; S = stapes. (From Calkins E, Davis PJ, Ford AB: The Practice of Geriatrics. Philadelphia: WB Saunders Co, 1986.)

mulative occupational noise exposure, arteriosclerotic vascular disease, drug usage, and heredity.
3. Higher sound frequencies are affected initially.
4. Hearing losses can range from mild to profound.
5. Hearing aids are of limited benefit for sensorineural hearing loss because even with amplification, sounds are distorted. Distortion with some forms of sensorineural loss may make use of a hearing aid impossible.

Other Types

1. *Mixed hearing loss* occurs with a problem in the outer or middle ear and the inner ear. A conductive loss is superimposed on a sensorineural loss.
2. *Central hearing loss* occurs with damage or impairment to the nerves or nuclei of the central nervous system, either in the pathways to the brain or in the brain itself.

Predisposing Factors For Hearing Impairment

CERUMEN ACCUMULATION

1. Cerumen accumulation is one of the most common causes of mild to moderate conductive loss. When concomitant with other causes of hearing loss, the decrease may be significant.
2. Reduction in the number and activity of cerumen glands leads to drier cerumen with hearing loss or stuffiness and itching of the ear.
3. Cerumen impactions tend to be more frequent in older males because tragi (hairs in the ear canal) become imbedded with the dry accumulation of wax and prevent the natural outflow of the wax.
4. Removal of soft wax may be accomplished by irrigation of the ear canal with water at room temperature and a bulb syringe or a water pick (used gently).
5. Ceruminolytic agents, such as carbamide peroxide (Debrox), instilled in the ear at bedtime will soften dry wax and make successful irrigation possible in the morning. If there is no pathology, such as history of ear drainage or a perforated eardrum, this regimen of softening the wax and then irrigating with warm water should be followed one to three times a month at home to prevent wax impaction.
6. Hard impacted cerumen may have to be softened and extracted by a physician using a speculum and ear spoon.

7. The use of cotton swabs (e.g., Q-tips), bobby pins, or other sharp objects to clean the ears should be discouraged.

Presbycusis

1. Stiffening of the bones of the middle ear and thickening and decreased flexibility of the eardrum are associated with aging and conductive hearing loss with aging.
2. Beginning in middle to older age, the most detrimental changes take place in the inner ear with a slow, progressive bilateral sensorineural degeneration of auditory function.
3. There may be complex changes along the nerve pathways leading to the brain that slow down signals from ear to brain.
4. The disorder is complex, involving loss of speech processing and discrimination and perception of pure tones. The person's speech may lose quality and tone, as he fails to modulate because he does not hear himself.
5. Although presbycusis is usually attributed to aging, it does not involve everyone and some researchers attribute it to heredity, exposure to stress and noise, and circulatory problems.
6. Hearing losses associated with presbycusis are more difficult to compensate for with a hearing aid.
7. Hearing losses that cause difficulty in understanding speech and in discriminating conversation in a noisy environment cause many elderly to feel isolated even when they are surrounded by people. These problems are usually not helped by hearing aids.

Ototoxic Drugs

1. The high usage of prescription and over-the-counter (OTC) drugs and altered rates of metabolism and excretion for these drugs in the elderly increase the probability of ototoxicity.
2. The cumulative effect of ototoxic drugs, such as diuretics and aspirin, in use for chronic health problems may impair hearing.
3. Eighth cranial nerve damage by ototoxic drugs may be minimized by:
   a. Avoiding prescription and use of these drugs when possible.
   b. Alerting the client and family to possible side effects and appropriate interventions to prevent ototoxicity.
   c. Teaching the client and family to recognize and report subtle signs of hearing impairment.

EXCESSIVE NOISE

1. Lifelong occupational and recreational exposure to excessive noise can cause progressive and eventually severe sensorineural hearing loss.
2. Prolonged exposure or increased intensity of sound above 85 decibels greatly increases the chances of permanent hearing loss because the structures of the inner ear are affected.
3. Noises that often rise above this level are rock music, subways, lawn mowers, power tools, guns, factory machinery, airplanes, and some kitchen and home appliances.
4. Minimizing exposure to excessive noise and wearing protective equipment, such as ear plugs, aid in the prevention of further damage from exposure to high levels of noise.

OTHER CONDITIONS

Less frequently occurring conditions that diminish hearing in the aged are tumors, head trauma, otosclerosis, and otitis media.

THE EFFECTS OF HEARING IMPAIRMENT

1. The inability to hear environmental sounds leaves some elderly persons with an empty, dull, or isolated feeling, as they lose connectedness with their surroundings. They experience feelings of aloneness and abandonment, followed by despair and depression.
2. The inability to hear warning sounds, such as a car horn, places the elderly at great risk for physical harm or misfortune. The resulting feelings of insecurity often trigger withdrawal in all psychosocial dimensions.
3. Loss of the ability to receive and understand language on a symbolic and social level is especially threatening. Since what has been said remains unknown (because it has not been heard), the elderly are afraid of saying the wrong thing or of seeming inattentive or stupid.
4. Hearing loss may result in depression, with diminished performance on verbal tests of intellectual ability.
5. The hearing-impaired use the following coping mechanisms:
   a. Pretending to understand what is being said, they try to bluff their way. The problem may not be concealed at all, and communication is not improved.

    b. Practicing alertness to cues from other senses (especially visual) increases the chance for understanding.

    c. Using prior agreement, a non–hearing-impaired companion will cover for the hearing-impaired person in certain situations, such as ordering dinner in a restaurant. This arrangement avoids embarrassment, but the issue of dependency and control arises.

    d. Denial, repression, and rationalization may be used in a situation that is felt to be threatening even by those who usually deal with hearing impairment realistically. Avoidance mechanisms delay learning positive ways of managing.

    e. Rather than dealing with hearing loss, and recognizing and accepting a permanent change in oneself, the hearing-impaired may accuse others of not speaking clearly and may attempt to avoid contact with society. The loneliness, depression, and social isolation that follow may trigger the onset of paranoia.

6. Time is essential for working through the stages of grieving to enable the hearing-impaired to accept the loss, to admit the problem, to deal with their own attitudes and the attitudes of others, and to finally develop effective means of coping. The elderly who successfully accomplish the grieving process demonstrate effective coping in a variety of situations by:

    a. Admitting the problem.

    b. Exploring devices that may be helpful.

    c. Explaining to others what help will facilitate communication.

    d. Learning to accept and tolerate much higher levels of loneliness and isolation than most adults experience.

    e. Joining in small-group activities.

    f. Involving themselves in more handiwork.

    g. Including more hearing-impaired persons among their friends.

    h. Relying more on other people in social situations.

    i. Joining a support group.

    j. Interacting with a counselor.

ASSESSMENT FOR HEARING IMPAIRMENT

Signs and Symptoms

Alertness to signs and symptoms of hearing loss can lead to early diagnosis. Signs and symptoms include:

1. Behaviors during conversation, such as:

  a. Failure to respond when spoken to.
  b. Inappropriate interpretation.
  c. Inappropriate response.
  d. Frequent requests for repetition.
  e. Strained facial expression.
  f. Tilting head or turning one ear toward speaker.
2. Difficulty in following and participating adequately in conversation.
3. Dulled or increased sensitivity to environmental sounds.
4. Diminished ability to hear higher-pitched voices of women and children.
5. Tendency to avoid social activities involving communication.
6. Loss of expressive quality of voice; speech too soft or too loud.
7. The following in addition with sensorineural loss:
  a. Ringing in the ears (tinnitus).
  b. Difficulty in understanding conversation when there is background noise.

History

Health history is reviewed for ear infections, ear drainage, previous ear surgery, tinnitus, head trauma, excessive exposure to noise, familial history of hearing loss, or use of ototoxic medications.

Physical Assessment

1. An otoscope should be used for visualizing the inner ear canal and the eardrum when checking for cerumen, redness, swelling, drainage, lesions, or scales.
2. Auditory acuity may be screened by using a whispering technique as described in physical assessment guides. Using the ticking of a watch is not recommended, as the sound is usually higher pitched than a human voice and the elderly first lose high-frequency sounds.
3. The Weber test and the Rinne test (see reference book on physical assessment) may be used in screening to compare hearing in both ears and to differentiate between conductive and sensorineural hearing loss.

Audiometric Evaluation

The client should undergo an audiometric evaluation, consisting of an audiogram and a speech discrimination test, when there are subjective or objective findings that suggest a hearing loss.

1. An audiogram is used to measure the client's threshold for hearing pure sound by air and bone conduction in each ear.
   a. A hearing sensitivity threshold of 15 decibels or less at any given frequency is considered normal.
   b. An average hearing sensitivity threshold of 30 decibels or less in the speech frequencies (500 to 3000 Hz) usually meets average listening needs, but amplification should be considered if psychosocial or employment needs necessitate better hearing.
2. Understanding, or speech discrimination, is tested by administration of a standardized list of monosyllabic words to the client at a comfortable listening level. Correct repetition of only 70 to 80% of the words indicates difficulty in speech discrimination.
   a. In hearing-impaired elderly with a pure tone hearing loss, the speech discrimination test usually reveals more difficulty in understanding speech than would be expected from the amount of pure tone hearing loss.
   b. This loss in speech discrimination ability is thought to be age-related, with generalized cerebral atrophy resulting in decreased auditory processing in the temporal lobes.
   c. Speech discrimination tests are therefore required to accurately assess hearing and to determine what benefits might be derived from a hearing aid.

COMMUNICATION AND HEARING IMPAIRMENT

Strategies for the Hearing-Impaired to Improve Communication with Hearing People

Teach the hearing-impaired person to:
1. Tell the hearing person how he can most effectively verbally communicate with him.
2. Request the speaker to rephrase a misunderstood sentence, clarify meaning by repeating an important word, spell a word not understood, or repeat a long number digit by digit.
3. Engage in conversation in an area that is well lighted and quiet when possible.
4. Plan ahead to minimize difficulties in the environment that interfere with communication (e.g., a hearing-impaired person should request a restaurant table in a corner that is away from the traffic pattern).

5. Come early to a presentation to get a seat close to the speaker.
6. Request a change of room or the installation of an assistive listening system if the room has poor acoustics.
7. Be alert to voice and visual cues.
8. Focus on the speaker.
9. Be assertive in admitting hearing loss and requesting assistance.
10. Request written cues when needed.
11. Become familiar with a program or the text of a play before a performance.
12. Listen to the flow of the conversation without interrupting to gain more meaning.
13. Communicate to the speaker how well he is doing.
14. Ask questions if he does not understand rather than trying to bluff.
15. Defer discussion to later if he is too tired to concentrate.
16. Identify conditions at home that cause problems and plan how to minimize these problems without disrupting the household. For example, hearing-impaired persons and their families or significant others should agree always to communicate face to face rather than from another room, keeping background noise to a minimum.

Strategies for Hearing People to Improve Communication with the Hearing-Impaired

Teach family and friends of the hearing-impaired person to:
1. Wait until they have the attention of the person before speaking. If necessary, family or friends should touch the hearing-impaired person to first gain his attention.
2. Avoid speaking directly into the person's ear, as the message may be distorted and visual cues will not be discernible to the person.
3. Emphasize the visual as they face the person directly from a distance of about 3 to 6 feet and to maintain eye contact.
4. Speak slightly louder than normal, but not to shout.
5. Speak at a moderate rate.
6. Avoid chewing gum, smoking, or covering the mouth while talking.
7. Use facial expressions and gestures to clue the person into the topic being discussed and when changing the subject.
8. Change their communication into shorter, simpler sentences if it seems that the person does not understand, and avoid repeating the same words that are not being understood.
9. Highlight facial features to assist the hearing-impaired person in speech reading.
10. Minimize competing or background noise that tends to inferfere with communication.

11. Ask what they can do to make communication easier.
12. Note that, as the elderly often experience loss of ability to hear sound in the high-frequency range, they may have more difficulty hearing women and children.
13. Remain positive, relaxed, and patient even if the response is slow.
14. Talk directly to the person, not about him.
15. Communicate respect to help build self-esteem and confidence.
16. Encourage participation in group activities and increased social communication.
17. Encourage the appropriate use of available assistive devices.
18. Refer the person to an audiologist if his hearing aid is not working.
19. Encourage regular audiologic follow-up.
20. Attend aural rehabilitation classes with the client if needed for improved communication.
21. Assist with maintenance of a hearing aid or assistive devices as necessary.
22. Note that touch may be threatening to the elderly with hearing loss. A person should use a handshake that is benign and provides an opportunity for the client to signal acceptance or rejection.

Aural Rehabilitation

FACTORS INFLUENCING AURAL REHABILITATION

1. Client characteristics.
   a. Self-image.
   b. Motivation.
   c. Health status.
   d. Alertness.
   e. Adaptability.
   f. Attitude toward assistive devices.
   g. Hand and finger motility.
   h. Eyesight.
2. Inclusion of family and significant others.
3. Physical and cost availability of recommended assistive device.

COMPONENTS

1. An audiologist uses an audiometric examination to determine:
   a. Extent and type of hearing impairment.
   b. Associated communication problems.

    c. Need for aural rehabilitation to develop maximum communi-
cation.
2. Recommendations include:
    a. A plan for rehabilitation.
    b. A personal listening system and other assistive devices appro-
priate for use in the client's living environment.
3. Counseling for the hearing-impaired client and family involves:
    a. Changing attitudes and orientation.
    b. Assisting personal adjustment.
4. Teaching the client and family includes the following topics:
    a. How aging affects hearing.
    b. How hearing loss affects communication.
    c. Problems associated with hearing loss.
    d. Optimum use and care of hearing aid and assistive devices. (Di-
rections should be made available with equipment.)
    e. Simple ways to improve communication.
    f. Knowledge for recognizing fraudulent claims.
    g. Social, education, technologic, and financial resources available
for assisting the hearing-impaired.

FOLLOW-UP

It is essential to monitor the client for:
1. Consistent use and appropriate care of hearing aid and assistive
devices.
2. Changes in communication abilities.
3. Social, emotional, and psychologic adjustment to hearing impairment and hearing-aid use.
4. Adjustment problems that may indicate need for referral to a psy-
chiatrist, psychologist, or psychiatric social worker.

Communication Systems

1. The hearing-impaired elderly frequently use speech reading for
communication in addition to speaking and writing.
2. Speech reading includes not only lip reading but receiving visual
cues for all lip movements, facial expressions, body gestures, and
the surrounding environment.

   a. Visually impaired elderly have great difficulty distinguishing lip movements, facial expressions, and gestures.

   b. Training in speech reading is an ongoing process.

AIDS FOR THE HEARING-IMPAIRED

Alerting Devices

A variety of visual and tactile devices for use in daily life have been developed and are available:
- Telephone amplifiers
- Burglar alarms
- Baby criers
- Doorbell signalers
- Fire/smoke alarms
- Answering machines
- Pagers
- Telephone signalers
- Telecast decoders
- Bed vibrators
- Wake-up alarms

Hearing Dogs

1. Hearing dogs signal events and provide companionship and aid to the hearing-impaired.
2. Hearing dogs are used infrequently by the elderly hearing-impaired because elderly individuals often lack the stamina for the training period with the dogs and also tend to be unable to assume the physical responsibility for their care.

Personal Listening Devices

HEARING AIDS

1. Electric hearing aids are miniature amplifiers of acoustical energy whose purpose is to deliver sound to the ear with as little distortion as possible.
   a. Each model is acoustically different but can be individualized to meet the changing needs of the user.
   b. Adaptive compression of sound, which enables the user to un-

derstand the spoken word in a background noise situation, is available in some hearing aids.

2. Electric hearing aids consist of:
   a. A microphone that converts sound waves into electric energy.
   b. An amplifier that increases the intensity of the electric impulses.
   c. A receiver that converts the energy back into sound waves.
   d. A power source (batteries) that runs the system.
   e. A volume control switch.
   f. A microphone switch (M switch).
   g. A telecoil magnetic induction system (T switch), an optional feature that allows the hearing aid to be used for picking up signals from television or any of the communication access systems.

TYPES OF HEARING AIDS (FIG. 8–2)

1. *Postauricular hearing aids* are bone-conduction receivers and are worn behind the ear against the skull. They are most commonly recommended for neat appearance, wide application, and versatility of fit.
2. *Body hearing aids* have higher visibility, as they contain large wires that connect an ear piece to an amplifier worn on the chest. They are capable of providing greater power for more severe hearing

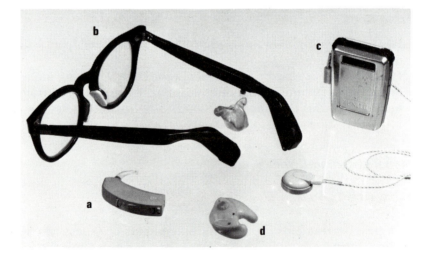

Figure 8–2. *Types of hearing aids: a, Postauricular (behind-the-ear); b, eyeglasses hearing aid; c, body aid; and d, all-in-the-ear hearing aid. (From Calkins E, Davis PJ, Ford AB: The Practice of Geriatrics. Philadelphia: WB Saunders Co, 1986.)*

losses. Body hearing aids are preferable for handicapped elderly because less manual dexterity is required.

3. *Eyeglass hearing aids* are convenient, as they comprise eyeglasses and a hearing aid in one piece of equipment and the hearing aid may not be visible. Servicing may present a problem because the client may be temporarily deprived of both his vision aid and hearing aid.

4. *All-in-the-ear hearing aids* are air-conduction receivers with miniaturized circuitry. An ear mold, a custom-fitted plastic insert, directs the amplified sound from the hearing aid into the external auditory canal. These aids generally are helpful only for mild to moderate hearing loss.

5. *Binaural hearing aids* may be used when pure tone loss is bilaterally symmetrical within an approximately 15-decibel loss of each ear and speech discrimination scores are within 16 to 20% of each ear.
   a. Binaural aids help localize sound, provide increased sound intensity, and generally improve speech discrimination.
   b. Use on a trial basis after fitting allows the client to decide whether binaural aids are helpful.
   c. The expense for two hearing aids is higher than that for one.

CHOOSING A HEARING AID

1. Criteria for selection of the hearing aid model include:
   a. Type and degree of hearing loss.
   b. How much hearing improvement is needed.
   c. Which frequencies require the most amplification.
   d. The upper limit of sound that can be tolerated by the client.
   e. Personal preferences, including cosmetic wishes.
   f. Manual dexterity, tactile sensitivity, and vision present for placement and management of controls.
2. Problems using a hearing aid, such as discomfort, difficulty inserting the hearing aid, problems with acoustic feedback, and other types of unsuspected difficulties, may be caused by age-related changes in the outer ear.
   a. Identification of the following problematic changes, selection of the appropriate hearing aid, and appropriate supportive intervention may markedly reduce problems:
      (1) Changes in skin resiliency, tissue structure, and muscle tonicity.
      (2) Increased cerumen.
      (3) Increased hair in the ear canals.
      (4) Increased tendency for prolapse of ear canals.
      (5) Decreased tactile sensation in the outer ear.

3. Auditory training for orientation and evaluation of the hearing aid includes:
    a. Special listening sessions in which a client wears a hearing aid and practices listening to speech and environmental sounds.
    b. Hearing tests performed as the client wears different types of hearing aids.
    c. Comparison of hearing test scores and the client's subjective evaluation of each aid.
    d. Recommendations indicating whether a hearing aid will benefit the client.
    e. Teaching the client to listen in a new way and to adjust to amplified sounds.
    f. Instruction in use and maintenance of hearing aids and assistive devices.
    g. Counseling on realistic expectations and limitations of hearing aids.
    h. Development of a schedule for use to promote gradual adjustment to the use of the hearing aid.
    i. Guidance for family, co-workers, and significant others for interacting effectively with the hearing-impaired.
4. A trial period with a hearing aid should be available for 30 days after purchase to:
    a. Allow time for the client to become oriented to the hearing aid.
    b. Determine whether the client can learn to operate controls and tolerate sounds that he is no longer accustomed to hearing.
    c. Protect against poor fit and incorrect selection.

GUIDE TO ASSIST THE CLIENT BEGINNING TO USE A HEARING AID

Provide the client with the following instructions:
1. Set the hearing aid in the "off" position.
2. Test the battery with a battery tester. Insert the battery with the ($\pm$) side of the battery next to the ($\pm$) side of the battery compartment of the aid.
3. Before a mirror, put the hearing aid in position and the ear mold in the ear. Insert by holding the ear mold between the thumb and forefinger so that the canal portion is pointing into the ear canal. Gently push and twist so that the ear mold fits snugly in place.
4. Turn the hearing aid on slowly, adjusting the volume between one third to one half. If "whistling" (feedback) occurs, move the ear mold around for better fit. Fitting the ear mold snugly in the ear should stop the whistling.
5. Ask someone to talk 3 to 4 feet away in a regular voice and adjust

the hearing aid for comfort. Talk about familiar topics, look at the speaker, use good lighting, and minimize noise.

6. Once the hearing aid is adjusted, leave it alone. Do not try to adjust it for each different situation.
7. Listen and identify sounds, but avoid all loud sounds.
8. Turn on the radio or television to a newscast and try listening with the volume at a normal level.
9. Some discomfort may be experienced at first, but the hearing aid should not be taken off or turned down.
10. Use the hearing aid for ½ hour the first day. Each day ½ hour should be added. By the end of the week, the hearing aid should be worn 4 to 5 hours a day.
11. If you feel nervous or irritated, take the hearing aid off and put it back on later.
12. *Do not give up!* Becoming accustomed to the use of a hearing aid is often a frustrating experience, as the unaccustomed noise is difficult to deal with. Gradually increase the time wearing the hearing aid.
13. After wearing the hearing aid 4 to 5 hours a day at home, try to use it with a small group and then in other situations, such as when in stores. Until you are comfortable in these situations, avoid using the hearing aid where there are large numbers of people, as in a theater or at large parties. Usually by the end of the third week, the hearing aid may be worn 8 to 10 hours a day.

CARE OF HEARING AID

Provide the client with the following instructions:
1. Shut off the hearing aid when not in use, remove the battery, and store the hearing aid in a clearly marked container.
2. Be careful not to drop the hearing aid on a hard surface. Work over a bed or a similar soft area when handling the hearing aid.
3. Do not knot, wiggle, or twist the cord or unnecessarily disconnect it.
4. Check the ear mold for cracked or rough edges that may be irritating. Pain from the ear mold should be reported to the audiologist.
5. Clean the tip of the ear mold with a pipe cleaner to remove the wax that can impair the conduction of sound.
6. Use only the type of batteries recommended by the audiologist or hearing-aid dealer.
   a. Silver batteries are the most expensive and powerful.
   b. Zinc batteries last about twice as long as mercury batteries.
   c. Rechargeable batteries are available.

    d. Extend the life of extra batteries by storing them in a cool, dry place.
7. Cleanse the battery and remove corrosion of the battery case by rubbing it gently with a pencil eraser, knife, or fine sandpaper. If corrosion is difficult to remove, the case should be taken to the audiologist or dealer. Dry the contacts of a damp battery with a cotton swab.
8. Take the batteries out of the hearing aid and store them if the hearing aid is not going used for a day or longer.
9. Prevent moisture in the hearing aid by not wearing it in the bathtub, in the rain, or during activities that cause excessive perspiration.
    a. Avoid exposing the hearing aid to steam vaporizers.
    b. Use an airtight container with a silica-gel pack for storage.
10. Do not use any sprays on or near the head, as they may clog the microphone in the hearing aid.
11. Protect the hearing aid from excessive heat or cold.
12. Carry an extra battery and cord in case of breakdown.
13. The ear mold of an all-in-the-ear hearing aid should be cleaned daily. *The ear mold must be removed from the hearing aid before cleaning it.*
    a. Clean an ear mold by disconnecting it from the hearing aid.
    b. Rotate a pin, needle, or small crochet hook into the hole in the center of the ear mold to remove any wax plugging the mold.
    c. Wash the ear mold in warm soapy water in a container. Do not use alcohol, as it may dry or crack the ear mold.
    d. Rinse and dry the ear mold thoroughly before reconnecting it to the aid. Use an ear mold blower to blow out any excess water in the mold to prevent water droplets in the connecting tubing from entering the hearing aid and damaging it.

PROBLEMS WITH FUNCTION OF HEARING AID

Provide the client with the following information:
1. Check that the switch on the hearing aid is in the M (microphone) position for hearing aid and not the T position.
2. Check that the volume control is set properly.
3. Replace the battery, checking that it is the right type and that the terminals are not corroded.
4. Check the hearing aid for wax, cracks, loose fit, or loose connections.
5. Examine the cord and its connections for damage. Replace a damaged cord.
6. Take the hearing aid for servicing if the opening that leads to the microphone is clogged by dirt.

7. If whistling occurs that is stopped by pressing a finger against the mold but returns when the pressure is released, the mold may be removed and reinserted. Whistling may originate in the hearing aid itself or may result from a poorly fitting mold that may need to be adjusted or replaced.

8. Strange noises with a body hearing aid are often created by clothing rubbing against the hearing aid or some loose part of the hearing aid rubbing against the case.

9. Behind-the-ear models worn by eyeglass wearers may tap against the eyeglass frame with every step. Gluing a soft piece of cotton on the eyeglass frame at the point of contact may eliminate this problem.

10. When the T switch on the hearing aid is being used, a "hum" may be prevented by avoiding being near any operating electrical devices, such as a television, fluorescent light, or electric motor, during telephone conversation.

11. The hearing aid should be guaranteed at time of purchase to be free from all defects in materials and workmanship for a period of time, and any defects that do appear during the guarantee period should be repaired at no charge. Exclusions from coverage may be listed. The hearing aid should be checked and serviced at least yearly by the dealer.

Personal Sound-Enhancement System

1. A personal sound-enhancement system is composed of a small microphone, receiver, and amplifier to transmit an amplified speech signal directly from the microphone to the listener's aided or unaided ear.
   a. The device is housed in a small unit measuring approximately 3 inches by 2 inches, which may be worn on a cord around the neck or attached to a belt worn around the waist.
   b. Some devices are hard-wired (a wire connects the device worn by the user to the sound source located near the person speaking), while others are wireless and allow for various degrees of freedom of movement.

2. These systems are useful in situations involving a few other people or in noisy environments in which listening may be difficult. For example, a hearing-impaired television viewer can adjust the volume on a hearing aid set on T switch without disturbing the other television viewers in the room.

3. Consideration of the advisability and practicality of a personal listening system is a part of aural rehabilitation.

Telephone Aids

1. A telephone handset wired with an amplification device may increase power by 30% for the listener. Phones equipped with amplified handsets in public places are becoming more accessible and are identified by a blue rubber piece between the receiver and the cord.
2. Hearing-impaired persons may use devices that strengthen a telephone's auditory signal. Before purchase of amplifiers or adapters, compatibility with certain types of phones should be checked.
3. The newer phones have an "L" coil, which cannot be used with a hearing aid. The telephone company must be requested to provide an older phone with the "U" coil if a hearing aid is to be used.
4. Telecommunications devices for the deaf (TDDs) may be leased or purchased from the telephone company.
   a. A TDD allows a person to communicate directly with anyone who has a similar device.
   b. Two callers with compatible TDDs can communicate over regular phone lines. The conversation is typed by the caller. It appears on the receiver's display panel, and the receiver of the message types back a reply.
   c. When a user wants to communicate with a hearing person who does not have a TDD, a TDD message-relay operator serves as a bridge between the two parties. The message is received by the hearing operator, who contacts the third party and conveys the message from the hearing-impaired caller. The operator then relays the response from the third party back to the hearing-impaired by TDD.
   d. There are a variety of TDDs on the market that allow the buyer choices in models, features, and accessories.

Communication-Access Systems

1. Communication-access systems for groups and large rooms consist of a transmitter that sends signals and a receiver that picks up signals and transmits them at increased sound levels to the hearing aids of hearing-impaired persons.
   a. The speaker holds or clips to his clothing a microphone.
   b. The speech signal is amplified and transmitted either to a receiver, which then amplifies and delivers the signal into the ears (via headphones), or to the hearing aids of the hearing-impaired people in the audience.
2. If there is an amplification system, the hearing-impaired person should look around to find where the speakers are located.

a. The person should sit close to the speakers but not right under them, or the sound will move right over his head.
b. The person should avoid sitting next to poles or walls, as the sound reflects off of them and makes listening difficult. The person should also avoid sitting under balconies.
3. Communication-access systems in public places such as theaters, classrooms, or churches are increasing in number as the public becomes more sensitive to the needs of the hearing-impaired.

Television and Film Access

1. Telecaption adapters (decoders) are built into televisions or may be purchased and attached to televisions to enable the hearing-impaired to view captioned programs.
2. Captioned Films for the Deaf is a loan service of theatrical and educational films for deaf viewers funded by the U.S. Department of Education. Information on distribution and membership is available from:
Captioned Films for the Deaf
Modern Talking Services, Inc.
500 Park Street North
St. Petersburg, FL 33709
1-800-237-6213

Financial Assistance

1. Medicare will pay for diagnosis and evaluation of hearing loss, but it does not pay for a hearing aid at this time.
2. Medicaid may cover some costs of a hearing aid.

Resources

American Speech-Language-Hearing Association
10801 Rockville Pike
Department AP
Rockville, MD 20852

The American Speech-Language-Hearing Association provides information on hearing aids or hearing loss and communication problems in the elderly. A list of certified audiologists in each state is provided on request.

Self Help for Hard of Hearing People (Shhh)
7800 Wisconsin Avenue
Bethesda, MD 20814

> Shhh is a national organization that publishes a biomonthly journal, *Shhh*, materials, and reprints for the hearing-impaired.

National Association for the Deaf
814 Thayer Avenue
Silver Spring, MD 20910

> With 50 state association affiliates, the NAD is a consumer advocate organization. The NAD works with other organizations representing the disabled. The NAD provides information on deafness and a list of local affiliates.

National Information Center on Deafness
Gallaudet College
800 Florida Ave NE
Washington, DC 20002

> Gallaudet College, a college for the deaf founded in 1857, is also the National Information Center on Deafness and provides information on all areas related to deafness.

Telecommunications for the Deaf, Inc.
814 Thayer Avenue
Silver Spring, MD 20910

> Telecommunications for the Deaf provides information on telecommunications devices for the deaf.

AT&T National Special Needs Center
20001 Route 46
Parsippany, NJ 07054

> The AT&T National Special Needs Center provides information on telephone adapters, TDDs, and visual and tactile devices.

The local telephone company will provide information on what equipment and services they offer especially for the hearing-impaired.

References

Anderson RG, Meyerhoff WL: Otologic disorders. In Calkins E, Davis PJ, Ford AB, eds: The Practice of Geriatrics. Philadelphia: WB Saunders Co, 1986.
Anderson RG, Simpson K, Roeser R: Auditory dysfunction and rehabilitation. Geriatrics 38(9):101–112, 1983.

Bate HL: Aural rehabilitation of the older adult. Family Forum May/June 1986, pp. 21–23.

Bates B: A Guide to Physical Examination. Philadelphia: JB Lippincott, 1974.

Butler R, Gastel B: Hearing and age. Annals of Otology, Rhinology and Laryngology. 88:676–683, 1979.

Dipietro L, Williams P, Kaplan H: Alerting and Communication Devices for Hearing Impaired People: What's Available Now. Washington, DC: Gallaudet College/National Information Center on Deafness and the American Speech-Language-Hearing Association, 1984.

Lawson PK: Helping Geriatric Patients, Nursing Photobook. Springhouse, Pa: Intermed Communications, Inc, 1983.

Luckmann J, Sorensen KC: Medical-Surgical Nursing. Philadelphia: WB Saunders Co, 1987.

Madell JR: You and your hearing aid. New York League for the Hard of Hearing.

McCann J, Rodnick J, Ruben R: Problems of the ears, nose, and throat. In O'Hara-Devereaux M, Andrus LH, Scott CD, eds: Eldercare. New York: Grune & Stratton, 1981.

Podoshin L, Fradis M, Ben-David J, Levy S: Hearing and old age. Geriatric Medicine Today 3(11):22–29, 1984.

Wax T, DiPietro LJ: Managing Hearing Loss in Later Life. Washington, DC: Gallaudet College/National Information Center on Deafness and the American Speech-Language-Hearing Association, 1984.

Williams PS: Hearing Loss: Information for Professionals in the Aging Network. Washington, DC: Gallaudet College/National Information Center on Deafness and the American Speech-Language-Hearing Association, 1984.

9

Sexuality and the Elderly

SEXUAL ACTIVITY
DRUG THERAPY AND SEXUALITY
STRATEGIES TO PREVENT SEXUAL
   DYSFUNCTION
SEXUAL DYSFUNCTION
SECONDARY CHANGES AND SEXUALITY

1. The expression of sexuality provides individuals of all ages with a means of meeting needs for safety, security, love, belonging, and self-esteem.
2. Sexual needs for intimacy, excitement, and pleasure persist throughout life.
3. The elderly express intimacy, caring, and love by touching, caressing, fondling, embracing, and coitus.
4. All of these forms of sexual expression can help the elderly cope with losses and enhance feelings of self-worth.
5. A pattern of regular sexual activity (which may include masturbation) helps preserve sexual ability.
6. The elderly are capable of maintaining active and satisfying sex lives, although primary aging changes in the physical and psychosocial dimensions may alter sexual expression.
7. Contrary to the negative stereotype of the elderly as asexual beings, a large proportion of the elderly engage in sexual activity and an even greater proportion report continuing interest in sexual activity.
8. However, for some elderly the myth of the sexless years of old age, held when they were younger, becomes a self-fulfilling prophecy as they negate their own sexuality.
9. Misinterpretation about the meaning of primary aging changes in

the sexual response cycle may curtail or prematurely terminate sexual relationships that might have continued until death.

10. Discussion with the elderly about changes in the sexual response cycle may help promote healthy sexuality and prevent sexual dysfunction.

11. Losses in the psychosocial dimension and high exposure to drugs that may affect sexuality increase the vulnerability of the elderly to sexual dysfunction.

12. Often, sexuality is ignored in the elderly, as it is threatening to professionals and to the elders' children.

13. Sensitivity of the health care provider to her own and to her clients' attitudes and value system regarding sexuality increases her personal comfort and enables her to assist the elderly in considering alternatives and making choices.

14. The continuing sexuality of the elderly needs recognition in a society that too often denies the elderly the opportunity for sexual pleasure and intimacy.

SEXUAL ACTIVITY

1. Sexual activity and interest appear to gradually diminish with age, possibly because of cultural expectations that become self-fulfilling prophecies.
   a. Patterns of sexual activity remain relatively stable through middle and late adulthood.
   b. From 60 to 65 years of age, about 70 to 75% of individuals are sexually active.
   c. By age 80, the percentage of sexually active individuals is decreased to about 20 to 25%.
   d. Sexual interest and activity may continue into the nineties regardless of actual physiologic potency.
2. Sexual activity is reduced more in frequency and vigor than in type.
3. Although the desire for orgasm may not be as strong in elderly individuals as when they were younger, the elderly continue to find orgasm pleasurable.
4. The ability to continue sexual function depends on how successfully the elderly adjust to primary and secondary aging changes in the physical and psychosocial dimensions.

SEXUAL ACTIVITY IN ELDERLY WOMEN

1. Sexual activity with the opposite sex diminishes largely as a result of lack of available men engendered by the disparity in life expectancy between the sexes.
2. After 65 years of age, the frequency of coitus decreases for unmarried and divorced or widowed women, but the prevalence of masturbation is higher than among married women of similar age.

SEXUAL ACTIVITY IN ELDERLY MEN

1. The important determinant of the level of sexual activity appears to be the level of sexual activity in earlier adulthood.
2. Men tend to maintain relatively high or low rates of sexual activity.
3. Sexual activity is higher for men than women at all ages.
4. As they age, men demonstrate a growing disparity between the number of individuals still sexually interested and those still sexually active.
5. Older men can maintain an erection and make love for a longer time before coming to orgasm. They are capable of providing more prolonged stimulation during the lengthened excitation and plateau phase.
6. Decline in sexual activity is related to aging changes in the male rather than to diminished sexual capacity of the female.
7. In the Baltimore Study on Aging (1984), elderly men who were not fully potent but had other resources for maintaining self-esteem appeared to function sexually at a level they desired and did not show signs of emotional trauma.

CHANGES IN THE SEXUAL RESPONSE CYCLE WITH AGING

1. See under "Primary Aging Changes, Genitourinary Tract" in Chapter 1. Also, see Table 9–1.
2. Delay in sexual arousal may precipitate sexual dysfunction.
   a. The lengthened time required after loss of erection for a man to achieve another erection is associated with normal aging but may cause an elderly man to fear he is becoming impotent and thus lead to performance anxiety.
   b. Pain on intercourse (dyspareunia) resulting from lack of vaginal lubrication may lead a woman to avoid sexual activity with her partner.
   c. The delay in the male partner's sexual response cycle may be

Table 9–1. Changes in the Sexual Response Cycle with Aging

Female Response	Male Response
Excitement Phase	
Breasts do not increase in size with sexual arousal but sensitivity to stimulation continues	More direct stimulation is needed for a longer time to achieve erection that is less firm than in young people
Sex flush occurs less often and less extensively	Sex flush and breast changes occur less frequently and less extensively
Decrease in muscle tone during arousal may explain reduced intensity of orgasm by some women	Decrease in muscle tension occurs
The clitoris and surrounding tissue may be atrophied but the sensation from stimulation is not decreased	Testes elevate more slowly and only partly up the perineum
Decrease in vaginal expansion occurs as a result of decreased elasticity of the vagina	
Lubrication begins more slowly and is somewhat less; dryness and discomfort may result	
Labia do not become engorged and may continue to appear as limp folds	
Plateau Phase	
Plateau phase may be prolonged	Plateau phase usually is prolonged
	Increase in control occurs
Orgasmic Phase	
Orgasm may be of shorter duration and less intense	Decrease in intensity of orgasm occurs
Multiorgasmic ability remains intact	Orgasm is more diffuse and less centered in the genitals
	Orgasm remains pleasurable
	Decrease in frequency of physical need to ejaculate occurs
	Amount of semen decreases
	Force of ejaculation decreases
	Pre-ejaculatory seepage is usually absent
	Nonorgasmic, nonejaculatory intercourse may occur
	Decrease in period of ejaculatory inevitability occurs, though period of direct penile stimulation needed for ejaculation lengthens
Resolution Phase	
Resolution phase is rapid	Erection is rapidly lost
	Increase in refractory period (time after erection is lost until the male can attain another erection) occurs, ranging from several to 24 hours

misinterpreted and lead to feelings of inadequacy in the female partner.

ALTERNATIVE SEXUAL ACTIVITY

1. Sexual activity is not restricted to, and should not be measured just by, coital behavior. Stroking, lying side by side, masturbation, oral sex, and manual stimulation continue.
2. Solitary sexual activities, such as masturbation and nocturnal dreams to orgasm, gradually increase until the fourth decade, remain constant to the sixth decade, and then gradually decline.
3. Masturbation is practiced more in single and divorced or widowed women.
4. Older individuals tend to disapprove of bisexuality, but this may change in the future as younger cohorts age.
5. Senior Action in a Gay Environment (SAGE) in New York City reports that gays and lesbians experience discrimination due to both age and sexual choice.
   a. Among elderly homosexuals, age appears to have little to do with sexual preference.
   b. Studies have described close, long, satisfying relationships between homosexuals.
   c. The surviving partner in a homosexual relationship often has no one to share his feelings with, as the need for support for the loss of lover is not recognized by society. A bereavement support group may be helpful.

Factors Influencing Sexual Activity

The following factors influence sexual activity in the elderly:
- Health of self
- Age
- Past sexual enjoyment
- Loneliness
- Boredom
- Health status of partner
- Loss of partner
- Fear of failure
- Lack of privacy
- Potency
- Marital status
- Use of alcohol or drugs
- Depression

- Overeating
- Previous sexual activity
- Religious beliefs
- Loss of cognitive function
- Self-image

DRUG THERAPY AND SEXUALITY

As there is a paucity of data on drug-related sexual dysfunction in women, the following data reflect findings on the male sexual response to drug therapy.

1. Although many prescribed drugs may affect sexuality, sexual dysfunction may be due to the client's physiologic condition, psychologic state, and his anticipation of effect of the drug (placebo effect).
2. There may be difficulty differentiating between previous sexual adjustment, the effect of depression, and the reaction to drug therapy.
3. Drugs that affect sexual function may increase libido, but usually tend to depress libido, cause impotence, and impair orgasm.
4. Depression in libido may be due partially to generalized drowsiness and easy fatigability, which are often side effects of the drug.
5. Antidepressants in small doses have been known to increase libido as anxiety is relieved. However, these drugs may cause paradoxical sexual dysfunction as the depression starts to lift.
6. Barbiturates in small doses may relieve sexual dysfunction by reducing inhibition.
7. Certain drugs, such as anticholinergics, by their very nature cause sexual problems that are difficult to alleviate by dose adjustment.
8. Increase in drug dosage may dramatically affect sexual function. For example, one gram per day of methyldopa (Aldomet) depresses libido and causes impotence in 10 to 15% of men. Doses of 2 g or more per day raise the proportion to about 50%.
9. Classifications of drugs that may (or may not) affect sexual function include:
   - Anticholinergics
   - Antidepressants
   - Antihistamines
   - Antianxiety agents
   - Antipsychotics
   - Sedative-hypnotics
   - Tranquilizers
   - Cardiovascular drugs

STRATEGIES TO PREVENT SEXUAL DYSFUNCTION

1. The nurse should make available to the elderly the following information to help reduce fear of failure, anxiety, and avoidance.
   a. The longer period of time needed for the male to achieve an erection results from age-related slower physical response to sexual arousal rather than to loss of attractiveness of the aging female.
   b. Because vasocongestion occurs more slowly, extension of foreplay promotes maximal stimulation for female lubrication and male erection before intercourse is initiated.
   c. The use of a water-soluble lubricant (e.g., K-Y Jelly) is helpful when vaginal lubrication is insufficient.
   d. Genital stimulation may require more pressure, as sensation is decreased as one ages.
   e. Maintaining and improving sexual activity are desirable as long as possible. Regular sexual activity helps maintain optimum physical health and response of the genital organs.
   f. Physical disability from painful joints or contractures may be circumvented by alternative techniques or positions (Fig. 9–1).
   g. Sexual problems that occur while a client is receiving drug therapy should be reported to the physician, who may be able to relieve these problems by adjusting dosage or by changing the drug regimen.
   h. Good communication between partners enhances sexual activity.
2. Refer the client for counseling or treatment for reported sexual difficulties if one of the partners is troubled by the changes and indicates a willingness to proceed. Sex therapy may be appropriate and is often helpful even when the sexual dysfunction is not clearly due to secondary changes.
3. Bring to public awareness the following:
   a. Continuity by those for whom sexual expression has been an important part of their lives in the past is desirable and should be encouraged to maintain self-esteem and personal well-being.
   b. Living arrangements for the elderly should provide privacy for sexual expression.
   c. Greater acceptance of the need for and the practice of solitary sexual expression is desirable, especially as many elderly do not have partners with whom to fulfill their sexuality.
   d. Remarriage between partners of similar values and with a history of a satisfactory marriage has an excellent chance of being emo-

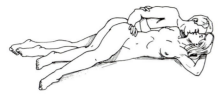

A Both partners lying on side. The man enters from behind. The woman can have a pillow between her knees. This position is good when the woman has hip involvement.

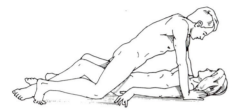

B The woman lies on her back, knees together, with pillow under hips and thighs. Notice that the male partner is supporting his own body weight on his hands and knees. This can be used when the woman has hip or knee involvement or is unable to move her legs apart.

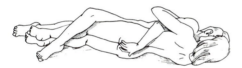

C Side position with partners facing each other. Can be used if man has back involvement. Notice that in positions C and G, the woman must provide most of the hip movement.

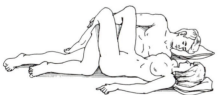

D The woman lies on her back with knees flexed. This can be used when the woman has severe contractures.

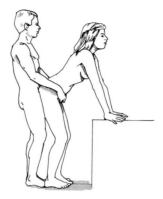

E Both partners are standing. The man enters from behind. The woman uses furniture at a comfortable height for support and balance.

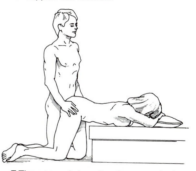

F The woman is kneeling, her upper body supported by furniture. Her knees can be supported by a pillow. May be helpful when woman has hip problems. Not good if shoulders are involved.

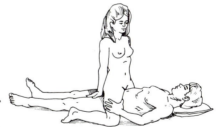

G The man lies on his back. He may use pillows for support. The woman can support her own body weight on her elbows and/or knees. This can be used when the man has hip or knee involvement.

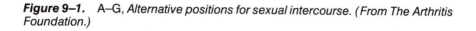

Figure 9–1. A–G, *Alternative positions for sexual intercourse. (From The Arthritis Foundation.)*

tionally, socially, and economically satisfying and tends to extend the life of the partners.

(1) Contrary to the fear of the elderly or the elder's children, social security benefits need not be lost or reduced by remarriage.

(2) Social security benefits can continue without any reduction in amount to a widow or surviving divorced spouse who remarries after age 60 or to a disabled widow or disabled surviving divorced spouse who remarries after age 50.

(3) If the new husband receives social security checks, the woman can take a wife's benefit on his record if it would be larger than her widow's payment.

SEXUAL DYSFUNCTION

1. Sexual dysfunction occurs when the ordinary physical responses of sexual functions are impaired.

2. The elderly are reluctant to discuss sexual matters and rarely seek help for sexual dysfunction. They are more likely to reveal their concerns during review of systems prior to a physical examination. The nurse should be alert to cues, gently inquire about the older person and his sex life, and invite discussion.

3. Sexual dysfunction in elderly women usually presents as one of the following:

    a. Dyspareunia, associated with dryness of the vagina as vaginal lubrication during the arousal phase begins more slowly and the quantities of lubrication are somewhat reduced. Diminished vasocongestion (related to low estrogen levels) in the walls of the vagina of older women may delay seepage of moisture across the vaginal lining.

    b. Vaginismus, characterized by involuntary spasm or constriction of the muscle around the vaginal outlet or outer third of the vagina.

    c. Loss of libido.

4. Sexual dysfunction in elderly men usually presents as one of the following:

    a. Loss of libido.

    b. Erectile failure, inability to attain or maintain an erection.

5. The causes of sexual dysfunction in the elderly may be:

    a. Organic, associated with secondary changes or drug usage.
    b. Psychogenic.

Assessment

1. To identify the problem, the nurse should begin by spending time with the client:
    a. Listen to a description of the situation.
    b. Determine the issue.
    c. Identify what aspects of sexual function the issue affects.
    d. Work with the client to identify what meaning the issue has in his life.
2. During the interview, the nurse should:
    a. Use words that the client both understands and feels comfortable with.
    b. Start with more general questions.
    c. Express concern about the problem.
    d. Ask in a thoughtful, concerned manner more specific questions involving particular areas of the problem.
    e. Communicate the intention of helping to resolve the problem.
    f. Provide periodic assurance that thinking and talking about sex are acceptable.
3. Include the assessment of partner interaction transferences, partner rejection, lack of trust, power struggles, contractual disappointments, sexual sabotage, and failure of communication.
4. Explore with the client his attitudes and value system that influence sexual function.
    a. A client may be closed and self-limited as a result of his value system. This is especially true for those whose sexual attitudes have been formed within the framework of a specific religious doctrine.
    b. A client may rethink his values and choose to be open and look at new values.
    c. An increase in self-awareness of one's own value system and choosing can lead to a sense of growth and increased self-esteem in the client.
5. Be alert to the development of a widow's or widower's syndrome.
    a. After prolonged illness or death of a partner and abstention for 6 to 12 months, the survivor attempts intercourse and fails. After one erectile failure or dyspareunia, there is a reluctance to repeat coitus.
    b. The prophecy is self-fulfilled as a result of a combination of

physical and psychologic problems, such as guilt feelings about having sex with another partner.

   c. Sexual dysfunction in a woman may be reversed with an understanding, nondemanding mate, using sensate focus, non-demand intercourse, and a water-soluble lubricant. Sexual dysfunction in the male can be reversed in days or weeks with a knowledgeable, patient partner.

   d. Widow's syndrome is reversible in 6 weeks to 3 months.

Strategies to Alleviate Sexual Dysfunction

1. The nurse should:
   a. Review interventions to prevent sexual dysfunction in the elderly.
   b. Check for drugs that may be causing sexual dysfunction. Use a current drug reference book.
      (1) Be alert to the client who reports feeling well on a drug but finds excuses for not taking the drug. He may be hiding the fact that it affects his sex life.
      (2) Ascertain the reason for noncompliance by direct questioning.
      (3) Assure the client that though sexual problems may occur, the physician can adjust his medication to relieve the problem and yet maintain therapy.
   c. Encourage elderly clients who constantly monitor their performance and experience performance anxiety to focus on sensate pleasure rather than "spectatoring."
   d. Reassure the client who fantasizes during sexual activity that sexual fantasies are basically no different from other fantasies and what is in the mind does not have to be acted on in reality. Fantasy can enhance pleasure during sexual activity and may broaden and deepen sexual experience.
   e. Respect religious commitment that may influence sexual expression, and work with the client to achieve alternatives that he can accept within his own framework.
2. Depending on the problem identified and her own comfort and expertise, the nurse may choose to provide in-depth therapy or may refer the client to an appropriate resource. Referral to a physician may be made.
   a. A history, physical assessment, and laboratory work are usually performed to rule out organic cause. A psychologic assessment is completed as indicated.
   b. Medical supervision may refer the "impotent" male client to a

sleep lab to differentiate between psychogenic and organic impotence.

    (1) Nocturnal penile tumescence (NPT) is recorded in the sleep lab. The tracings monitor the occurrence of nocturnal erections during rapid eye movement (REM) sleep and the quality of the erection.

    (2) Reduction in NPT indicates organic impotence.

    (3) Correction is done in accordance with a client's age, as NPT also declines with age.

3. Sex therapy may be indicated if the sexual dysfunction is not clearly organic. For those elderly couples willing to undergo sexual therapy, Masters and Johnson have demonstrated 50% improvement rates.

SECONDARY CHANGES AND SEXUALITY

Diabetes Mellitus

DIABETIC WOMEN

Results of studies on sexual function in women conflict as to the incidence of orgasmic response in diabetic women.

DIABETIC MEN

1. More than 50% of male diabetics suffer erectile impotence, and the prevalence of impotence increases with age.
   a. Libido may appear diminished with the decline in sex drive that occurs with aging and the emotional response to loss of function.
   b. Orgasmic and ejaculatory capacity may continue.
   c. Retrograde ejaculation may occur as a result of incomplete closure of the bladder sphincter.
2. Frequent causes of erectile impotence in diabetics include the following:
   a. Uncontrolled blood sugar. Impotence may be the presenting complaint in an undiagnosed male diabetic.
   b. Reduction in penile blood flow related to atherosclerosis, commonly associated with diabetes mellitus.
   c. Peripheral autonomic neuropathy, a complication of diabetes, which may reduce the ability of the parasympathetic nerves of the lower spine to dilate the penile arteries. More gradual and progressive organic impotence in compensated elderly clients is usually related to pelvic neuropathy.

    d. Acute metabolic decompensation with lack of control of diabetes. Metabolic decompensation usually causes the acute onset of erectile impotence within days or weeks.

3. Strategies to promote sexuality include the following:
    a. Assess for sexual dysfunction.
    b. Provide information. The client may not realize that sexual dysfunction is related to diabetic mellitus.
    c. Work with the client toward achieving optimum control of diabetes.
    d. Refer to a physician for further examination and treatment.

4. Treatment of sexual dysfunction includes:
    a. Identification of the cause of impotence.
    b. Control of diabetes.
    c. Counseling for the client regarding sexual dysfunction.
    d. Surgery to revascularize the penis to correct the effects of atherosclerosis.
    e. Insertion of a penile prosthesis (Fig. 9–2) or the use of a penile engorgement device. Although neurogenic impotence is permanent, these aids may assist the client in regaining a normal sex life.

Cardiovascular Disease

Because there are no data from studies available on the female with cardiovascular disease, the following data refer to males.

1. Impact of cardiovascular disease on sexuality.

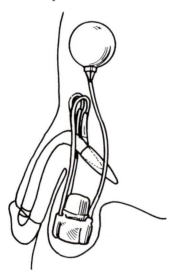

Figure 9–2. *A penile prosthesis is a medical device that a urologist implants in a man's body to help him to create an erection for sexual activities. It also allows him to make the penis flaccid for everyday activities. (Courtesy of American Medical Systems, Inc, Minnetonka, Minnesota.)*

a. The fear of precipitating angina or a heart attack, the effect of medications, or a change in self-image tend to decrease libido, increase impotence, and thereby reduce sexual activity.
b. Limited pulmonary ventilatory capacity and disabling dyspnea, which characterize some cardiopulmonary disorders, often lead to diminution of sexual intercourse, as it is too taxing.
c. Elderly people who can tolerate mild physical exertion, such as walking up two flights of stairs, can tolerate most forms of sexual activity. Contrary to fears, the occurrence of death associated with sexual intercourse is rare.
d. Most stable postcoronary clients are capable of resuming sexual activity in 2 to 4 weeks after discharge if capable of sustaining a maximum heart rate of 120 to 130 beats/minute for a short time or walking up two flights of stairs without discomfort.
e. Extramarital activities, non-routine sexual experiences, or sex after a meal or heavy alcohol consumption may be more physiologically stressful for the client.

2. Strategies to promote sexuality.
a. Dispel myths and relieve fears by counseling.
b. Include the client's partner in sessions, as the partner often may not believe reported advice and may be fearful of resuming sexual activity.
c. Counsel the client:
   (1) Recommend participation in a progressive exercise conditioning program, which, as it improves tolerance to physical stress, also tends to improve the frequency and quality of sexual performance.
   (2) Encourage continued sexual function when cleared by physician.
   (3) Encourage the client and his partner to use comfortable positions with which they are more familiar. No significant difference in physical exertion has been noted in the on-top or on-bottom positions. Standing or sitting positions may reduce attacks of angina (left ventricular end-diastolic volume is reduced).
   (4) Recommend avoidance of vigorous exercise or extremely long sessions of sexual activity.
   (5) Advise the client not to smoke.
   (6) Encourage clients with stable angina to use prophylactic nitroglycerin or long-acting nitrates prior to sexual activity to relieve both physical and psychologic stress.
   (7) Advise clients with more severe disease to avoid sex after a heavy meal or alcohol intake.

(8) Advise the client taking drugs that may affect sexual function, such as beta-blockers, diuretics, and antihypertensives, to report the occurrence of sexual dysfunction. Caution the client to discuss the problem with the physician and not to make medication adjustments on his own.

Stroke

1. The physical aspects of sexual function are rarely affected following a stroke.
2. Sexual erection is not likely to cause another stroke.
3. Sexual function may be maintained by adjusting position to either side-lying or with partner on top and by using medical devices that can help compensate for paralysis or weakness.

Prostate Surgery

1. Prostatectomy is usually performed on elderly men to relieve benign prostatic hypertrophy or prostatic cancer.
2. Difficulties in potency are rarely experienced following prostatectomy by transurethral resection or suprapubic or retropubic prostatectomy.
   a. Clients may experience retrograde ejaculation if the sphincter muscle of the bladder is cut or there is dissection around the bladder neck.
   b. Except for a lack of seminal fluid, sexual capacity and enjoyment should return to the presurgery level.
3. Potency after perineal prostatectomy is affected by the degree of radical dissection, usually performed to eradicate prostatic carcinoma.
4. Preoperative as well as postoperative counseling is strongly recommended. Counseling effectively reduces the incidence of postoperative impotence resulting from misinformation that for some men becomes a self-fulfilling prophecy.

Cancer

1. Receiving the diagnosis of cancer often results in depression, an altered body image, guilt, despair, and marital difficulties.
2. The client experiences an increased desire for physical closeness with a diminished interest in coitus.
3. Significant others should be counseled regarding the client's need for physical closeness and other expressions of love and caring.

CANCER OF THE BREAST AND MASTECTOMY

1. Impact of mastectomy on sexuality.
   a. Mastectomy creates psychologic conflicts for the woman, with fears of loss of attractiveness and of possible rejection by her sex partner.
   b. Reaction varies from relatively easy adjustment to depression, loss of sexual desire, or sexual dysfunction.
   c. The reaction of the partner in an ongoing relationship greatly influences adjustment.
   d. Nudity may cause self-consciousness for the woman or discomfort for her partner.
2. Strategies to promote sexuality.
   a. Counseling should begin early to avoid sexual dysfunction, characterized by reduction in coital orgasm and reduction in sexual function.
   b. Because self-image is linked with sexuality, various types of surgery should be discussed with the client.
   c. Assist the client in choosing the least disfiguring surgery recommended and encourage reconstruction.
   d. Assist with obtaining and using a prosthesis if reconstruction is delayed.
   e. If the client is married, encourage the husband to visit frequently and to participate in counseling and planning for surgery.
   f. Encourage the client and her husband to have him view his wife's body soon after surgery, as this appears to facilitate the relationship.
   g. After surgery, in addition to professional counseling, refer the client to a lay group, such as Reach for Recovery (sponsored by the American Cancer Society).

CANCER OF THE CERVIX OR UTERINE LINING

1. Impact on sexuality following surgery or radiation.
   a. Sexual dysfunction is common following surgery or radiation.
   b. Surgery appears to result in sexual dysfunction to a lesser degree than radiation, as it causes less scarring.
   c. Although hysterectomy does not usually cause negative effects on female function, some women experience impaired sexual responsiveness or decreased sexual interest, as their femininity is threatened.
2. Strategies to promote sexuality.
   a. Provide counseling for those women who feel they have been

damaged by hysterectomy or for men who consider their partners less feminine.
  b. Encourage consultation with the physician for assessment and treatment of complications that may cause sexual dysfunction following surgery or radiation.

Arthritis

1. Impact of arthritis on sexuality.
   a. Sexual activity is limited because of pain associated with active disease.
   b. Contractures and limitation of motion may impede active movement and the use of certain positions.
2. Strategies to promote sexuality. Counsel the client:
   a. Focus on issues of self-image and establishment of communication between partners.
   b. Discuss alternative methods of sexual expression if one partner is severely limited.
   c. Review various positions for coitus (see Fig. 9–1).
   d. Encourage the client and his partner to plan sexual activity when they feel the best.
   e. Advise taking pain medication at least ½ hour before coitus to minimize discomfort during intercourse.
   f. Advise a warm shower or bath before sexual activity to relax muscles and relieve stiffness.

Endocrine Disorders

1. Impact of endocrine disorders on sexuality.
   a. Endocrine disturbances threaten impotence with catastrophic effects on sexual self-image, self-esteem, and feelings of intactness.
   b. Alterations in function of the pituitary, thyroid, or adrenal gland are commonly associated with decreased libido, orgasmic difficulties, and erectile dysfunction (see under "Diabetes Mellitus," previously).
2. Strategies to promote sexuality.
   a. Explain about the endocrine disorder.
   b. Encourage compliance with replacement therapy.
   c. Provide reassurance that the replacement hormones will relieve sexual dysfunction and associated problems.

Resources

Sex Information and Educational Council—Resource Center and Library
32 Washington Place
New York, NY 10011
(212) 673-3850

Provides library, computer searches, and bibliographies as needed.

Senior Action in a Gay Environment (SAGE)
208 West 13th Street
New York, NY 10011
(212) 741-2247

Provides literature on gay and lesbian aging, social services, and recreational activities for elderly homosexuals and outreach services to the frail isolated gay and lesbian elderly.

References

Applegate WB: Sexuality and the elderly. In Calkins E, Davis PJ, Ford AB, eds: The Practice of Geriatrics. Philadelphia: WB Saunders Co, 1986.

Berger R: Realities of gay and lesbian aging. Social Work January–February, 1984, pp. 57–62.

Brown MA: Human sexuality. In Longo DC, Williams RA, eds: Clinical Practice in Psychosocial Nursing Assessment and Intervention. New York: Appleton-Century-Crofts, 1978.

Busse EW, Pfeiffer E: Behavior and Adaptation in Late Life. Boston: Little, Brown & Co, 1977.

Fuentes RJ, Rosenberg JM, Marks RG: Sexual side effects. RN 46(2):35–41, 1983.

Labby H: Aging's effects on sexual function. Postgraduate Medicine 78(7):32–43, 1985.

Living and Loving: Information about Sex. Atlanta: Arthritis Foundation, 1982.

Masters WH, Johnson VE, Kolodny RC: Masters and Johnson on Sex and Human Loving. Boston: Little, Brown & Co, 1986.

Normal human aging: The Baltimore Longitudinal Study on Aging. Chapter 5: Cross-Sectional Studies of Aging in Men. NIH No. 84-2450. Washington, DC: US Government Printing Office, 1984.

Stanford D: All about sex after middle age. American Journal of Nursing 77(4):608–610, 1977.

Walbroehl GS: Sexual changes in aging. Geriatric Medicine Today 3(9):29–32, 1984.

10

Maintaining Oral Health

CHANGES IN THE AGING MOUTH
  AND UNDERLYING BONE
FACTORS THAT PRECIPITATE
  ORAL HEALTH PROBLEMS
PREVENTIVE ORAL HYGIENE PRACTICES
SIGNIFICANT ORAL PROBLEMS
SOURCES OF ASSISTANCE FOR PROBLEMS
  WITH TRAVEL OR ACCESS

1. Primary and secondary changes in the oral tissues of the mouth, dentition, and underlying bone interfere with well-being in the physical and psychosocial dimensions.
2. Many elderly who grew up without the benefit of fluoridated water or fluoride products are more likely to have experienced dental decay and to have required fillings.
3. Almost 44% of the elderly 60 years or older who grew up without regular dental care and the benefit of fluoride are edentulous.
4. Pessimistic attitudes toward tooth retention as well as dental fears and anxiety cause many elderly to ignore oral health and to accept toothaches, bleeding gums, clicking dentures, and sore spots in their mouths.
5. Preventive oral hygiene, examinations, and professional prophylaxis are essential for a healthy mouth and for early discovery of oral cancer and other disease processes.
6. A lifestyle that includes good mouth care and appropriate nutrition is of utmost importance in maintaining and improving integrity of oral tissues and in retaining dentition.
7. Education of the elderly as to the benefits of regular oral care and

advocacy for the provision of accessible, affordable dental care are urgently needed for promotion of optimum oral health.

CHANGES IN THE AGING MOUTH AND UNDERLYING BONE

Oral changes affecting the elderly are summarized in Table 10–1.

FACTORS THAT PRECIPITATE ORAL HEALTH PROBLEMS

1. Primary changes of the underlying bone, the neural appratus, the immune system, and the glandular mechanisms affect the vital func-

Table 10–1.   *Oral Changes in the Elderly*

Structure	Change
Teeth	Become worn, develop caries, and are lost.
Oral mucosa	Becomes thinner as it atrophies with resorption of roots.
Tongue	Loses tastebuds, thus resulting in a decline in taste sensation.
Lips	Commonly become cracked, dry, and chapped. Angular cheilosis may occur. As teeth that supported the lip musculature are lost, overclosure of the jaw produces a fold at the corner of the mouth where saliva collects.
Jaw bones and temporomandibular joint	Undergo degenerative changes. Bone loss occurs at a younger age in women than in men and is presumably related to postmenopausal loss of steroid production, especially estradiol. Research is in progress on the relationship of alveolar bone loss in the elderly and osteoporotic bone changes that occur elsewhere in the body.
Muscles of mastication	Decrease in bulk and strength; biting force may be reduced, and swallowing may require greater effort.
Tooth pulp	Atrophies, and regression occurs with diminished sensory levels.
Touch, pressure, temperature, and pain threshold	Increase.
Salivation	Decreases. Ptyalin content is reduced. As the mucin content increases, saliva becomes more viscous and ropy.
Supereruption of teeth	Occurs as a result of loss of opposing teeth.

tions of the mouth, such as chewing, tasting, swallowing, speaking, tonal expression, and guarding against infection and injury.

2. The loss of teeth, altered lip position, diminished salivation, or dysfunctional tongue movements may impair chewing efficiency and may lengthen the time needed for preparing food for swallowing.

3. Bacterial invasion by specific gram-negative anaerobes leads to periodontal (gum) disease.

4. Genetic immunocompetency or acquired changes in immunocompetency of the mouth reduces the ability of oral tissue to withstand the assault of bacterial invasion.

5. Stress interferes with nutritional intake, assimilation of food, and immunocompetency, which are essential to oral health.

6. Secondary changes that may cause problems include those that are local and affect oral tissue and those that are systemic with possibly severe debilitating symptoms that preoccupy the family and medical care giver to the exclusion of oral effects and the need for appropriate oral hygiene. Examples of such secondary changes are:

   a. Autoimmune processes, such as Sjögren's disease (primary sicca syndrome characterized by dry eyes and dry mouth, or xerostomia).

   b. Disorders of mood and behavior.

   c. Metabolic diseases, such as diabetes and osteoporosis.

   d. Degenerative and debilitating conditions, such as Parkinson's disease, Alzheimer's disease, poststroke, and posttrauma syndromes.

7. Chronic pain may interfere with practicing oral hygiene.

8. Medications may cause oral side effects.

   a. Phenothiazines (e.g., thioridazine hydrochloride [Mellaril], chlorpromazine hydrochloride [Thorazine]) may cause excessive dryness of the mouth and uncontrolled mouth and tongue movements.

   b. Cholinergic blocking agents (e.g., atropine sulfate, tincture of belladona) may cause dry mouth.

   c. Phenytoin (Dilantin) may cause gingival hyperplasia.

   d. Antihistamines (e.g., meclizine hydrochloride [Antivert]) and diuretics (e.g., furosemide [Lasix]) may cause dehydration of tissues.

   e. Acetylsalicylic acid (aspirin) may cause chemical burns of mucosa when placed on tissues and teeth.

9. Deficient nutrition can result in oral health problems.

   a. Diets low in calcium, protein, iron, zinc, folic acid, vitamin B complex, and vitamin C are reflected in oral tissues by:

      (1) Reduced metabolism of cells.

  (2) Reduced cohesiveness and integrity of epithelial layer.
  (3) Increased friability of epithelium.
  (4) Slower healing of connective tissue.
  (5) Canker sores, traumatic ulcers, and angular cheilosis.
  (6) Abnormal burning and taste in mouth (occurs in postmenopausal women).
  (7) Faster progression of periodontal disease.
  b. Causes of nutritional deficiencies include the following (see also Chapter 4, "Meeting the Nutritional Needs of the Elderly"):
  (1) Changes in taste as a result of primary aging, medications, or illness.
  (2) Avoidance of meat, raw vegetables, and fresh fruits because of inability to chew or swallow caused by painful teeth, poorly fitting dentures, dry mouth (xerostomia), or changes in facial muscle performance.
  (3) Lack of finances or transportation for purchasing food.
  c. Strategies for improved nutrition can be provided. Teach the client to:
  (1) Eat cooked oat or wheat cereals or cold high-fiber cereals for breakfast and use whole grain breads for sandwiches, if raw fruits and vegetables are hard to chew.
  (2) Eat snacks that promote dental health: meat, poultry, fish, nuts, peanut butter (without sugar), milk, cheese, plain unflavored yogurt, raw vegetables, toast, sugarless gum or candy.
10. Lack of education and motivation to maintain good oral hygiene contribute to the delay or lack of preventive dental care.
11. Lack of accessibility to services and money for payment further contributes to neglect of oral health.

PREVENTIVE ORAL HYGIENE PRACTICES

Brushing

  1. Brushing removes plaque from outside, inside, and chewing surfaces of the teeth.
  2. Teach the client to:
  a. Hold the toothbrush beside the teeth with the bristle tips at a 45-degree angle against the gum line (Fig. 10–1A).
  b. Move the brush back and forth several times, using short (half-

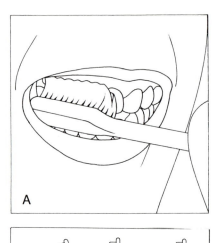

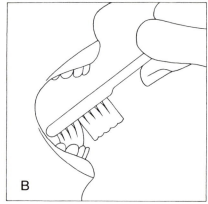

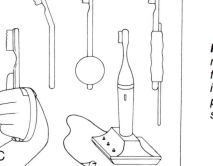

Figure 10–1. A, B, *Brushing techniques.* C, *Toothbrush adaptations for easier use. (Adapted from Keeping Your Smile in Later Years. Compliments of the American Dental Association, Chicago, 1985.)*

a-tooth-wide) strokes in a gentle scrubbing motion. Frequently change the position of the toothbrush, until the outer, inner, and chewing surfaces of each tooth are cleaned.

c. Brush the inside of the front teeth by tilting the brush vertically and making several up-and-down strokes with the front part of the brush (see Fig. 10–1*B*).

d. Brush the tongue and roof of the mouth to freshen breath and to remove bacteria.

e. Use a toothpaste that contains fluoride and has the seal of the Council of Dental Therapeutics of the American Dental Association (ADA).

f. Use a brush with soft end-rounded bristles. The toothbrush should be replaced when the bristles become frayed or worn. A soft-bristle brush used correctly—at least once a day for 2 to 4 minutes—will wear out after about 6 weeks.

3. The nurse should teach the following strategies to clients who have problems with a hand, arm, or shoulder that make it difficult to brush their teeth (see Fig. 10–1C):
   a. Attach the toothbrush to the hand with a wide elastic band.
   b. Enlarge a brush handle with a sponge, rubber ball, or bicycle handgrip. Wrapping the handle tightly with an elastic bandage, adhesive tape, or aluminum foil may be helpful.
   c. Lengthen the handle with a piece of wood or plastic, such as a ruler or wooden tongue depressor.
   d. Run hot water over a plastic toothbrush handle and then bend the handle for an easier grip.
   e. Use an ADA-approved electric toothbrush, as recommended.

Irrigating

1. As a supplement to regular oral hygiene, a dental irrigator may be used to dislodge any food particles and toxic materials that brushing or flossing does not remove.
2. A dental irrigator may be especially beneficial to those who wear braces or who have permanent bridgework.
3. The model selected should be one that is judged by the ADA to be safe for unsupervised use.
4. Individuals with poorly controlled diabetes or chronic rheumatic heart disease should check with their dentist and their physician before using an electric irrigator.

Flossing

1. Flossing daily removes plaque between the teeth and under the gum-line areas where a toothbrush cannot reach.
2. Teach the client to:
   a. Break off about 18 inches of floss. Wind most of it loosely around the middle finger of one hand. Wind the rest around the same finger of the other hand (Fig. 10–2A).
   b. Use the thumbs and forefingers. With an inch of floss between them, gently guide the floss between the teeth (see Fig. 10–2B).
   c. At the gum line, curve the floss into a C shape and slide it into the space between the gum and tooth until resistance is felt (Fig. 10–2C).
   d. Scrape the floss up and down against the side of the tooth.
   e. Take up the soiled floss on one hand and release an inch of clean floss from the other.
   f. Repeat this procedure for each tooth.

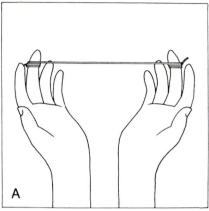

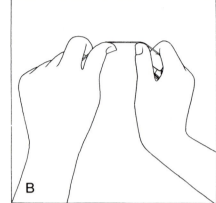

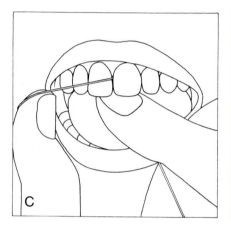

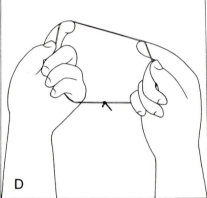

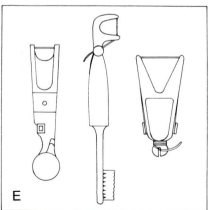

Figure 10–2. A–D, *Flossing techniques. E, Types of dental floss holders. (Adapted from Keeping Your Smile in Later Years. Compliments of the American Dental Association, Chicago, 1985.)*

g. If finger dexterity is lacking, a loop of floss may be helpful (see Fig. 10–2D) or a commercial floss holder (see Fig. 10–2E) may be easier to use.

SIGNIFICANT ORAL PROBLEMS

Dental Caries

In the elderly, dental caries (cavities) often occur between the teeth; on the roots; or beneath fillings, crowns, or clasps (Fig. 10–3). The first evidence of significant disease may be loss of enamel segments.

CAUSES

1. Decay results from the presence of bacterial infection, plaque, and carbohydrates in a susceptible tooth.
2. Caries are primarily attributed to the production of acidic metabolites by oral bacteria when carbohydrates become available for metabolism.
   a. As foods that contain sugars or starches are ingested, the bacteria in plaque (a thin colorless, sticky film of bacteria and their by-products constantly forming on the teeth) produce acids that can destroy the tooth.
   b. Sticky plaque holds these acids onto the teeth for at least 20 minutes after the client eats unless oral hygiene is carried out.

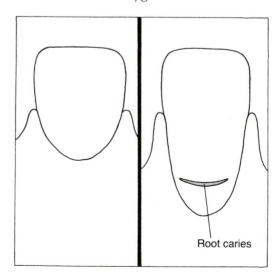

Figure 10–3. Evidence of dental caries. (Adapted from Keeping Your Smile in Later Years. Compliments of the American Dental Association, Chicago, 1985.)

Root caries

3. Root caries are likely to occur in adults who have receding gums resulting from periodontal disease. As the gum recedes, the softer root surface becomes exposed and decays more easily.

STRATEGIES FOR PREVENTION

Teach the client to:
1. Practice good oral hygiene.
2. Obtain regular dental examinations at least twice a year. As the elderly are less sensitive to pain of tooth origin, they tend to seek care when the problem is more advanced than do younger individuals.
3. Eat sugar-containing foods as part of a meal, as they are then less likely to be harmful to teeth than when eaten alone as a snack.
4. Avoid foods with high sugar content. Check labels for sugar content of foods (i.e., dextrose, sucrose, honey, corn syrup, and so on). Labels list ingredients in descending order by weight, meaning that the ingredient first on the list is present in the highest quantity.
5. Limit snacking between meals.

Xerostomia

Saliva protects and preserves oral tissues by lubricating the mouth, washing food away from around the teeth, and neutralizing acids produced by bacteria in plaque. When the supply of saliva is greatly reduced, xerostomia occurs.

CAUSES

1. Primary and secondary changes.
   a. Atrophy of the cells lining the intermediate ducts of the salivary glands, which decreases salivary flow.
   b. Autoimmune conditions such as Sjögren's disease.
   c. Blockage of salivary ducts as a result of tumors, ductal stones, or infection.
2. The treatment of primary and secondary changes.
   a. Over 400 over-the-counter drugs and prescription drugs known

to be associated with causing xerostomia, including sedatives, barbiturates, antihistamines, and drugs for muscle control.
   b. Radiation therapy to the head and neck.

SIGNS AND SYMPTOMS

1. Abnormal taste sensation.
2. Persistent sore throat or a burning sensation in the oral tissues, tongue, and throat.
3. Difficulty in chewing and swallowing food.
4. Difficulty in speaking related to soreness.
5. Frequent arousals from sleep by a hoarse throat and dry nasal passages.
6. Dry, smooth, translucent oral mucosa.
7. A thick, white, foul-smelling coating of bacteria on the tongue.
8. Cheilosis (cracking or bleeding of lips and corners of mouth).
9. Increased discomfort and inability to retain dentures because the thin coat of saliva that acts as adhesive, cushion, and lubricant is not present.

STRATEGIES TO RELIEVE XEROSTOMIA

Teach the client to:
1. Frequently sip water or sugarless carbonated drinks.
2. Increase fluid intake. When speaking, stop often to drink some liquid.
3. Chew sugarless gums.
4. Suck on sugarless mints or hard sugarless candies. Cinnamon and mint are most likely to stimulate flow of saliva.
5. Suck on a small piece of lemon rind.
6. Place a glass of water by the bed to relieve dryness during the night or on awakening.
7. Increase the humidity of the environment, particularly during the winter in heated areas.
8. Use artificial saliva, if necessary, to help lubricate the mouth. Several commercial artificial salivas are available over the counter.

Periodontal Disease

Inflammatory disease of the gingiva and periodontium (supporting structures) progresses slowly without pain (Fig. 10–4).
1. Periodontal disease accounts for the most loss of teeth in the elderly,

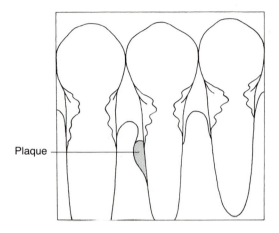

Figure 10–4. Periodontal (gum) disease. (Adapted from Keeping Your Smile in Later Years. Compliments of the American Dental Association, Chicago, 1985.)

Plaque

with about two thirds of those over age 64 experiencing some stage of the disease.

2. The longer undetected or uncontrolled periodontal disease exists, the more destruction occurs.
3. The major cause of periodontal disease is bacterial plaque.
   a. If plaque is not removed by daily flossing and brushing, it irritates the gums.
   b. The gums may become red, tender, and swollen and may bleed easily.
   c. The unremoved plaque hardens to calculus (tartar), which contains irritants that after a time destroy the tissue that attaches the gums to the teeth. Calculus can be removed only by a dentist or dental hygienist.
   d. As the gums pull away from the teeth, small pockets are formed that fill with more plaque, which accumulates along the roots of the teeth and eventually destroys the supporting structures.
   e. Without treatment, the affected teeth become loose, fall out, or require extraction by a dentist.

WARNING SIGNS

1. Bleeding, red, swollen, or tender gums.
2. Gums that have pulled away from teeth.
3. Pus appearing between teeth and gums when gums are pressed.
4. Loose teeth or teeth moving apart.
5. Changes in the way teeth fit together when mouth is closed.

6. Changes in the way partial dentures fit.
7. Bad breath or bad taste in mouth.

STRATEGIES TO PREVENT OR CONTROL PERIODONTAL DISEASE

Teach the client to:

1. Adhere to a daily regimen of effective tooth brushing, flossing, and mouth rinsing. Daily flossing is necessary to remove germs and pieces of food from between the teeth and near the gum line.
2. Obtain periodic assessment and prophylaxis by a dentist or dental hygienist (usually every 3 months).
3. Practice good nutrition to maintain tissues.
4. Be alert to and report side effects of medication regimen and drug interactions. (For example, periodontal disease may flare because immunosuppressant therapy may further depress immunocompetence of oral tissues.)
5. Use stress-management techniques to counteract negative effects of stress on nutrition and immunocompetency.

III-Fitting Prostheses

EDENTULOUSNESS AMONG THE ELDERLY

1. About 44% of adults aged 60 years and older have none of their natural teeth remaining.
2. By age 75, 66% of people have lost all of their teeth.
3. Elderly individuals who have been without teeth for a long time and who do not desire dentures may get along very well nutritionally and may manage better than those with inadequate dentures. If facial appearance is not important to them and being edentulous does not alter their personalities, the wish of these elders to do without dentures should be accepted.
4. Prosthetic replacement may be done with bridges, partial plates, or by refitting or replacing old dentures.

OBJECTIVES OF DENTURES

1. Maintenance of health.
2. Restoration of facial appearance.
3. Restoration of masticatory function.

4. Promotion of clear speech.
5. Provision of oral comfort.

CAUSES OF DENTURE FAILURE

1. Diminished strength in masticatory and facial muscles causes sagging of facial muscles and imbalance. The difficulty of learning to manipulate flaccid facial muscles often leads to rejection and claims that the dentures are uncomfortable and "don't fit."
2. Weight loss and the diminution of the ridge of the alveolar bone affect the fit of the prosthesis and may cause the dentures to move around too much while the client is eating or talking.
3. The inability to accept that dentures are less efficient than natural teeth may lead to rejection.
4. Poor tissue tolerance is associated with inadequate nutrition following poor appetite and reduction in senses of smell and taste. Taste acuity is further reduced by dentures that cover secondary taste sites in the upper palate.
5. Enlargement of the tongue (possibly resulting from transfer of some masticatory and phonetic functions to the tongue) interferes with denture retention.
6. Pain caused by the denture compressing nerve endings of the atrophied mandibular ridge discourages use of the denture.
7. The physical and emotional health of the patient affects coping abilities and may make the oral environment nonconducive to denture use. Examples of conditions affecting denture usage are:
    a. Exacerbation of metabolic problems, such as diabetes.
    b. Xerostomia caused by drugs, such as diuretics.

STRATEGIES FOR PROMOTING DENTURE USE

Support and encouragement during the breaking-in period of new dentures are essential as manipulation and retention of dentures are acquired, temporary discomfort is experienced, and adjustment to a new body image occurs.

The nurse should provide the client with instructions in the following areas.

1. *Oral care.*
    a. Clean the mouth daily. With piece of damp gauze, gently brush or wipe mouth surface, tongue, and roof of mouth.
    b. Rinse the mouth vigorously to remove food deposits (especially seeds) after eating.
2. *Adjusting to dentures.*

    a. Use the cheek and tongue muscles to hold dentures in place when speaking or eating.

    b. Cut food into small pieces, and chew on both sides of mouth.

    c. Eat small amounts of soft food frequently, taking small bites and chewing carefully and thoroughly.

    d. Avoid seeds and sticky or hard foods until adjustment to dentures is complete.

    e. Cook fruits until they are soft, and strain them, if necessary.

    f. Cook foods by steaming to soften them and to retain nutrients.

    g. Be alert to temperature of foods and liquids before eating, as dentures tend to reduce sensitivity to heat.

    h. Check food for bones or other harmful objects that may not be as readily noted with dentures in place.

3. *Insertion and removal of dentures.*

    a. Place water or a towel in the bottom of the sink to prevent dentures from breaking if dropped.

    b. Insert the wet top denture first by applying gentle pressure on both sides to work the denture into place. Then insert the wet lower denture.

    c. Remove a full upper denture grasping the front surfaces on both sides of the denture and pressing with the forefingers until the seal between the denture and the gum is broken, and pull out the denture.

    d. Remove a full lower denture by grasping the front and lingual (tongue) surface with thumb and forefinger.

    e. Remove a partial denture by exerting equal pressure on both sides of denture close to the gum.

    f. Avoid removing a partial denture by lifting clasps because this may bend or break clasps.

    g. Remove dentures at night to allow mouth tissues to rest.

DENTURE MAINTENANCE

Teach the client to:

1. Clean dentures daily to remove plaque, calculus, food debris, and stains and to prevent lesions, infections, discomfort, and bone loss.

2. Brush dentures after each meal and before going to bed when possible. At least rinse with water after eating, especially if food with seeds is eaten.

3. Remove dentures nightly and soak them in a covered container in fresh water (not hot water).

4. Follow procedure for cleaning dentures:

    a. Use a brush for cleaning dentures, as a brush cleans more effectively because the bristles conform closely to the shape of the denture (Fig. 10–5). A regular, soft-bristle toothbrush may be used.

  b. For clients with unsteady or weak hands or limited range of motion, the nurse or family may:

    (1) Attach the brush handle to the hand with a wide elastic band.

    (2) Enlarge the handle by attaching it to a sponge, styrofoam ball, or similar object.

    (3) Attach suction cups to a nail brush or a vegetable brush, and fasten the brush to the inside of the sink. Then the client may rub dentures on bristles of brush (see Fig. 10–5a).

    (4) Provide a fingernail brush with handles (see Fig. 10–5b).

  c. Clean removable partial dentures carefully around the clasps with a special clasp brush.

  d. Before brushing, put water or a towel in the bottom of the sink to prevent dentures from breaking if dropped.

  e. Remove dentures from mouth.

  f. Rinse with tepid water.

  g. Apply a cleaning agent to a moist brush and brush thoroughly. Do not apply hard pressure, as the plastic may be damaged.

  h. Rinse the dentures.

  i. For removal of calculus, soak dentures in one tablespoon of white vinegar to 8 ounces of water or in a commercial denture cleaner such as Denalan or Kleenite. *Do not use bleach for cleaning dentures.*

  j. Use Denalan or Kleenite for soiled dentures until the dentures

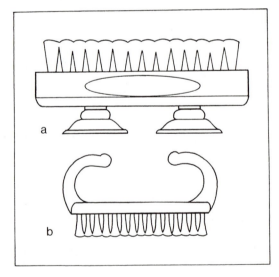

Figure 10–5. *Denture brushes for the handicapped. (Adapted from Keeping Your Smile in Later Years. Compliments of the American Dental Association, Chicago, 1985.)*

are clean; then use a commercial product, such as Polident, to maintain clean dentures.

5. Care for loose dentures.

   a. Dentures should not be changed with do-it-yourself kits, as the denture may be irreparably damaged and may further irritate oral soft tissues. A dentist or a denturist (a dental laboratory technician) should be consulted who may recommend soft denture liners or a new prosthesis. Dentures should be re-examined periodically by dental personnel.

      (1) Hardening of the soft denture liners is slow and often barely noted by the elderly. When the soft liner loses resiliency, it should be relined, rebased, or replaced.

      (2) Soft denture liners may be ideal for providing comfortable use of dentures by the very ill or terminally ill.

   b. OTC glues often contain chemicals that can damage the plastic material of dentures.

   c. Correct alignment by an untrained person is almost impossible and can lead to poor fit and possible harm to oral tissues.

   d. If regular use of the adhesive seems necessary to stabilize the denture or to make it feel comfortable, the denture may need to be relined (have the tissue-bearing surface replaced).

   e. Denture adhesives mask infection and cause bone loss in the jaw and should therefore be used only in an emergency until dental personnel can be seen.

   f. If denture adhesive is used, advise the client to:

      (1) Apply a light coat of powered adhesive to moistened denture bases or a light coat of paste to dry denture bases.

      (2) Clean the denture twice a day with a soft brush and rinse the denture well under lukewarm water.

      (3) Clean adhesive material from mouth with a piece of damp gauze and rinse the mouth before reinserting dentures.

      (4) Refrain from adding more and more adhesive.

      (5) Avoid sleeping with dentures to which adhesives have been applied.

Oral Cancer

1. Oral neoplasms occur in about 4% of the adult population and have a greater tendency to be malignant in the older client.

2. The elderly should be carefully assessed for precancerous conditions and for oral cancer, as early detection increases the prospect for cure.

3. Oral cancer in the elderly usually appears as a squamous cell carcinoma of the lower lip or lateral border of the tongue.
4. Intraoral cancers may occur in any soft tissue area but tend to occur more in areas of chronic, frequent irritation from cigarettes, cigars, and pipe stems.

WARNING SIGNS

1. A sore on oral tissue that does not heal within 2 to 3 weeks.
2. White, scaly patches on oral tissue.
3. Unexplained numbness or pain in the mouth.
4. Bleeding episodes in the mouth without known cause.

STRATEGIES FOR PREVENTING ORAL CANCER

Teach the client to:
1. Obtain regular oral assessments.
2. Maintain good nutrition.
3. Avoid materials that cause chronic irritation of the oral mucosa, such as cigarettes, cigars, and pipe stems.
4. Use sun screens on lips if directly exposed to the sun.
5. Obtain medical supervision for lesions that persist over 2 weeks.

SOURCES OF ASSISTANCE FOR PROBLEMS WITH TRAVEL OR ACCESS

1. Financial.
   a. Medicaid is available for dental care in some states.
   b. Local dental associations sponsor access programs for the needy.
   c. Prepayment systems, such as dental insurance, may be available.
2. Travel or access to service.
   a. The local community may offer travel assistance.
   b. Programs may be offered by dental colleges or local health departments.

Resources

Dental health services are listed under the local public health department in the telephone book.

The American Society of Geriatric Dentistry
1121 W. Michigan Street
Indianapolis, IN 46202

American Dental Association
211 E. Chicago Avenue
Chicago, IL 60611

National Foundation of Dentistry for the Handicapped
1250 14th Street, Suite 610
Denver, CO 80202

National Institute of Dental Research
National Institutes of Health
Bethesda, MD 20205

References

A Research Agenda on Oral Health in the Elderly. Washington, DC: Veterans Administration, 1986.

Bennett J, Creamer H, Fontana-Smith DJ: Dentistry. In O'Hara-Devereaux M, Andrus M, Scott CD, eds: Eldercare. New York: Grune & Stratton, 1981.

Keeping Your Smile in the Later Years. Chicago: American Dental Association, 1985.

Lawson PK: Helping Geriatric Patients. Springhouse, Pa: Intermed Communications, Inc, 1983.

Winkler S, Massler M: Oral aspects of aging. In Calkins E, Davis, PJ, Ford AB, eds: The Practice of Geriatrics. Philadelphia, WB Saunders Co, 1986.

Zach L, Trieger N: The oral cavity. In Rossman I, ed: Clinical Geriatrics. Philadelphia: JB Lippincott, 1986.

11

Supporting the Client
With Arthritis

ARTHRITIC CONDITIONS
STRATEGIES FOR PREVENTION
   OR LIMITATION OF DAMAGE
   TO TISSUES BY ARTHRITIS
COMPONENTS OF A COMPREHENSIVE
   TREATMENT PROGRAM
ASSISTIVE DEVICES

1. Arthritis and rheumatic diseases are terms used for a group of disorders that affect not only joints but also supportive connective tissues, including muscles, tendons, ligaments, and protective coverings of internal organs, throughout the body.
2. Although each of the rheumatic diseases differs in potential causes, course, and prognosis, arthritis is usually chronic, lasts a lifetime, and is a leading cause of disability in the elderly.
3. More than one third of the 37 million Americans affected with arthritis are 65 years of age or older.
4. Arthritic changes often affect overall lifestyle by:
   a. Decreasing mobility.
   b. Causing pain and depression.
   c. Altering self-image and sexual expression.
   d. Reducing ability to work.
5. Early diagnosis of rheumatic disease and treatment are important for preventing or limiting damage to tissues.
6. Therapy is best designed to meet the needs of the individual client in an effective self-management program with maximum benefit and minimal risk.

7. Continued assessment, instruction, and monitoring for compliance are important for the success of a therapeutic program.
8. A well-planned treatment program properly carried out is beneficial, but great patience and confidence are essential because exacerbations occur and improvement is slow.

ARTHRITIC CONDITIONS

1. The most common arthritic (rheumatic) conditions in the elderly are osteoarthritis, rheumatoid arthritis, and gout.
2. The joint is the focus of the degenerative process in all three conditions, with local cartilage and bone disruption the most prominent features (Fig. 11–1).
3. Symptoms usually include painful joints, possible tenderness, swelling, and compromised range of motion.
4. All types of arthritis cause joint and muscle pain, but the amount of inflammation in the joints varies a great deal from none at all to severe.
5. There is no clear relationship between the amount of pain and the extent of damage. Some clients with advanced joint changes have few complaints, whereas others with only apparent minimal changes experience severe pain.

Osteoarthritis

1. Osteoarthritis (degenerative joint disease or "wear and tear arthritis") is the most common arthritic process in the elderly with an incidence as high as 80 to 90% (based on x-ray studies of joints).

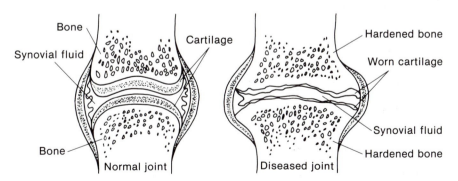

Figure 11–1. *Normal joint and diseased joint. (From* Learning to Live with Osteoarthritis, *© 1983 by Medicine in the Public Interest, made possible by a grant from Pfizer Pharmaceuticals.)*

2. The vast majority of people with osteoarthritis never experience aching, pain, or stiffness.
3. Pain that is experienced is described as one of three types:
   a. A deep, boring pain focused in the involved joint that frequently occurs at night.
   b. A sharp, jarring pain that occurs while the person is walking or placing the affected joint under stress.
   c. Referred pain that is not experienced in the involved joint but is experienced elsewhere.
4. Pathologic changes seem to be exaggerated manifestations of the aging process. Wear and tear are a major cause, but the infrequency of arthritic changes in the weight-bearing joint of the ankle and the common occurrence of changes in the distal fingertips suggest other causes of a traumatic, metabolic, or immunologic nature.
5. Osteoarthritis primarily affects the cartilage of joints, causing it to fray, wear, ulcerate, and in extreme cases disappear entirely, leaving a bone-on-bone joint.
   a. The exposed bone may thicken and become hard and dense.
   b. Spurs (little jagged lumps that are proliferations of bone and cartilage) may form at the edges of the joint, but they do not usually cause discomfort.
   c. Heberden's nodes (bony knobs) often appear between the last two joints of the fingers (distal interphalangeal [DIP]), and Bouchard's nodes appear in the middle joints (proximal interphalangeal [PIP]). These nodes are painful at first during formation (about 6 months). After the nodule is formed, pain often goes away.
   d. The inflammatory changes (soft tissue swelling and tenderness of the synovium) are much less than in rheumatoid arthritis but do occur to some degree with osteoarthritis.
6. Muscles give support to joints and help them move.
   a. With arthritis, muscle fatigue occurs fairly regularly, as the muscles surrounding affected joints are physically stressed to work harder.
   b. Muscles surrounding affected joints may become tense and contract in response to pain. These contractions, or spasms, tend to foster non-use of the joint. The result is loss of the joint's natural shape and ability to move.
   c. Muscles that support painful joints may become weakened from lack of exercise or incorrect use.
      (1) Joints surrounded by these weakened muscles then become more painful than those surrounded with strong muscles, which can share the stress.

(2) These unprotected joints are more susceptible to further cartilage injury or to tiny bone breaks with spur formation.
7. Table 11–1 summarizes the major distinguishing characteristics of osteoarthritis.

Rheumatoid Arthritis

1. Rheumatoid arthritis (RA) affects about 7 million people in the United States. Among the elderly, the incidence is increased, with 30 to 50% or more of the elderly demonstrating symptoms of RA.
2. Rheumatoid arthritis is a chronic inflammatory disease of unknown cause usually characterized by polyarthritis (monoarticular rheumatoid arthritis may occur) of the diarthrodial (hinged) joints.
3. The principal tissue involvement of RA is the synovium of the joint lining, which becomes inflamed, rough, granulated, and swollen.
   a. Cells such as lymphocytes, plasma cells, and macrophages (elements of the body's immune, or disease-fighting, apparatus) are visible in samples of the tissue. This finding suggests that RA may be a virus-initiated disease.
      (1) The antigen, which may be a virus in the synovial tissue, stimulates the immunologic reaction. In the effort of rejection, pain and swelling occur and result in synovial destruction.
   b. The immunologic reaction that characterizes RA appears to stimulate a second reaction in connective tissue (or granulation tissue), which proliferates and invades the joint cartilage.
      (1) Pannus, or aprons of granulation tissue, grows across and between both bones in the joint. The pannus may invade and destroy bone and ligaments.
      (2) Relatively symmetrical swelling appears on both sides of the joints with the disease.
      (3) Tenderness of the involved joints is the most sensitive physical sign.
   c. The progressive, symmetrical, inflammatory process is potentially crippling.
4. During remission, medication may be decreased or discontinued. The cause of remission is unknown.
5. The majority of elderly clients with long-standing RA have survived to old age with less crippling disease and fewer constitutional manifestations than those for whom the disease was fatal at a younger age.
   a. In about 75% of patients with late-onset RA the onset is insidious

with mild systemic symptoms but potentially crippling joint in-volvement.

   (1) The disease process is usually more benign than in early adult-onset types, but remissions are less frequent and the client is subject to a mild but continuously active form of arthritis.

  b. In about 25% of late-onset RA cases in the elderly, the onset is precipitous and stormy with severe systemic symptoms. In most of these cases, RA is self-limited, and the client experiences a spontaneous remission within several months.

6. Table 11-1 summarizes the major distinguishing characteristics of rheumatoid arthritis.

Gout

1. The incidence of gout (gouty arthritis) increases with age.
  a. Primary gout peaks at between 48 and 53 years of age.
  b. Postmenopausal women demonstrate an increase in serum urate levels.
  c. Drugs used by the elderly, such as thiazides, tend to elevate serum urate levels.
  d. Surgery and trauma, which both tend to occur with increased frequency in the elderly, appear to be antecedents of gouty arthritis.

2. When the excretion of uric acid is slowed or the production is excessive, the level of uric acid in the body rises to the point of supersaturation.
  a. Precipitation of sodium urate acid crystals then occurs with deposition upon cartilage or in synovial fluid.
  b. This deposition of crystals causes abrupt and painful joint inflammation, often in the great toe joint.
  c. A slower build-up of precipitated urate in bone, cartilage, or even skin (e.g., great toe, ear lobes, olecranon bursa, ankles, heels, wrists, and hands), which gradually enlarges (usually without pain) into lumps called tophi, may be disfiguring and disabling.
  d. Tophi rarely occur now, as effective medication for prevention is available.

3. Table 11-1 summarizes the major distinguishing characteristics of gout.

Table 11-1. *Major Distinguishing Characteristics of Arthritic Conditions Most Common in the Elderly**

Parameters	Osteoarthritis	Rheumatoid Arthritis	Gout
Age at onset	40 to 60	20 to 60	20 to 60
Sex	Affects mostly females over age 45; affects mostly males under age 45	Affects mostly females	Affects mostly males
Joint pain	1+ to 4+†	1+ to 4+	1+ to 4+
Joint swelling	0 to 2+ Usually lasts 10 to 30 minutes	2+ to 4+ May last 1 to 2 hours	2+ to 4+
Morning stiffness	1+ to 2+	1+ to 4+	WNL
Major joint sites involved	DIP, knee, hip, MTP, CMC, spine (usually asymmetric joint involvement)	PIP, cervical spine, cricoarytenoid, knee, ankle (polyarticular symmetric joint involvement)	MTP, tarsal
Nodules	Heberden, Bouchard	Subcutaneous	Tophi
Systemic symptoms	None	Fever, muscle wasting, anemia, pleuritis, vasculitis, neuropathy, Sjögren's syndrome, episcleritis, ocular nodules, pericarditis, presence of HLA-B27 antigen in blood	Tophi on the ears, fingers, hands, and feet; hyperuricemia, nephrolithiasis
Course prognosis	Slow mild joint destruction; may require replacement surgery to restore function	Intermittent with remissions or rapid or low disabling, destructive disease; prognosis varies depending on individual course and treatment	Excellent with adequate treatment

*Modified from Evens RP, Hawkins DW: Bone and joint disorders. In Covington TR, Walker JI, eds: Current Geriatric Therapy. Philadelphia: WB Saunders Co, 1984.
†Symptom scale: (none) to 4+ (severe).
Abbreviations: CMC = carpometacarpal; DIP = distal interphalangeal; MTP = metatarsophalangeal; PIP = proximal interphalangeal; WNL = within normal limits.

STRATEGIES FOR PREVENTION OR LIMITATION OF DAMAGE TO TISSUES BY ARTHRITIS

The nurse should teach the elderly and the family:
1. To report early warning signs of arthritis.
   a. Swelling in one or more joints.
   b. Early morning stiffness.

    c. Recurring swelling, pain, or tenderness in any joint.
    d. Inability to move a joint normally.
    e. Redness and warmth in a joint.
    f. Unexplained weight loss, fever, or weakness combined with joint pain.
    g. Symptoms like these that persist for more than 2 weeks.
2. The goals of the individualized treatment program.
3. How to comply with the individual treatment program.
    a. Explain the purpose, limits, contraindications and hazards of each modality.
    b. Provide helpful guidelines to promote compliance with the treatment program.
    c. Demonstrate therapeutic activities.
    d. Check for safe performance by observing the client perform therapeutic activities.
    e. Instruct in several modalities so that the client may replace one with another when conditions change (e.g., switch from a hot to a cold modality with a joint flare; shower for pain in several joints rather than using a pack for each joint).
    f. Provide written instructions with appropriate modifications.

COMPONENTS OF A COMPREHENSIVE TREATMENT PROGRAM

Goals of Program

1. Reduction of predisposing factors.
2. Relief of pain and discomfort.
3. Reduction of inflammation.
4. Maintenance or restoration of joint function.
5. Prevention of joint deformities.
6. Promotion of an optimal lifestyle.

Emotional Support

1. Living alone, suffering psychologic isolation, increasing inactivity, and losses in functional capacity decrease expectations for improvement and lead to depression, noncompliance, and susceptibility to quackery.
2. Emotional trauma and strain appear to influence the degree of

symptoms and possibly the course of the disease by exacerbating muscle tension and interfering with free, relaxed joint motion.

3. Guidelines for providing emotional support to the arthritic client include:
   a. Attempting to give the client confidence that something can be done and therapeutic possibilities are ahead.
   b. Reducing emotional stress by explaining fully the disease pathology and the likelihood of gradual control with therapy.
   c. Fostering self-management of arthritis by emphasizing the need for compliance with the total long-term therapy program.
   d. Assisting the client in adjusting to changes in lifestyle. (See under Arthritis and Sexuality, Chapter 9.)

Nutritional Counseling

1. Gear nutritional counseling to:
   a. Providing energy.
   b. Maintaining muscle strength.
   c. Reducing weight in the overweight client.
2. See Chapter 4, "Meeting the Nutritional Needs of the Elderly."

Rest

Guidelines for promoting rest include:
1. Planning with the client for a balance between rest and exercise, which is essential to control fatigue and joint inflammation.
2. Planning with the client for extra sleep at night and short rest periods during the day.
3. Encouraging correct posture in either a sitting or supine position to help the client derive maximum benefit from rest.
4. Promoting compliance with joint rest techniques, splints, and assistive devices to protect inflamed or swollen joints (see Fig. 11–8).
   a. Rest is more important than exercise during inflammation to lessen the inflammation, deformity, and pain.
   b. Permanent loss of joint mobility does not result from rest or splinting of an inflamed joint.
5. Encouraging the use of relaxation and stress-reduction techniques to help with the stress of pain and chronic disease.

Good Posture

Teach the client guidelines for maintenance of good posture.
1. Avoid positioning a painful joint in a bent position (even though it

may feel comfortable), for the bent position usually leads to stiffness and loss of joint motion and finally deformity.

2. Avoid carrying packages or other articles. If some things must be carried, the weight should be evenly distributed into two packages that allow for both arms being used.
3. Use a lightweight shoulder bag rather than a handbag if possible.
4. When standing, position the body in good alignment that allows the arms to swing freely at the sides and the weight to shift easily from side to side.
5. For sitting, use a straight-backed chair (preferably with arm-rests) with a firm seat high enough for arms and hands to reach work easily and naturally and for the feet to rest flat on the floor.
6. For lying in bed, use a firm mattress (preferably with a board underneath). Lie flat with the arms and legs straight and only a small pillow under the head. Never place a pillow under the knees.
7. Extend legs whether sleeping or sitting to prevent knee contractures.

Thermotherapy

1. Contraindications for thermotherapy are:
   a. Poor circulation.
   b. Decreased sensation (especially of scar tissue).
   c. Cold or heat hypersensitivity.
   d. Sedation.
   e. Decreased alertness.
   f. Skin infection.
   g. Reduced cardiac and respiratory reserves associated with less tolerance for heat.
   h. Vasculitis, Raynaud's phenomenon, cryoglobulinemia, and paroxysmal cold hemoglobinuria.
2. Considerations in the choice of modality for thermotherapy include:
   a. Patient preference.
      (1) Heat is often the first choice, as clients tend to dislike cold.
   b. Ease of use.
   c. Expense.
   d. Availability of equipment.
   e. Current disease process.
      (1) Cold is often more effective for acute pain and hot, inflamed joints.
      (2) Heat is often more effective for subacute or chronic joint problems.
   f. Benefit of the modality.

(1) Differences in the benefit of superficial and deep heat have not been demonstrated.
   (a) Superficial heat is obtained by the use of moist heat packs and paraffin baths.
   (b) Deep heat to the joints by diathermy and ultrasound is contraindicated for acutely inflamed joints, as increased temperature accelerates cartilage destruction.
   (c) Ultrasound is particularly effective as an adjunct to exercise to increase range of motion when periarticular and capsular tightening is present.
(2) Dry heat is better tolerated at higher temperatures, but wet heat penetrates more deeply than dry heat at the same temperature.
   (a) Similar degrees of deep tissue healing may occur, but moist heat is often reported to be more effective.
(3) Hydrotherapy, by immersion of all or parts of the body, provides the buoyancy and viscosity of water that eases joint motion and muscle functioning in therapeutic water exercise.
   (a) Immersion of large parts of the body causes systemic effects, such as increased pulse and decreased blood pressure, that may contraindicate use, especially for the frail elderly.
   (b) Spa therapy with whirlpool, hot tub, and sauna is more expensive but has not been demonstrated to be more effective than warm tub baths.
   (c) Mineral and mud baths have no effect on arthritis, and mud may cause a rash.
   (d) Hot packs are used for treating a single joint while large parts of the body are immersed in water when two or more joints are involved.
3. Safety precautions should be emphasized in the use of thermotherapy, as the elderly client is particularly susceptible to adverse reactions to thermal changes.

Light Massage

Light massage may help reduce stiffness and muscle spasm, but it should not be used on inflamed joints.

Transcutaneous Electrical Nerve Stimulation

1. Transcutaneous electrical nerve stimulation (TENS) may be ordered by the doctor to relieve chronic pain by electrical stimulation.

2. The TENS device is made up of a small box measuring about 2 inches square with a battery and two to four electrodes that are taped to the skin.
3. Assistance may be needed in applying electrodes.
4. The unit may be attached to a belt or carried in a pocket.
5. When the device is turned on, the electrical current activates the large, more rapidly conducting fibers and causes a tingling or vibratory sensation as the incoming pain signal is blocked.
6. Overall efficiency in clients with chronic pain is about 25%.

Therapeutic Exercise

1. An exercise program is specifically helpful for:
   a. Preventing or improving the range of motion of joints.
   b. Maintaining a useful pattern of joint motion.
   c. Preventing joints from freezing in position.
   d. Achieving maximum function of upper and lower extremities.
   e. Preventing muscle atrophy and increasing muscle bulk.
   f. Restoring and strengthening muscles around joints that provide support and stability to the joint, thereby reducing pain and making movement easier. For example, an exercise program may help to relieve backache by strengthening the abdominal muscles.
2. In collaboration with the health care team, a physical therapist best designs and implements a realistic individual exercise program that addresses the specific joint problems, capabilities, and lifestyle of the elderly client.
3. Teach the client guidelines for an exercise program.
   a. Optimally, carry out an exercise program three times a day.
   b. Perform exercise slowly because rapid movements fatigue muscles quickly and a sudden jerk may damage joints.
   c. Initially move joint only as far as it feels comfortable and not to the point where it really hurts. If a joint is still painful an hour or so after exercise, probably too much has been done.
   d. Perform each exercise only a few times a day to start. The number of repetitions should be increased gradually.
   e. Seek professional assistance and decrease activity if there is an increase in joint or systemic symptoms.
   f. Apply heat before exercise to help reduce pain and ease movement.
   g. Wear warm clothing to help reduce aching in joints and to allow for more comfortable movement.
   h. Arrange for ongoing assessment of ambulation, transfer, posture, and performance of the exercise program.

    i. Continue exercise sessions as part of daily activities even when flares necessitate modification.

    j. Avoid putting too much pressure on the back when lying down to exercise by bending the knees until the feet are flat or tucking a pillow under the thighs against the buttocks.

    k. When exercising the joints of the lower extremities, exercise one leg at a time so that both legs have an equal workout. When both legs are done together, there is a tendency to concentrate on the affected leg.

    l. Counteract stiffness that often occurs on standing by limbering up both knees by flexing and extending them before standing.

4. Range of motion (ROM) exercises help to maintain or increase joint movement by moving joints through their full range of motion.

    a. ROM exercises may be active or active-assisted.

    b. Activities of daily living are insufficient for maintenance because they do not move joints through full range of motion. As a result, motion may be easily lost and may be difficult or impossible to regain.

    c. One to two full joint ROM exercises per day will maintain motion.

    d. Two to three repetitions of ROM per day are needed to regain lost range of motion.

    e. Excessive repetitions are contraindicated, as they may increase joint temperature and accentuate inflammation.

    f. See Figures 11–2 through 11–6 for basic exercises aimed at increasing ROM.

5. Isometric (static or "muscle-setting") exercises are one form of strengthening exercises that help to increase the power and work ability of muscles.

    a. Isometric exercises are particularly suitable for clients with swollen and painfully inflamed or severely damaged joints.

    b. Muscle-setting exercises are performed with a body part remaining fixed in one position as the client contracts a muscle without moving the joint or part.

        (1) The muscle is held tense for a count of 6 seconds and then relaxed for a count of 10 seconds. The cycle is repeated several times.

        (2) When performing isometric exercises, the client should be instructed to:

            (a) Count out loud to six during each isometric exercise.

            (b) Hold the muscle tense.

            (c) Continue breathing.

            (d) Avoid performing the Valsalva maneuver.

Do these exercises while lying on your back. To reduce the pressure on your back, bend your knees and keep your feet flat or tuck a pillow under your thighs.

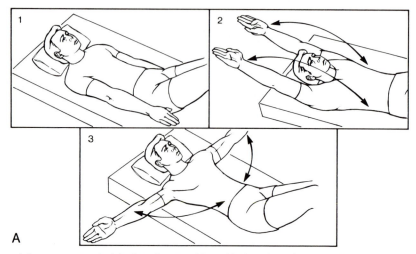

1, Lay your arms straight down by your sides, with the palms of your hands down. *2*, Keeping your elbows straight, raise your arms over your head as far as possible and return them to your sides. *3*, With your elbows still straight, move your arms away from your sides and return.

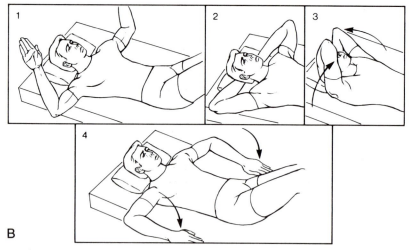

1, Stretch your arms out to the side and bend the elbows so that your hands point up. *2*, Move your arms to your head and put your hands under your head, with the backs of your hands flat on the bed. *3*, With your hands behind your head, try to bring your elbows together. *4*, Return to the first position with your arms out to the side and your elbows bent; move your forearms forward until the palms of your hands are flat on the bed by your sides.

Figure 11–2. A–C, *Exercises for shoulder and elbows. (From* Learning to Live with Osteoarthritis, *© 1983 by Medicine in the Public Interest, made possible by a grant from Pfizer Pharmaceuticals.)*

234

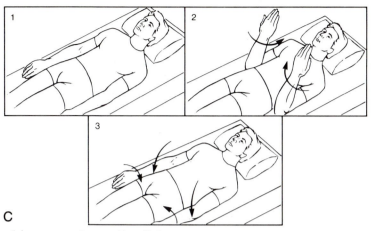

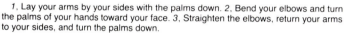

C

1, Lay your arms by your sides with the palms down. *2*, Bend your elbows and turn the palms of your hands toward your face. *3*, Straighten the elbows, return your arms to your sides, and turn the palms down.

Figure 11–2 Continued.

   c. Quadriceps-setting should be encouraged because the quadriceps muscle assists in rising and then in standing.
     (1) Quadriceps-setting should be done on a regular basis both with the leg elevated and with the knee bent at a right angle and the foot on the ground.
6. Stretching exercises may be needed if the joint is too stiff to move through a normal range of motion.
   a. Stretching exercises are to be done only under the supervision of a physician or a physical therapist.
   b. Stretching exercises cannot be done for a joint that is fused.
7. Functional exercises (movements and motions that are involved with the activities of daily living) should be encouraged even though they be difficult for the client (e.g., buttoning clothes).
   a. An occupational therapist may best design and implement a program to help an individual learn to do activities of daily living comfortably and effectively.

Joint Protection

1. Joint protection is particularly geared to:
   a. Helping rest inflamed joints.
   b. Preventing or possibly correcting joint deformities.
   c. Protecting joints from stress.
2. Splints are used for joint protection (Fig. 11–7).

Do these exercises while sitting at a table or other flat surface. Be sure to exercise both hands.

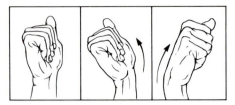

With your hands relaxed, bend your wrist back and forth as far as possible. You can rest your forearm gently on the table or hold your arm up while doing this exercise.

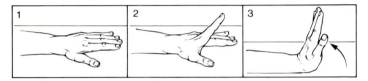

1, Place your hand and forearm down as flat as possible on a table or flat surface. Spread your fingers apart. *2,* One by one, lift each finger as high as it will go, keeping the rest of your hand flat. Relax. Do this with your thumb, too. *3,* With your fingers straight and your lower arm flat, bend your wrist and lift your whole hand as far back as you can. Relax.

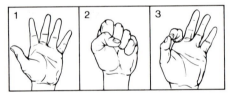

Rest your arm gently on the table or hold your arm up. *1,* Open your hand, spreading your fingers and thumb wide. *2,* Close your hand into as tight a fist as possible. Relax. *3,* With your hand open, touch the tip of your thumb to the tip of your index finger, making an O. Open your hand and spread your fingers wide. Continue touching the tip of each finger with your thumb, spreading your fingers wide in between each step. If necessary, use your other hand to push your fingers closer together.

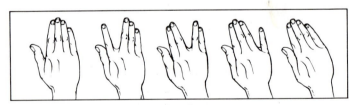

Place your hand on a table with your palm down. Move the thumb out to the side. Bring your index finger over to the thumb. Then, one by one, bring the other fingers over, closing the gap, until all your fingers are together. Relax.

Figure 11–3. A–D, *Exercises for wrist and fingers. (From* Learning to Live with Osteoarthritis, *© 1983 by Medicine in the Public Interest, made possible by a grant from Pfizer Pharmaceuticals.)*

For these exercises, sit comfortably in a chair. Do them in your stocking feet or in bare feet. Do them all several times for each foot or leg.

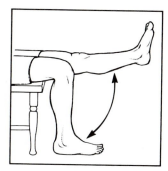

Raise your leg. Straighten it out as far as it will go. Lower it.

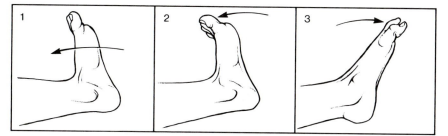

1, With your leg out straight, bend your ankle and point your foot toward you. *2*, Curl your toes toward you. *3*, Straighten the ankle and curl your toes away from you. Relax and lower your leg. You may find it more comfortable to do this exercise while lying down or with your leg propped up on a footstool or in front of you on a sofa.

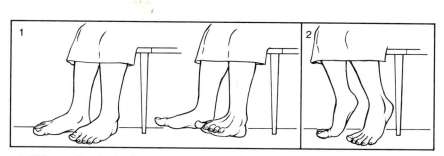

1, With your feet flat on the floor, curl your toes up as far as possible, keeping your heels flat. Relax. *2*, With your toes flat on the floor, lift your heels as far as they will go. Relax.

Figure 11–4. A–C, *Exercises for legs, ankles, and toes. (From* Learning to Live with Osteoarthritis, *© 1983 by Medicine in the Public Interest, made possible by a grant from Pfizer Pharmaceuticals.)*

These exercises will help the knees. The first one will also help the hips and the lower back. The second one is also good for the hips. Do both legs, gently and slowly. When working on knees, you don't want to add any more stress than necessary. Therefore, always lie down when doing knee exercises. Repeat each exercise several times.

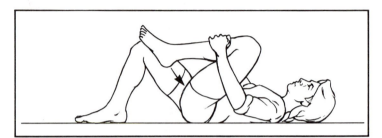

Lie on your back with both knees bent slightly and your feet flat. Raise one leg and bend the knee as far as it will go. Try to touch your buttock with the heel of your foot, pulling very gently with your hands to help. Hold this position for a few seconds and then relax.

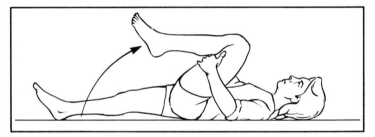

Raise one leg and put your hands under your thigh. Bring the knee as close to your chest as possible, pulling with your hands. Hold this position for a few seconds and then relax.

Figure 11–5. A, B, *Exercises for knees. (From* Learning to Live with Osteoarthritis, © *1983 by Medicine in the Public Interest, made possible by a grant from Pfizer Pharmaceuticals.)*

    a. A resting splint stabilizes and immobilizes the joint in a desired position when the client does not need use of the joint.

    b. A functional splint stabilizes the joint in use. Individualized lightweight thermoplastic splints are made and adjusted by physical or occupational therapists.

    c. General guidelines for use of splints are as follows:

        (1) Initially, the splint should be worn for no more than 2 hours at a time.

Do these exercises while lying down. The first one increases sideways hip motion. The second exercise helps with the rotation motion.

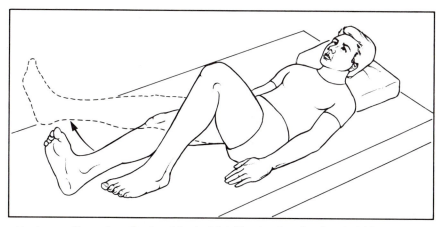

Lie down, with one knee bent and the foot flat. Keeping the other leg straight, stretch it out to the side as far as possible. Coax it just a little farther. Bring it back. Do this an equal number of times with both legs.

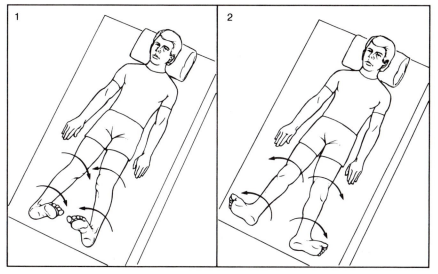

1, Lie down with your legs straight in front of you, about 12 inches apart. Roll your legs toward each other, so that your knees and toes point together. Return. *2,* Roll your legs away from each other, so that your knees and toes point outward.

Figure 11–6.   A, B, *Exercises for hips. (From* Learning to Live with Osteoarthritis, © *1983 by Medicine in the Public Interest, made possible by a grant from Pfizer Pharmaceuticals.)*

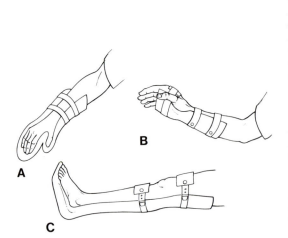

Figure 11–7. Types of splints.
A, Resting splint for hand and wrist. Used during periods of rest and sleep, this splint is helful in preventing hand and wrist deformities. Muscle-setting exercises can be done while the splint is worn.
B, Functional wrist splint. This splint rests and supports an inflamed wrist and at the same time lets the fingers move so that routine work can be done while it is worn. The splint is removable.
C, Long leg splint. This splint rests the knee. It can be effective in preventing a knee from becoming stiff in a bent position. It is also sometimes used temporarily to support and protect the knee joint when standing or walking. Muscle-setting exercises can be done while this splint is worn.

    (2) After each use of the splint, the skin should be checked for redness or soreness.

    (3) With increased tolerance, daily wearing time may be gradually increased until the splint can be worn for 6 to 8 hours.

    (4) Compliance is improved when instructions are provided for the client about when to wear the splint, how to store the splint, how to clean it, problems to look for, and to whom to report problems.

    (5) Encouragement and support are essential for appropriate use and care of the splint.

  3. Many types of equipment are used to reduce stress on the joints.

    a. Canes, crutches, and walkers are recommended for ambulation for clients with pain in the hip, knee, or ankle.

    b. Cervical collars, braces, corsets, prescribed shoes, and shoe inserts are recommended for clients with pain in the neck, back, and feet.

    c. Assistive devices, such as grab bars, handrails, extended and built-up handles, and elevated chairs and toilet seats, reduce weight-bearing and stress on involved lower extremities.

    d. Use of home traction may be prescribed for chronic neck pain. The traction is designed to carry the weight of the skull for a

period of time so that the neck muscles can be relaxed and gentle exercises can be undertaken.
   (1) When head traction is prescribed, the kit may be obtained from a pharmacy or medical supply house.
   (2) The apparatus should be attached to the ceiling or to a door-way.
   (3) The client should sit in a relaxed position with the head positioned slightly forward.
   (4) The amount of weight can be regulated by filling the bag to the desired level (5 to 7 pounds is usually sufficient).
   (5) Traction should be used for 30 minutes three times a day.
   (6) Relief should occur within 4 to 6 days if the procedure is beneficial for the individual client.
4. Teach the client guidelines for joint protection.
   a. Avoid activities that cause pain an hour or two later.
   b. Use the largest muscles and strongest joints when possible. For example, carry a shoulder bag instead of a handbag.
   c. Alternate between light and heavy work.
   d. Take frequent rest breaks. For example, intersperse hand activities with periodic resting of the hands.
   e. Schedule activities to avoid general fatigue and joint pain.
   f. Prevent extra stress and deformity by using appropriate joints for a task. For example, leaning on the palm of the hand straightens fingers, while leaning on the back of the hand pushes fingers into a deforming position.
   g. Shift position frequently when doing a task to reduce strain on muscles, ligaments, tendons, and joints.
   h. Use lightweight equipment and assistive devices to make work easier.
   i. Conserve energy by eliminating unnecessary tasks and reducing the number of times needed to climb stairs.
   j. Maintain good posture.
   k. Use warm, swollen joints as little as possible and put them through range of motion only once a day.
   l. When walking, plan to incorporate a 10-minute rest period into the outing. Stop to rest before pain is experienced.
   m. Sit rather than stand for doing tasks when possible.
   n. Ask for help and understanding from family and friends.

Medication

ANALGESICS

Analgesics are used to control pain without inflammation.
1. Nonsteroidal anti-inflammatory drugs (NSAIDs), such as aspirin

and ibuprofen (e.g., Motrin), provide analgesia at lower doses and anti-inflammatory action at higher doses.

2. Aspirin continues to be the drug of choice among NSAIDs because all the drugs are equally effective and aspirin is the least expensive.
   a. Intolerance to aspirin commonly occurs, requiring a change to another NSAID.
   b. Aspirin should be taken with meals, or a type with an enteric coating should be taken.
   c. More than eight to ten tablets of aspirin a day is contraindicated for the elderly, as elders are more susceptible to central nervous system manifestations and gastrointestinal irritation.
   d. Watchfulness is essential for the occurrence of major side effects involving the gastrointestinal (gastric intolerance), hematologic (bleeding), and otologic (tinnitus and deafness) systems.
   e. Because of primary hearing changes that have occurred, the elderly are less likely to report tinnitus and deafness (early warning signs of toxicity). As a result, these elders are more vulnerable to eighth cranial nerve damage.
      (1) Serum salicylate levels should be checked more frequently in the elderly. A range of 12 to 18 mg/dl is the goal.
3. Acetaminophen (Tylenol) and propoxyphene hydrochloride (Darvon) are also used for relief of noninflammatory pain.

Nonsteroidal Anti-Inflammatory Drugs

NSAIDs are used for pain with inflammation.
1. NSAIDs are similar to each other in pharmacologic, therapeutic, and toxicologic actions.
2. The irritating effect of NSAIDs on the gastrointestinal tract makes the elderly arthritic client susceptible to gastric ulceration.
3. NSAIDs are used at doses appropriate to the progression of the disease. Higher doses are used to treat inflammation.
4. Chronic daily dosage should be continued even during quiescent periods of the disease.
5. Night-time dosage is helpful for reducing nocturnal pain and additional morning stiffness.
6. Indomethacin (Indocin) and phenylbutazone (Azolid, Butazolidin) do not demonstrate greater therapeutic efficacy than other NSAIDs and are the most toxic of the NSAIDs.

Corticosteroids

1. Oral corticosteroid therapy is indicated only for treatment of very resistant arthritic disease that is unresponsive to NSAIDs and disease-modifying drugs.

    a. Short courses of oral corticosteroids, such as prednisone, are used to control severe attacks in multiple joints.

    b. Alertness to the occurrence of the many potential toxic effects of oral corticosteroids is essential.

2. Intra-articular injections of corticosteroids are indicated when single, asymmetric, acutely inflamed arthritic joints do not respond to NSAIDs and impair mobility.

    a. After intra-articular injection of corticosteroids, clients should be instructed to rest the joint for several days.

    b. A joint should not be injected more frequently than every 4 months.

    c. If no benefit occurs after an injection, repeat injections are unlikely to succeed.

REMITTING AGENTS

Remitting agents (disease-modifying drugs) are used for active progressive arthritic disease that has failed to respond to NSAIDs.

1. The client receiving remitting agents must be closely monitored, as the drugs are highly toxic.

2. The client should be informed that treatment is prolonged and that response to therapy may not be apparent for 6 months.

3. Gold is the drug of choice among remitting agents. Use of gold is now more convenient because therapy has become available in oral form.

4. Penicillamine (Cuprimine) may also be administered orally.

5. Antimalarial drugs, such as chloroquine (Aralen) and hydroxychloroquine sulfate (Plaquenil), are also used if gold or penicillamine therapy is unacceptable.

6. NSAIDs, at full dosage, may be continued with the remitting agents.

IMMUNOSUPPRESSIVE THERAPY

Immunosuppressive therapy is used when there is a lack of response to remitting agents and the possibility of serious disability exists.

1. Immunosuppressant drugs are used to limit the inflammation and to stop the disease progression, if possible.

2. Serious side effects of immunosuppressants restrict their use.

MUSCLE RELAXANTS

Muscle relaxants, such as cyclobenzaprine hydrochloride (Flexeril) and methocarbamol (Robaxin), are cautiously used to reduce muscle spasm adjacent to osteoarthritic joints.

ANTI-GOUT DRUGS

1. Uricosuric drugs produce an increase in the excretion of uric acid by preventing renal tubular reabsorption of tubular secretion at the proximal renal tubules.
2. Anti-gout drugs used for long-term gout control are allopurinol (Zyloprim) and colchicine, which can be used for maintenance as well as acute attacks.
3. NSAIDs are also used for treatment of acute gout.
4. Adjunctive therapy is recommended with uricosuric drugs.
   a. Hydration with at least 2 to 3 liters/day is considered optimal.
   b. The urine should be made less acid (pH 6.0 to 6.5) but not alkalinized to prevent formation of uric acid stones. See urinary alkalizers in Chapter 5.
   c. Reduced intake (but not elimination) of high-purine foods, such as sardines, anchovies, sweetbreads, beer, liver, kidney, yeast, and herring, is indicated.

PRINCIPLES OF DRUG USE FOR THE ARTHRITIDES

1. Selection of a drug includes considerations of cost, efficacy, tolerability, safety, flexibility of dosage, range of therapeutically active doses, and frequency of administration.
2. No one drug is best for all clients. A period of trial with several agents, in serial fashion or in combinations, may be used to establish an optimum regimen.
3. A client starting a new drug should be alerted to possible side effects.
4. The client must understand that NSAIDs are to be taken at prescribed dosage to achieve and maintain blood level for anti-inflammatory action. There is a tendency for the client to reduce dosage when pain relief is experienced.
5. Parameters should be monitored to assess efficacy of therapy.
6. Gastric intolerance can be minimized by dosing with meals.
7. Compliance is improved with agents that need to be administered only once or twice daily.
8. The duration of drug therapy should extend long enough for the onset of peak action to have been experienced before therapy is changed (e.g., about 1 to 4 weeks for NSAIDs and 3 to 6 months for disease-modifying drugs).
9. Age over 50 years, hypertension, diabetes, congestive heart failure, and concomitant use of diuretic agents increase the risk factors for nephrotoxicity associated with use of NSAIDs.
10. Increased incidence and severity of side effects of NSAIDs are re-

lated to secondary changes experienced by the elderly, such as peptic ulcer, cardiovascular disease, and chronic constipation.
11. The client with arthritis and diabetes must be alert to the interactions that may occur between hypoglycemics (drugs that lower blood glucose) and drugs used for treating arthritides.
    a. NSAIDs (including aspirin) have a blood sugar–lowering effect when used in conjunction with hypoglycemics that may require adjustment of dosage.
    b. Oral hypoglycemics raise the level of aspirin in the blood.
    c. Corticosteroids raise the blood sugar level and interrupt diabetic control.
12. Degree of pain relief may be assessed by asking the client to evaluate the degree of pain on a scale from one to 10 before instituting therapy and then after therapy has been instituted.
13. A complete discussion of drug therapy for the arthritides is beyond the scope of this book. See a drug reference book for complete pharmacologic information on individual drugs used for the arthritides.

Surgery

Surgery is another option for clients suffering from severe crippling arthritis.

ORTHOPEDIC SURGICAL PROCEDURES FOR ARTHRITIC JOINTS

1. *Debridement* is used successfully for elbow, shoulder, and hand joints. The procedure involves the removal of inflamed synovium, loose bodies, fragments of cartilage, and other tissues.
2. *Osteotomy* involves realigning joints that are not aligned correctly by cutting and wedging the bone back together.
    a. By correcting malalignment and eliminating abnormal joint stress, the progression of disease is slowed.
    b. Osteotomy is rarely used for the elderly, as the associated immobilization is contraindicated.
3. *Arthrodesis* usually involves fusion of an ankle or foot joint to relieve pain but alters function by elimination of motion of the joint.
4. *Arthroplasty* involves the removal or replacement of a damaged joint with an artificial joint.
    a. Arthroplasty may be used for all joints except the DIP joint, for which arthrodesis is done.

b. The most common and successful procedures are arthroplasty of the hip and the knee.
c. Total hip replacement is performed by an orthopedic surgeon.
   (1) The head of the femur is replaced with a steel ball on a stem.
   (2) The acetabulum is replaced with a high-density polyethylene cup.
   (3) Implants are secured to the living normal bone with a fast-hardening methyl methacrylate glue–like substance.
   (4) Results are immediate, with clients who previously were un-

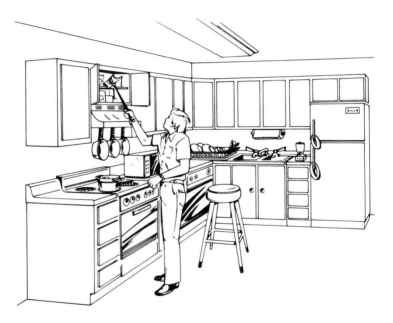

Kitchen

- long-handled reacher
- built-up faucet handles
- cloth loops on refrigerator door
- stool to sit on while cooking, washing dishes
- double-handled strainer basket
- appliances stored within easy reach
- built-up saucepan handles

Figure 11–8. *Assistive devices in the kitchen. (From Taking Care: Protecting Your Joints and Saving Your Energy. Atlanta, Arthritis Foundation, 1986.)*

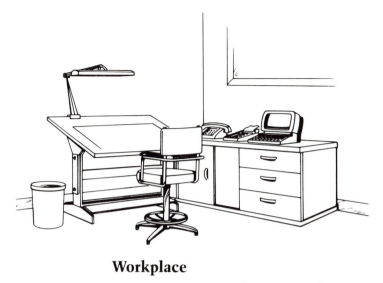

Workplace

- necessary items within easy reach
- swivel chair, adjustable, with good back support
- work surface at a comfortable height to avoid strain

Figure 11–9. *Assistive devices in the workplace. (From Taking Care: Protecting Your Joints and Saving Your Energy. Atlanta, Arthritis Foundation, 1986.)*

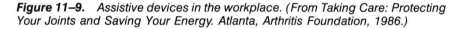

able to walk because of extreme pain able to walk out of the hospital free of pain at time of discharge.

ASSISTIVE DEVICES

1. Using self-help assistive devices and making home surroundings functional increase the independence of the arthritic client (Figs. 11–8 through 11–12).
2. Information is available that identifies equipment aids and clothing for the handicapped that can be designed at little expense from materials usually found in the home or in hardware stores and in building-supply companies at low cost.
    Extension Publication HE 137
    The North Carolina Agricultural Extension Service
    North Carolina State University at Raleigh
    Raleigh, NC 27695

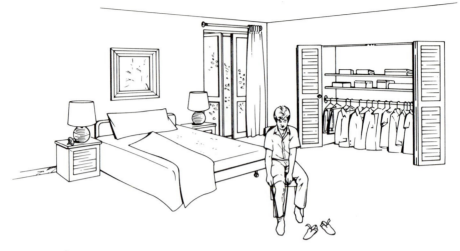

Bedroom

- "velcro" closures on shoes
- cloth loops on socks to put on with long-handled hook
- shelving and storage within easy reach
- sit to dress

Figure 11–10. *Assistive devices in the bedroom. (From Taking Care: Protecting Your Joints and Saving Your Energy. Atlanta, Arthritis Foundation, 1986.)*

> *Physically Handicapped: Aid to Self Help in Homemaking, Grooming, and Clothing*

3. Sources for additional information on homemaking and grooming are:

The Institute of Rehabilitation Medicine
New York University Medical Center
400 East 34th Street
New York, NY 10016
A Manual for Training the Disabled Homemaker
Meal-Time Manual for the Aged and Handicapped

4. Catalogues on aids for the handicapped may be ordered from:

Aids for Arthritis, Inc.
3 Little Knoll Court
Medford, NJ 08055

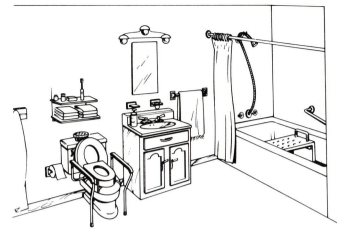

Bathroom

- built-up faucet handles
- built-up toothbrush
  (or electric toothbrush)
- suction mat on stool
- raised toilet seat
- towels within easy reach

Figure 11–11. *Assistive devices in the bathroom. (From Taking Care: Protecting Your Joints and Saving Your Energy. Atlanta, Arthritis Foundation, 1986.)*

Fred Sammons, Inc.
Box 32
Brookfield, IL 60513

Shalik's Rehab Aids
Box 826
Miami, FL 33143

5. Information about clothing for the handicapped is available.
   a. Ready-to-wear garments for the physically handicapped may be
      ordered from:
      Fashion-ABLE
      Rocky Hill, NJ 08853

      Vocational Guidance and Rehabilitation Services
      2239 East 55th Street
      Cleveland, OH 44103

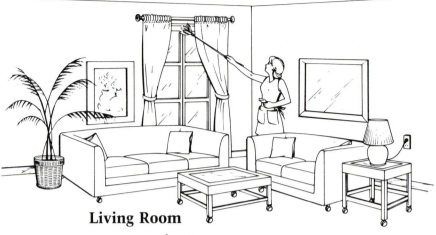

Living Room

- casters on furniture
- long-handled feather duster
- apron with pockets for carrying cleaning supplies

Figure 11–12.   *Assistive devices in the living room. (From Taking Care: Protecting Your Joints and Saving Your Energy. Atlanta, Arthritis Foundation, 1986.)*

Solve Garments, Inc.
Box 123-B
Bayport, MN 55003

Ziegler Medical Supply
Special Products for People with Special Needs
703 Ferry Street, Box 53
Buffalo, NY 14222

b. For additional information on clothing for the handicapped, see:
Superintendent of Documents
US Government Printing Office
Washington, DC 20402
Flexible Fashions: Clothing Tips and Ideas
for the Woman with Arthritis

Resources

Arthritis Foundation
1314 Spring Street
Atlanta GA 30309

Provides publications and list of local chapters (also available in telephone book).

Medicine in the Public Interest, Inc.
65 Franklin Street, Suite 304
Boston, MA 02110
(617) 482-3288
Learning to Live with Arthritis

Information Specialist
Arthritis Information Clearinghouse
P.O. Box 9782
Arlington, VA 22209
(703) 558-8250

The Arthritis Information Clearinghouse is a service of the National Institute of Arthritis, Diabetes, and Digestive and Kidney Disorders, Department of Health and Human Services.

References

Arthritis, rheumatic diseases, and related disorders. National Institute of Arthritis, Diabetes, and Digestive and Kidney Diseases. NIH Pub No. 85-1983. Washington DC: US Government Printing Office, May 1985.

Becker MA: Hyperuricemia and gout. In Rakel RE, ed: Conn's Current Therapy. Philadelphia: WB Saunders Co, 1986.

Calkins E, Papademetriou T, Challa HR: Musculoskeletal diseases in the elderly. In Calkins E, Davis PJ, Ford AB, eds: The Practice of Geriatrics. Philadelphia: WB Saunders Co, 1986.

Dickinson GR, Gorman TK: Adult arthritis: The assessment. American Journal of Nursing 83:262–265. 1983.

Evens RP, Hawkins DW: Bone and joint disorders. In Covington TR, Walker JI, eds: Current Geriatric Therapy. Philadelphia: WB Saunders Co, 1984.

Hamerman D: Rheumatic disorders. In Rodman I, ed: Clinical Geriatrics. Philadelphia: JB Lippincott, 1986.

Koerner M, Dickinson GR: Adult arthritis: A look at some of its forms. American Journal of Nursing 83:253–261, 1983.

Luckmann J, Sorensen KC: Medical-Surgical Nursing. Philadelphia: WB Saunders Co, 1987.

Podolsky S: Diabetes and arthritis. Diabetes Forecast 36(4):35–37, 1983.

Porter SF, Dapper MJ, Foran C: Adult arthritis: Hand splints. American Journal of Nursing 83:276–278, 1983.

Sharp JT: The locomotor system. In Rakel RE, ed: Conn's Current Therapy. Philadelphia: WB Saunders Co, 1986.

Simpson CF: Adult arthritis: Heat, cold, or both? American Journal of Nursing 83:270–272, 1983.

Simpson CF, Dickinson GR: Adult arthritis: Exercise. American Journal of Nursing 83:273–274, 1983.

Strand CV, Clark SR: Adult arthritis: Drugs and remedies. American Journal of Nursing 83:266–269, 1983.

Alterations in Glucose Metabolism

GLUCOSE METABOLISM IN THE ELDERLY
ACUTE COMPLICATIONS OF DIABETES
LONG-TERM COMPLICATIONS OF DIABETES
MONITORING DIABETIC CONTROL
TREATMENT PROGRAM

1. Diabetes is a chronic disease in which the body does not produce or properly use insulin to convert sugar, starches, and other foods into energy.
2. With advancing years, there is a marked increase in glucose intolerance and frank diabetes.
3. Estimates are that 10 to 30% of the elderly over 65 years of age have some form of abnormal glucose tolerance and that 15 to 20% have diabetes mellitus.
4. Diabetes with its complications is a major public health problem that is the third most common cause of death by disease in the United States each year.
5. The causes of impaired glucose tolerance (IGT) of aging have not been established, but research suggests that the most significant causes are:
   a. Alteration in the action of insulin at the receptor, postreceptor, or intracellular level.
   b. Reduction in synthesis of insulin or secretion by the pancreas.
6. Additional factors contributing to IGT in the elderly are related to:
   a. Changes in body composition as muscle mass decreases and fat deposits increase.
   b. Changes in diet with poor nutrition.

    c. A genetic pattern often linked to obesity.
    d. Reduction in physical activity.
    e. Acute illness.
    f. Endocrinopathies.
    g. Drugs used by the elderly, such as diuretics, corticosteroids, estrogen, beta-blockers, and antianxiety agents.

7. Acute complications associated with diabetes that are most likely to be experienced by the elderly are hypoglycemia, hyperglycemia, and hyperosmolar coma.

8. Long-term complications of diabetes that may develop over a period of 20 to 30 years lead to blindness, kidney disease, amputations, heart disease, and stroke.

9. Most clients over age 40 who develop the disease usually have non–insulin-dependent diabetes (NIDDM), which may be controlled by diet, exercise, and oral medication.

10. Screening is advisable in the elderly, as the gradual, undramatic onset of diabetes over age 40 results in missed diagnosis until the development of a life-threatening complication.

11. Diabetic clients should be encouraged to plan and comply with a therapeutic program to:
    a. Maintain normal blood glucose levels.
    b. Prevent complications if possible.
    c. Build resistance against infection.
    d. Support a feeling of well-being (by easing stress and depression).

12. Dietary intervention and regular exercise are essential to normalize blood glucose in diabetic clients, although oral medication and insulin may also be required.

13. Control of diabetes necessitates that the client and family have a thorough understanding of the nature of the disease and actively participate in the day-to-day management.

GLUCOSE METABOLISM IN THE ELDERLY

Impaired Glucose Tolerance

1. Elderly clients who have elevated postprandial blood glucose levels but normal fasting plasma glucose levels are classified as having IGT.

2. Criteria for the diagnosis of impaired glucose tolerance (National Diabetes Data Group [NDDG], 1980):
    a. Fasting plasma glucose level below 140 mg/dl.

    b. Two-hour plasma glucose level above 140 mg/dl and below 200 mg/dl with one intervening value above 200 mg/dl following a 75-gm glucose load.
3. IGT in elderly clients (hyperglycemia of aging) is predominantly attributed to primary aging changes in insulin-receptor sites.
    a. The fasting plasma glucose level appears to increase about 2 mg/dl per decade after the age of 30 to 40.
    b. The 1- to 2-hour postprandial blood glucose level appears to increase 8 mg/dl to 20 mg/dl per decade after the age of 30 to 40.
4. Adhering to an appropriate diet and exercise program often results in reversal to normal glucose tolerance.
5. IGT may "worsen to diabetes" (10% of individuals develop diabetes within the next 5 years), revert to normal, or remain impaired.
6. IGT does not put the client at risk for microvascular complications, but it does pose a risk for macrovascular complications when associated with other risk factors, such as hypertension, hyperlipidemia, obesity, and cigarette smoking. Applicability of these findings after the seventh decade has been established.

Diabetes Mellitus—Adult

1. Diabetes mellitus occurs when the body is unable to convert nutrients properly into energy necessary for daily activity.
2. Criteria for the diagnosis of diabetes—adult (NDDG, 1980):
    a. Unequivocal elevation of plasma glucose level (above 200 mg/dl) and classic symptoms of diabetes, including polydipsia, polyuria, polyphagia, and weight loss.
    b. Fasting plasma glucose level above 140 mg/dl on two occasions.
    c. Fasting plasma glucose level below 140 mg/dl and 2-hour plasma glucose level above 200 mg/dl with one intervening value above 200 mg/dl following a 75-gm glucose load (oral glucose tolerance test [OGTT]).

Presentation of Diabetes in the Elderly

1. Because the elderly may be asymptomatic (with an absence of classical symptoms) (Table 12–1), they should be periodically screened for glucose intolerance and for the presence of diabetic complications.
2. Predominant symptoms may be lethargy and subtle mental changes.
3. Undetected elderly diabetics often present with the following conditions:

Table 12–1. *Classification of Diabetes Mellitus—Adult*

Type and Prevalence	Characteristics
Insulin-Dependent (IDDM) 10–15%. Dependent on exogenous insulin to sustain life.	Classical symptoms: Abrupt onset of weight loss Frequent urination Excessive thirst Extreme hunger Fatigue and weakness Nausea and vomiting Insulinopenia Proneness to ketosis
Non–Insulin-Dependent (NIDDM) 85–90%. Not dependent on exogenous insulin to sustain life. May require insulin if hyperglycemia cannot be controlled by diet or oral drugs Onset usually in those over 40 years of age and overweight.	Classical symptoms may be absent and onset insidious. Fatigue, itching, or blurred vision may be noted at onset. Low, normal, or high insulin levels may be present. Tissues are insulin-resistant. Prone to hyperosmolarity rather than ketosis.

    a. Decreased vision associated with diabetic retinopathy, cataracts, or glaucoma.

    b. Pruritus vulvae associated with monilia vaginitis.

    c. Intermittent claudication caused by peripheral vascular disease.

    d. Painless ulceration or numbness of lower extremities resulting from peripheral neuropathy.

    e. Weakened thigh muscles as muscle atrophies.

4. A middle-aged elderly client who is usually mildly diabetic may present suddenly with hyperosmolar nonketotic coma or lactic acidosis.

5. Lactic acidosis, possibly as a result of cellular anoxia, may suddenly present precipitated by shock, hemorrhage, and exacerbations of chronic obstructive lung disease.

Goals of Therapy

1. Control of blood glucose levels in or near normal range in an attempt to mitigate or even prevent the complications attributed to hyperglycemia is a primary goal. (Prevention or reduction in severity of complications by tight control of blood glucose levels has not as yet been demonstrated in human studies but has been hypothesized from animal studies.)

2. Elimination of risk factors with control of blood glucose levels may delay or possibly even reverse complications (Table 12–2).

Table 12–2. *Risk Factors for Diabetes and Diabetic Complications*

Risk Factors	Effect	Strategies
Hypertension	Increased risk of vascular damage	Be alert to effects of drug therapy on the diabetic client: Diuretics may cause hypokalemia, which may cause hyperglycemia. Beta-blockers may cause impotency and orthostatic hypotension and may precipitate gangrene in the presence of peripheral vascular disease.
Smoking (cigarettes)	Increased risk of coronary heart disease 4 times and intermittent claudication	Stress the importance and benefit of immediate cessation of smoking. Assist client in choosing the appropriate help to stop smoking.
Obesity	Decreased sensitivity to insulin	Refer to nutrition counselor for development of appropriate diet. Encourage behavior modification.
Hypercholesterolemia	Increased risk of atherosclerosis	Same as for obesity.
Hypertriglyceridemia	Increased risk of atherosclerosis	Same as for obesity.

ACUTE COMPLICATIONS OF DIABETES

Hypoglycemia

1. Although hypoglycemia is mainly a problem for type I clients with insulin-dependent diabetes mellitus (IDDM), it may occur in type II elderly with NIDDM who are treated with oral antidiabetic agents.
2. Precipitating factors are:
   a. Eating less or missing meals so that medication is not covered by sufficient food intake.
   b. Unexpected or unusual exercise without eating additional food.
3. Warning signs of hypoglycemia require eating or drinking something containing simple sugars (such as regular ginger ale, orange juice, corn syrup, or honey).
   a. Early symptoms:
      • Sweating*
      • Tiredness
      • Weakness
      • Headache

---

*May be absent in elderly.

- Tingling sensations
- Shakiness
- Palpitations
- Tachycardia
- Hunger
- Slurred speech
- Double or blurred vision
- Lethargy*
- Depression*

b. Symptoms at night:
- Nightmares
- Difficulty sleeping
- Sweating
- Morning headache or fuzziness
- Seizures or cognitive impairment

c. Symptoms of prolonged hypoglycemia:
- Confusion
- Appearance of drunkenness
- Irritability
- Unusual behavior†
- Unconsciousness
- Coma

4. IDDM individuals with frequent insulin reactions are advised to carry glucagon (for releasing glycogen from the liver) with them. A family member or friend should be taught when and how to inject the medication to counteract the hypoglycemia.

Hyperglycemia

1. Precipitating factors:
   a. Poor compliance with diet, exercise, and/or medication regimen.
   b. Infection.
   c. Surgery.
   d. Extreme emotional stress.
   e. Use of drugs that raise blood glucose level.
2. Warning signs of hyperglycemia that require adjustment of insulin or oral medication:
   a. High levels of sugar present in blood and urine tests.
   b. Symptoms:
      - Excessive thirst

---

*In the elderly.
†For example, may resist treatment.

- Frequent urination
- Headache
- Drowsiness
- Stomach pain
- Nausea and vomiting
- Blurred or dim vision
- Dry skin*
- Rapid breathing
- Fruity smell on breath†
- Loss of consciousness

  c. Coma, usually preceded by 24 to 48 hours of high blood glucose levels and progressive cognitive impairment.

     (1) Acidosis or ketoacidosis develops in IDDM elderly experiencing severe hyperglycemia as fat is broken down for energy when there is insufficient insulin to convert blood glucose into energy.

        (a) Ketones are released into the blood stream. Acetone (one of the ketone substances) is present.

        (b) Ketoacidosis requires immediate hospitalization for treatment.

     (2) NIDDM elderly rarely experience ketoacidosis, but they may experience hyperosmolar nonketotic coma, which requires immediate medical care.

3. The elderly type II client experiencing hyperglycemia is particularly susceptible to the following problems:

  a. Increased incidence of superficial skin infections (in men and women) and candidal vulvovaginitis (in women) related to the reduced ability of leukocytes.

     (1) Healing of infections and wounds is often delayed because of poor circulation.

  b. Osmotic diuresis (marked fluid loss) with dehydration and salt depletion.

  c. Hypokalemia is especially likely if the client is taking a non–potassium-sparing diuretic. In addition to causing cardiac irregularities, hypokalemia may further inhibit insulin secretion.

  d. Exacerbation of hyperglycemia may lead to greater fluid loss, thrombotic events, and postural hypotension with subsequent increased risk of injuries and fractures.

  e. Polyuria and dehydration, leading to osmolality with more water

---

*Absence of sweating.
†Sign of ketoacidosis.

lost than solutes, intracellular dehydration, and finally hyperglycemic, hyperosmolar, nonketotic coma (HHNK).
   (1) Hyperosmolar state in the elderly carries a mortality rate of 15 to 20%. Elderly clients living alone are at the highest risk for hyperosmolar state.
   (2) Early recognition and treatment of symptoms are important for prevention of coma.
   (3) Thirst, polyuria, dehydration, and progressive cognitive impairment precede coma.
   (4) Focal and generalized seizures may also occur prior to coma.
   (5) Therapy for hyperosmolar coma in the hospital is directed toward restoring normal plasma volume and reducing the blood glucose level.

LONG-TERM COMPLICATIONS OF DIABETES

1. The major long-term complications associated with diabetes mellitus are:
   a. Microvascular changes that occur when the basement membranes of smaller blood vessels throughout the body gradually thicken, narrowing the lumen and reducing its ability to carry blood.
   b. Macrovascular changes that cause:
      (1) Atherosclerosis (deposits of fatty plaques).
      (2) Arteriosclerosis (hardening of the arteries).
   c. Neuropathies that are partially caused by high levels of glucose that alter Schwann cells surrounding peripheral nerves. This alteration possibly delays neural conduction time and may aggravate or contribute to the causation of symmetric diabetic neuropathy.
2. Because the diabetic elderly are living longer, they are more likely to experience long-term complications.
3. Diabetic neuropathies are many and range from mild to severe with different etiology, prognosis, and treatment. They are characterized by remissions and exacerbations.
4. Because the early symptoms of autonomic neuropathy are subtle, only by questioning about changes in sweating, sexual function, bowel habits, and postural hypotension is early neuropathy uncovered and treated.
5. For long-term complications of diabetes, pathology, signs and symptoms, and strategies, see Table 12–3.

Text continued on page 267

Table 12–3. *Long-Term Complications of Diabetes*

Complication	Pathology	Signs/Symptoms	Strategies
I. Diabetic Vascular Changes			
A. Microvascular changes	Gradual thickening of basement membranes of smaller blood vessels throughout the body, narrowing the lumen and reducing its ability to carry blood.		Teach the client and family to: Aim at maintaining blood glucose levels as normal as possible. More rigorous control may be attempted by multiple daily injections or by use of an insulin pump.
1. Diabetic retinopathy	(See under "Diabetic Retinopathy" in Chapter 7)		
2. Diabetic nephropathy	Glomeruli thicken, start to leak, and are unable to adequately perform filtration to maintain homeostasis.	Pus cells, blood casts, and protein in the basement membranes in urine; edema of feet and ankles; constant fatigue; yellowing of skin; and hypertension.	Anticipate assessment for remaining kidney function. Control blood pressure. Screen for and seek early medical treatment for urinary tract infections. Reduce salt intake and increase protein intake to replace protein lost (in accordance with medical protocol). (Hemodialysis or kidney transplant may be required in severe kidney failure.)
B. Macrovascular arteriosclerosis	Hardening of the arteries and deposits of fatty plaques occur earlier in diabetics.	Kidney function reduced; incidence of heart disease and stroke in diabetic clients doubled.	Prevent or delay macrovascular changes by elimination of risk factors and by controlling blood sugar. Decrease use of saturated fats. Substitute unsaturated fats when fats are needed. Aim for optimal body weight. Control blood pressure. Avoid smoking. Exercise regularly. Avoid stress or learn appropriate methods for stress reduction.

II. Diabetic Neuropathies			
A. Peripheral neuropathies	Sensorimotor neuropathy affecting the limbs and the cranium.	Pain more marked at night in neuropathies.	Control blood sugar to minimize and possibly reverse conditions.
1. Milder neuropathies	Decreased stimulation to the blood vessels, resulting in decreased blood supply.	Pain bilaterally symmetric and more severe at night and predisposes to depression and anorexia. Decreased reflexes in extremities. Decreased surface sensation and decreased blood supply, predisposing to foot gangrene, ulcers, loss of balance, and Charcot's joint (neuropathic arthropathy resulting in a painful joint).	Check peripheral pulses regularly for early detection of occlusive peripheral vascular disease. (Therapy such as bypass surgery may be required to prevent loss of a limb.) Relieve pain with minor analgesia, and try walking to get blood moving through blood vessels affected by innervated nerves. Practice daily foot care. Inspect skin of feet daily for alterations that may not be felt because of reduced sensation.
	Peripheral nerve degeneration may occur 10 to 15 years after development of diabetes.	Lack of ability to perceive pain.	Protect feet from injury. The smallest feet cut should be treated with antibiotics. Check feet, particularly toenails, for external lesions. Cut toenails straight across and not too near the nail base. Trim toenails frequently enough to prevent curling, thickening, and development of self-inflicted wounds on feet. Wash feet daily in warm water. Dry feet well, particularly between toes; apply a moisturizing lotion; and wear clean, dry socks. Wear properly fitting shoes and maintain linings to prevent friction.

Table continued on following page

Table 12–3. Long-Term Complications of Diabetes Continued

Complication	Pathology	Signs/Symptoms	Strategies
2. Acute neuropathies a. Painful symmetric neuropathy	Develop quickly. Often follows stress. May be due to rise in blood sugar.	Pain more severe. Depression and loss of appetite. Pain feels like electric shock, toothache, or burning sensation.	Use warm foot baths and massage. Try aspirin or aspirinlike pain medication for relief unless contraindicated.
	May occur after insulin therapy is initiated.	Pain symmetrical, usually occurring in the legs and persisting for 6 to 18 months and then stopping.	Request other medication for pain if aspirin is not helpful. Codeine, phenytoin (Dilantin), carbamazepine (Tegretol), amitriptiline hydrochloride (Elavil) and fluphenazine hydrochloride (Prolixin) have been used for analgesia. Exercise to aid in optimal blood glucose control. Recognize that the condition is usually limited to 6 to 18 months with good blood glucose control.
b. Diabetic neuropathic cachexia	Ill health, malnutrition, and wasting syndrome. Occurs usually in men in their sixties with mild or possibly undiagnosed Type II diabetes.	Emaciation syndrome. Pain similar to painful symmetrical neuropathy, but this syndrome may be more painful. Syndrome usually disappears in 6 to 8 months. Weight loss may be up to 100 pounds.	Use supportive measures to relieve pain and to maintain nutritional status. Recognize that the condition is self-limited and usually resolves in 6 to 12 months. Be alert to other symptoms that may be indicative of other causes for the cachexia.
c. Diabetic amyotrophy	Muscular atrophy usually occurs in older NIDDM men after severe stress.	Severe pain, paralysis, and shrinking of thigh muscles.	Engage in as much exercise as tolerable. Use pain medication appropriately.
d. Mononeuropathies	Motor nerves on one side of the body are affected. Asymmetrical, usually involving only one nerve.		

(1) Eye paralysis	May affect the third, fourth, and fifth cranial nerves.	
	Starts with pain on one side of face for 3 to 7 days followed by a loss of ocular control and diplopia. Usually resolves in 3 months. Often suspected to be a symptom of brain disease before identification as a diabetic mononeuropathy. Ptosis may occur.	Use pain medication appropriately. Recognize that the condition usually resolves in 3 months. Use an eye patch to minimize effects of double vision.
(2) Foot drop	Affects nerve to tibialis anterior muscle. Inability to flex foot.	Use a foot brace for a limited period of time, as needed.
(3) Truncal neuropathy	Involves nerves of chest or abdomen. Mimics pain of heart disease, appendicitis, or renal calculi. Resolves usually in 3 months.	Use pain medication appropriately. Recognize that resolution usually occurs in 3 months.
B. Autonomic neuropathies		
1. Cardiovascular neuropathy	Affects the vagal and sympathetic nerves. Postural hypotension with a fall of 30 mm Hg when rising from a supine position. Resting tachycardia: 90–130 beats/minute. Painless myocardial infarction; silent symptoms delay diagnosis and lead to increased myocardial damage.	Be alert to symptoms of myocardial infarction in the elderly. See Chapter 13.
2. Visceral neuropathy a. Gastroparesis	Usually occurs during acidosis or acute stress. Dysphagia and heartburn occur as a result of esophageal pathology. Delayed gastric emptying. Vomiting, anorexia, early satiety, bloating, abdominal pain, persistent feeling of distention. A temporary reversal may occur after 12 months but is not permanent.	Comply with drug regimen when prescribed to stimulate upper gastrointestinal motility. Drugs most commonly used are metoclopramide hydrochloride (Reglan) or bethanechol chloride (Urecholine) (contraindicated with cramps). Narcotic agents are contraindicated for severe pain, as slowing gastric motility will only worsen the delayed gastric emptying.

Table continued on following page

263

Table 12–3. *Long-Term Complications of Diabetes Continued*

Complication	Pathology	Signs/Symptoms	Strategies
			Closely monitor blood glucose to assure maintenance of a stable intake and absorption.
			Monitor dietary intake for missing carbohydrates and replace with food that can be tolerated, such as juice or cola.
			Delay testing blood glucose for at least 20 to 30 minutes after drinking juice, as slowed gastric emptying slows absorption.
			Rub honey directly onto oral mucosa for rapid absorption to speedily treat hypoglycemia.
			Attempt dietary management of mild gastroparesis with six small meals a day.
			Substitute more concentrated foods, such as juice for whole fruits, in the diet.
b. Intestinal neuropathy	Neuropathy affects motility.	Constipation most frequent; diarrhea (20 to 30 loose, watery stools a day) may alternate with constipation. Fecal incontinence usually worse after meals and at night. No generalized malabsorption; severe weight loss uncommon. Spontaneous remission may occur.	For constipation, follow a high-fiber diet.
			Increase fluid intake.
			Exercise.
			(See under "Constipation" in Chapter 3.)
			For diarrhea, comply with a prescribed drug regimen of opiates (e.g., codeine) or diphenoxylate hydrochloride with atropine sulfate (Lomotil) to slow motility.
			Use a dietary water-soluble fiber (e.g., oatmeal) or Metamucil to increase stool bulk.
			Continue with the antibiotic therapy for at least 2 weeks after a positive hydrogen breath test that indicates bacterial over-

3. Genitourinary neuropathy			
a. Neurogenic bladder	Lack of response to bladder filling; atonic bladder.	Long periods between voiding. Large volume of morning voiding. Frequent urinary tract infection. Starts with straining to void, weak stream of urine, incomplete bladder emptying, increased residual volume, and finally overflow incontinence.	Void every few hours regardless of whether bladder feels full. Tighten the abdominal muscles and use Credé's method to help empty the bladder completely. Cholinergic drugs, such as bethanechol chloride (Urecholine), may be prescribed to stimulate contractions strong enough to empty the bladder. Carry out intermittent self-catheterization. Note early signs of urinary tract infection and the need for prompt treatment. Test urine for white blood count with a dipstick to detect infection. Monitor blood glucose if possible because urinary retention causes urinary tests to be even more unreliable. (See under "Diabetes Mellitus" in Chapter 9.)
b. Impotence	Reduced ability of the parasympathetic nerves of the lower spine to dilate penile arteries.	Reduction in penile blood flow, resulting in inability to achieve or maintain an erection.	
4. Neuropathy involving sweat regulation			
a. Anhidrosis	Neuropathy of sweat glands.	Diminished sweat, usually over feet and legs, resulting in cracking of skin.	(See under "Strategies for Skin Care" in Chapter 3.)
b. Hyperhidrosis	Involving head and trunk, as lower part of body has diminished ability to dissipate heat as a result of anhidrosis.	Profuse sweats of head, face, and neck, particularly after eating spicy foods (gustatory sweating).	Avoid use of foods that normally bring on salivation, such as cheese or spicy foods. (See under "Strategies for Skin Care" in Chapter 3.)

Table continued on following page

Table 12-3. Long-Term Complications of Diabetes Continued

Complication	Pathology	Signs/Symptoms	Strategies
5. Hypoglycemic unawareness	Failure of sympathetic response to hypoglycemia.	Absence of diaphoresis, nervousness, weakness, palpitations, and hunger (the warning signs that usually accompany hypoglycemia). Episodes of sudden untreated hypoglycemia.	Avoid use of beta- or ganglionic blockers, as these drugs mask and alter hypoglycemia. Family should be prepared to administer glucagon to client in hypoglycemic coma. Monitor blood glucose closely especially before sleep, driving and increased exercise. Eat at least 10 gm carbohydrate before each hour of activity.
III. Skin Disorders A. Pruritus	Caused by anhidrosis.	Generalized itching, cracking of skin with increased susceptibility to infection.	(See under "Strategies for Skin Care" in Chapter 3.)
B. Dupuytren's contracture	Contracture of palmar fascia.	Bending of the third and fourth fingers so that they cannot be extended.	Splint to limit contracture.
IV. Eye Disorders A. Cataracts	May develop at an earlier age and may mature earlier possibly as a result of osmotic swelling of the lens fibers secondary to the accumulation of sorbitol during hyperglycemia.		(See under "Cataracts" in Chapter 7.)
B. Diabetic retinopathy	(See under "Diabetic Retinopathy" in Chapter 7.)		

MONITORING DIABETIC CONTROL

1. Monitor for symptoms of hypoglycemia and hyperglycemia (see symptoms under "Acute Complications of Diabetes," previously).
2. Most diabetic clients are instructed to test for ketones (strips used) only when there is a sudden change in urinary glucose on two successive tests.
3. Urine testing for glucose is particularly unreliable in the elderly because of the necessity of dealing with both the lag time between blood glucose rise and urine spill and an age-related rise in the threshold for urinary glucose excretion that may delay glycosuria until plasma glucose exceeds 300 mg/dl.
4. The blood glucose measuring systems are useful monitoring devices.
   a. Clients are taught how to use the system and to adjust insulin dosage, food, or activity in response to the reading.
   b. For blood glucose monitoring, the client must be taught how to prick the sides of the finger pads (the least painful site for pricking), to squeeze out a large drop of blood (by lowering the finger below the heart and milking down on it with the other hand), and to drop the sample of blood onto the strip for measuring.
   c. The AMES EYETONE, AMES DEXTRO SYSTEM, and the BIO-DYNAMICS STATTEK solid phase systems (blood tested on a solid pad) use reflectance (measuring) meters to provide an accurate numerical measurement of the amount of glucose in the blood sample on the reagent strip. Meters take 1 to 2 minutes to use and weigh less than a pound. See *A Consumer's Guide to Blood Testing.**
   d. Chemstrips or Visidex II can be read by most clients after training and practice without a meter even if the strips are cut in half longitudinally to reduce the cost. The ability of an elderly client with reduced color discrimination to use these strips accurately must be carefully and periodically evaluated.
   e. For some elderly, the expense of the blood monitoring system and the follow-through demands are too great; it is recommended, however, for clients with sufficient visual acuity, willingness to purchase the system, and ability to learn the procedure and to accept the responsibilities that go with it.
   f. Blood glucose monitoring may require the client to cope with renewed grieving as self-monitoring forces him to acknowledge the fact that he has a disease.
5. Fractional urine testing, though not as accurate an indication of

---

*Available from the American Diabetes Association (ADA); reprinted from Diabetes Forecast March–April 37(2):25–28, 1984. See Resources for address of ADA.

blood glucose level, continues to be used by those elderly unable to afford the systems with reflectance meters or unable or unwilling to learn the procedures and follow-through demands.

6. Periodic assessment of the client's or family's technique in blood or urine testing, additional teaching when needed, and encouragement are essential for accurate results.
7. Glycosylated hemoglobin levels are best measured in the laboratory every 2 or 3 months to monitor effectiveness of treatment, to assess for compliance, and to adjust diet or drug therapy.
   a. With elevated blood glucose, more glucose attaches to hemoglobin A. Because the glucose stays attached for the life span of the red blood cell (approximately 4 months), the Hb A_{1c} level provides an accurate picture of diabetic control over that time period.
   b. An Hb A_{1c} level of 10 to 12% is considered satisfactory.
   c. Chronic renal failure, hypoxia, and drug interactions may affect glycosylated hemoglobin levels.

TREATMENT PROGRAM

Guidelines for Developing a Treatment Program

1. Help the client and family to understand the disease and to accept involvement in day-to-day management.
2. Gear a plan to health promotion and prevention of complications by including diet, exercise, stress reduction, and medication (if required).
3. Promote optimal compliance by planning with the client a regimen that fosters self-care.
4. Consider primary and secondary changes in the physical and psychosocial dimensions that affect attempts to control the diabetic state.
5. Attempt blood glucose control with a simple, rational regimen that causes the least interference and discomfort to the client's lifestyle. Adapt the treatment regimen to the client's lifestyle rather than vice versa.
6. Aim at achieving a balance between good control of hyperglycemia and prevention of hypoglycemia.

7. Teach the client general guidelines for managing diabetes during treatment of common illnesses.
8. Refer the client and family to support groups as needed.

Nutrition

DIETARY RECOMMENDATIONS

1. The optimal dietary regimen for control of diabetes has not been established, but the emphasis now is on a well-balanced, individualized flexible higher-fiber diet (50 to 60%), low in saturated fats, with moderate salt restriction.
   a. IDDM clients require a consistent basic daily meal plan with synchronization of food intake and insulin action.
   b. Nonobese NIDDM clients who are not on a weight-reduction program require adequate spacing between meals, a balanced nutritional program, and use of fiber-rich foods.
   c. Obese NIDDM clients, in addition to requiring meal spacing, balanced nutrition, and high fiber, require caloric restriction to promote weight reduction and improved peripheral tissue sensitivity to insulin.
   d. Significant weight reduction in the obese type II diabetic client can lead to normalization of carbohydrate tolerance or conversion to an IGT state.
2. Carbohydrates in the diet should be mostly in the form of whole-grain breads and cereals, dry beans and peas, fruit, and low-fat dairy products.
3. The benefits of high fiber in the diabetic diet include the following:
   a. Reduces the speed at which glucose enters the blood stream by delaying carbohydrate absorption after meals.
   b. Improves glycemic control.
   c. Improves efficiency of endogenous insulin.
   d. Reduces the requirement for the amount of insulin or oral medications used.
   e. Promotes weight loss, as fresh vegetables, whole grains, and fresh fruit with fiber are not high caloric foods but give a feeling of fullness.
   f. Aids in controlling blood pressure.
   g. Influences lipid serum levels favorably.
   h. Prevents constipation when combined with six to eight glasses of water a day.
   i. May prevent diseases of the large bowel or colon.

4. The nutritionist and the client work out an individual meal plan that shows the number of food choices (exchanges) that can be eaten at each meal and snack.

    a. Dietary recommendations for diabetic clients utilize the *Exchange Lists for Meal Planning* of the American Diabetes Association (1986).

    b. Every food on each of the six Exchange Lists has about the same amount of carbohydrate, protein, fat, and calories in the amounts given.

    c. All choices on each list are equal and can be exchanged or traded for any other food on the same list.

    d. A copy of *Exchange Lists for Meal Planning* ($1.75) is available from the American Diabetes Association. (See Resources at the end of this chapter.)

5. Alcohol is best avoided, but small amounts may be permitted if the calories are calculated into the meal plan and the alcohol is taken with food.

    a. Pure alcohol in the body acts most like fat and does not require insulin for its metabolism by the liver.

    b. If drunk without adequate food intake, alcohol may precipitate hypoglycemia because the alcohol enhances the blood glucose–lowering action of insulin and interferes with the body's ability to produce its own glucose in response to falling blood glucose levels.

    c. Diabetics receiving insulin or oral hypoglycemic agents should not drink alcohol on an empty stomach, as these individuals are especially susceptible to hypoglycemia.

    d. Excessive alcohol intake can promote hypertriglyceridemia and hyperglycemia.

    e. Heavy drinking of alcohol is associated with the development of painful diabetic neuropathy.

    f. Diabetics using oral hypoglycemic agents may experience dizziness, flushing, and nausea when they drink alcohol.

    g. Sweet alcoholic drinks (e.g., cordials) should be avoided.

    h. Mixers for alcoholic drinks should be low in sugar or sugar-free, such as diet soft drinks, club soda, seltzer, or water.

STRATEGIES TO PROMOTE DIETARY CONTROL OF GLUCOSE INTOLERANCE

1. Obtain a dietary history.
2. Assess and refer for:

    a. Malnutrition. (See Table 4–6.)

    b. Dental problems that may interfere with nutrition.

    c. Financial need. (Refer for financial assistance from Supplemental Social Security for a special diet.)

3. Develop an individual meal plan with the client that:
    a. Is a balance between idealism and realism.
    b. Is palatable and acceptable to the client.
    c. Takes into account the client's occupation; age; body build; habits; personal, ethnic, and religious dietary preferences; and lifestyle.
    d. Is similar to that consumed by family, peers, and society. (Because carbohydrate constitutes 40 to 60% of calories consumed in Western societies, this diet would be acceptable with the restriction of simple sugar.)

4. Provide guidance in selection and in obtaining commercially prepared foods or more costly fresh fruits and vegetables.
    a. Special dietetic or diabetic foods add unnecessary expense and provide no advantages over standard products, except for water-packed fruit, artificially sweetened drinks, and artificially sweetened chewing gum.

5. Review the use of alternative sweeteners in the diet.
    a. *Saccharin* is the most common alternative sweetener used.
      (1) Estimated to be 350 times as sweet as sugar.
      (2) Virtually calorie-free.
      (3) Leaves bitter aftertaste.
      (4) Least expensive of artificial sweeteners.
      (5) Carries a warning mandated by the Food and Drug Administration (FDA) about possible risks.
    b. *Fructose, sorbitol* and *xylitol* are nonglucose carbohydrate nutritive sweeteners.
      (1) Are acceptable with no significant side effects with modest use.
      (2) Caloric value must be considered, as blood glucose affected by these sweeteners.
      (3) Sorbitol and xylitol may cause dose-dependent osmotic diarrhea.
      (4) Fructose and xylitol taste sweeter than sorbitol.
    c. *Aspartame* (e.g., Equal) is a noncarbohydrate nutritive sweetener.
      (1) Several times sweeter than sucrose, though it contains only 4 calories/gm.
      (2) Has no impact on glycemia and is the preferred sweetener, but is more expensive.

6. Advise the client how to minimize postprandial hyperglycemia.
    a. Meals should be spaced approximately 5 hours apart to permit

restoration of basal (preprandial) glucose levels before additional food is eaten.

b. IDDM clients should plan reasonably consistent meal schedules with avoidance of long delays.

c. Time between food intake should be shortened, with snacks timed for when exogenous insulin peaks. (See Table 12–5.)

d. Greater flexibility may be achieved with highly individualized regimens involving self-monitoring of blood glucose and the use of preprandial regular insulin or long-acting insulin by injection or by insulin pump.

e. Whole-grain products and other high-fiber foods should be included in the diet, as dietary fiber has been shown to cause a more moderate rise in blood sugar levels.

f. The use of purified fiber supplements to minimize postprandial hyperglycemia should be avoided.

7. Be aware of diet modifications required by other illness.

a. See "General Guidelines for Clients on Sick Days," later.

b. Sodium restriction is desirable for those with hypertension, congestive heart failure, or edematous states.

c. Protein restriction may be required by azotemia.

d. Hyperlipidemia, hyperproteinemia, ulcer, anemia, cholecystitis, functional bowel disorders, ulcerative colitis, and food allergies all require diet modifications that may be developed by the nutrition counselor with the client and family.

8. See Chapter 4 for more dietary information.

Exercise

BENEFITS OF CONSISTENT EXERCISE PROGRAM

1. Improves sensitivity to insulin and glucose tolerance.
2. Decreases need for insulin or oral hypoglycemic therapy.
3. Increases dietary compliance while helping in weight control.
4. Increases work capacity.
5. Increases high density lipoprotein (HDL) cholesterol levels that decrease risk of coronary heart disease.

STRATEGIES TO PROMOTE EXERCISE BY THE DIABETIC CLIENT

1. Work with the client and family.

a. Tailor the exercise program to the client's physical abilities.

  b. Take into account physical impairments and psychological capabilities.
  c. Consult a physiotherapist as needed.
2. Encourage walking. Regular walking in an indoor shopping mall may be best for the elderly, as the environment is protected.
3. Refer those with a history of cardiovascular disease to a cardiac rehabilitation exercise program.
4. Teach the client:
  a. Exercise after a meal when the blood glucose is rising rather than before a meal when the blood glucose is low. (The insulin-dependent client is most susceptible to hypoglycemia, but the client receiving oral antidiabetic therapy may also experience hypoglycemia in association with exercise.)
  b. Extra protein and starch before increased physical activity often prevent low blood glucose.
  c. Quickly absorbed carbohydrates, such as orange juice, sugar water, honey, or soda, should be taken to correct hypoglycemia.
  d. Keep in mind that increased activity requires either more food or less insulin.
  e. For spontaneous exercise, extra food is best to prevent hypoglycemia.
  f. Start the exercise program slowly.
  g. Avoid injecting insulin into a limb that will be actively exercised to prevent faster absorption of insulin with subsequent hypoglycemia. Injection into a subcutaneous area on the abdomen may be preferable if exercise is to occur shortly.
  h. Consult with a physician for guidance in adjusting medication and diet when exercising.

Oral Drug Therapy

1. The majority of elderly diabetic clients (NIDDM) are managed with diet alone or with diet in addition to oral hypoglycemics.
  a. Therapy with an oral hypoglycemic agent is recommended for the type II (NIDDM) client who has failed to achieve glycemic control by diet and exercise within a 3-month period.
  b. The convenience of taking a pill rather than an injection tends to improve compliance in the elderly diabetic client.
2. Sulfonylureas (oral hypoglycemic agents) are effective in more than 85% of appropriate clients by achieving nearly normal or greatly improved glucose tolerance (Table 12–4).
3. The mechanism of action of sulfonylureas is as follows:
  a. Stimulating endogenous insulin production by the pancreas.

Table 12–4. Time Course of Action of Oral Sulfonylurea Agents*

Generic Name	Brand Name	Daily Dosage Range (Mg)	Duration of Action (Hr)
Tolbutamide	Orinase	500–3000	6–12
Chlorpropamide	Diabinese	100–500	60
Acetohexamide	Dymelor	250–1500	12–18
Tolazamide	Tolinase	100–1000	12–24
Glyburide	Diabeta Micronase	2.5–30	up to 24
Glipizide	Glucatrol	5–40	8–12

*From Rakel RE, ed: Conn's Current Therapy. Philadelphia: WB Saunders Co., 1986.

  b. Reducing glucose production by the liver.
  c. Possibly increasing the number of insulin receptors.
  d. Possibly potentiating insulin action.
  e. Increasing insulin responsiveness.
 4. Therapy should be initiated with about half of the usual dose to avoid hypoglycemia, to which the elderly are particularly susceptible.
  a. Blood or urine should be monitored for glucose at least four times a day during the initiation or treatment period.
  b. The dosage is gradually increased until blood glucose levels are normalized.
  c. When therapy with an oral hypoglycemic agent is considered, the benefit versus cardiac risk and other complications should be weighed.
 5. Elderly diabetics may experience primary failure or secondary failure that indicates therapy with insulin may be necessary.
  a. Primary failure occurs when blood glucose levels remain high after therapy is instituted.
  b. Secondary failure usually occurs after a few months of positive response to therapy. Stress often precipitates secondary failure.
  c. Insulin therapy is usually considered if maximal dosage fails to control the fasting blood glucose below 180 mg/dl.
 6. Adverse reactions are generally few in number:
  a. Gastrointestinal reactions are generally relieved by reduction in dosage.
  b. Hypoglycemia is more likely to occur with omission of meals and snacks, weight loss, increased activity, or impaired renal and liver function.
  c. Other drugs by interaction may increase or decrease the effects of an oral hypoglycemic agent. (For example, medications, such as aspirin, that also bind to albumin may produce a heightened effect when sulfonylureas are started, or these medications may

displace the sulfonylureas and thereby increase the effect of the oral diabetic agents and cause hypoglycemia.
   d. A client using an oral diabetic agent will experience a reaction similar to that caused by disulfiram (Antabuse) if ethyl alcohol is consumed.
7. Therapy considerations include the following:
   a. Chlorpropamide (Diabinese) is less desirable for use in the elderly because 3- to 5-day hypoglycemic reactions may occur and remain undetected.
   b. Because of the importance of renal excretion, acetohexamide, tolazamide, and chlorpropamide are contraindicated in clients with renal insufficiency.
   c. Glipizide is preferable for use in the elderly, as the short serum half-life (2 to 4 hours) reduces the risk of prolonged or severe hypoglycemia in elderly clients, who have a lower metabolic rate than younger clients.

Insulin Therapy

1. Indications for use of insulin by elderly clients are:
   a. Type I IDDM.
   b. Type II diabetes mellitus uncontrolled by diet or oral medication when the client is compliant and functional.
   c. Renal or hepatic failure.
   d. Acute stress (e.g., major surgery or active inflammation).
   e. Persistent hyperglycemia during glucocorticoid therapy.
2. Individualized therapy may be initiated in the home with team work of the client, family, and health professionals.
3. Assessment of the client's or a family member's ability to comprehend the use of this potentially hazardous drug must be ascertained before therapy is instituted.
4. Determination that the likelihood of a severe hypoglycemic reaction is high should be reported to a physician, as therapy with insulin may then be contraindicated.

INSULIN REGIMEN

1. A trial of the most simple regimen should be used to initiate therapy (Table 12–5).
2. Mixtures of intermediate-acting and short-acting insulin may be used in the same syringe to avoid the use of two injections, but these mixtures must be used within 15 minutes of mixing.
3. Clients with considerable insulin secretory capacity may attain rel-

Table 12–5.   *Time Course of Action of Insulin Preparations**

	Onset of Action	Peak Action	Duration of Action
Short-acting			
Regular Iletin II (crystalline-zinc)	15–30 minutes	2–4 hours	5–7 hours
Actrapid	30 minutes	2.5–5 hours	8 hours
Velosulin	30 minutes	2–5 hours	8 hours
Humulin	30 minutes	2–5 hours	6–8 hours
Intermediate-acting			
Lente	1–2 hours	6–12 hours	18–24 hours
NPH	1–2 hours	6–12 hours	18–24 hours
Monotard	2.5 hours	7–15 hours	18–24 hours
Humulin	1–2 hours	6–12 hours	14–24 hours
Novolin	1.5 hours	4–12 hours	18–24 hours
Long-acting			
Ultralente	2–6 hours	18–24 hours	32–36 hours

*From Rakel RE ed: Conn's Current Therapy. Philadelphia: WB Saunders Co, 1986, p 444.

atively good control with twice-daily dosage of intermediate-acting insulin (two thirds at breakfast and one third in the evening).
4. Clients with poor insulin secretory capacity may achieve control with daily or twice-daily injections of a mixture of short-acting and intermediate-acting insulin, crystalline zinc (insulin injection) and NPH (neutral protamine Hagedorn [isophane insulin suspension]) or semilente (prompt insulin zinc suspension) mixed in the same syringe.

CONSIDERATIONS FOR INSULIN USE IN THE ELDERLY

1. Potential for error exists when filling the syringe because of improper use of old U-40 or U-80 syringes for U-100 (100 U/ml) syringes or vice versa. Elderly clients should be encouraged to discard all U-40 and U-80 syringes.
2. There is increased potential for improper filling of the syringe as a result of impaired sight, dexterity, or cognition.
3. Acute overinsulinization may cause profound hypoglycemia.
4. Chronic overinsulinization may cause increased hunger, weight gain, and more insulin resistance. Initially, larger doses of insulin may be required to overcome insulin resistance for some clients.
5. When insulin therapy is expected to be temporary, ultrapork insulin or human insulin of either recombinant or semisynthetic origin is recommended to prevent the occurrence of antibody formation and an increase in insulin resistance.

ADMINISTRATION OF MEDICATION

1. Insulin injection for the elderly may be difficult because of problems such as low vision, arthritic joints, and reduced subcutaneous fat.
   a. Information about devices for visually-impaired diabetics can be obtained from The Lighthouse. See Resources.
   b. For the client who has difficulty with the pain and adverse psychologic reactions to insulin injection, there are specialized injectors available. Information on these injectors may also be obtained from The Lighthouse. See Resources.
      (1) The Presto-injector (B&G Medical Devices): A hidden needle penetrates quickly.
      (2) Medi-jector (Derata Corporation): Jet pressure is used to administer insulin without a needle and syringe.
   c. Measuring and storing unmixed insulin in glass or plastic syringes for up to 2 weeks has been found to be safe and may be desirable for those clients who have difficulty measuring insulin.
   d. Storing mixed insulin mixtures is contraindicated, as changed activity of insulin mixtures may occur when a preparation of NPH is mixed with crystalline zinc insulin (CZI). Excessive protamine in the NPH may precipitate changed activity of the insulin mixture.
2. Old habits, such as storage of insulin, site rotation, and actual technique of administration, should be reviewed or observed periodically.

General Guidelines for Clients on Sick Days

Teach the client to:
1. Notify a physician when he experiences symptoms of hyperglycemia, such as vomiting, diarrhea, severe pain, shortness of breath, extreme thirst, dehydration, persistent high preprandial blood glucose tests, ketones in the urine, or high fever.
2. Continue taking insulin or oral diabetic medication even if he is unable to eat normally. Consult with a physician about adjustments of medication.
   a. Insulin or oral hypoglycemic medication is needed to counteract the glucose and ketones produced by the illness.
   b. Extra supplemental insulin doses are often recommended for control.
   c. Shorter-acting insulins or a different dose may be ordered.
   d. On a temporary basis, insulin injection my be required by

NIDDM elderly who normally control blood glucose by diet or by diet and oral hypoglycemics.

3. Follow meal plan as closely as possible.
   a. Smaller portions should be eaten at more frequent intervals to take in the usual number of calories.
   b. Plenty of fluids should be drunk (4 to 6 oz every 30 to 60 minutes).
   c. If client is unable to tolerate solid foods, exchanges in the meal plan should be replaced with carbohydrate-rich fluids.
   d. The physician should be notified if the client is unable to drink fluids, is vomiting, or has a fever.

4. Test blood or urine for glucose every 4 hours and test urine for ketones. Clients with type I or type II diabetes should monitor for ketones as well as for glucose.
   a. Very high glucose even if there is no acetone for 24 hours should be reported, especially if the client is feeling drowsy.
   b. The physician should be notified if both the glucose and acetone levels are high.
   c. It should be remembered that ketone tests may remain positive for several hours after blood glucose has returned to normal.

5. Keep accurate records of tests, food intake, temperature, medication, and untoward symptoms. Changes in body weight and respiratory rate provide further information for the physician.

6. Avoid using other medications that may interfere with glucose control.
   a. The client should check with the pharmacist about interactions caused by effects on glucose monitoring by over-the-counter (OTC) drugs and prescribed drugs.
   b. OTC decongestants should be used cautiously, as some may raise blood glucose but may also cause symptoms mimicking hypoglycemia.

Resources

American Diabetes Association
National Service Center
1660 Duke Street
Alexandria, VA 22314
(800) 232-3472
(703) 549-1500, in Virginia and Washington, D.C.
Diabetes Literature List
ADA Diabetes Forecast Reprint Series

On request, provides order form for publications.

Local affiliates of American Diabetes Association. (See telephone directory.)

National Diabetes Information Clearinghouse (NDIC)
Information Specialist
Box NDIC
Bethesda, MD 20205
(301) 468-2162

On request, provides publications on diabetes and diabetes-related materials.

Pfizer Pharmaceuticals
P.O. Box 3852 DIP
Grand Central Station
New York, NY 10163
Learning to Live with Diabetes

On request, will provide copies of publication, one in a series of patient information books.

The Lighthouse
The New York Association for the Blind
111 East 59th Street
New York, NY 10022
(212) 355-2200
An Evaluation of Devices for Insulin-Dependent Visually Impaired Diabetics

References

Albin J, Ross H, Rifkin H: Diabetes in the elderly. In Rossman I, ed: Clinical Geriatrics. Philadelphia: JB Lippincott, 1986.
Davis PJ, Davis FB: Endocrine diseases. In Calkins E, Davis PJ, Ford AB, eds: The Practice of Geriatric Medicine. Philadelphia: WB Saunders Co, 1986.
Franz MJ: Evaluating the glycemic response to carbohydrates. Clinical Diabetes November–December 1986, p 122–141.
Funnell MM, McNitt P: Autonomic neuropathy: Diabetics' hidden foe. American Journal of Nursing 86:266–270, 1986.
Joyce MS, Kuzich CM, Murphy DM: Those new blood glucose tests. RN 46(4):46–52, 1983.
Kreines K: Diabetes mellitus in adults. In Rakel RE, ed: Conn's Current Therapy. Philadelphia: WB Saunders Co, 1986.

Levandoski LA, White NH, Santiago JV: How to weather the sick-day season. Diabetes Forecast 36(6):30–33, 1983.

Lipson LG: Diabetes mellitus in the elderly: Special problems, special approaches. New York: Pfizer Pharmaceuticals, 1985.

Luckmann J, Sorensen KC: Medical-Surgical Nursing. Philadelphia: WB Saunders Co, 1987.

McDonald J: Whiskey or water? Diabetes Forecast November–December 33(6):17–20, 1980.

National Diabetes Data Group: Classification and diagnosis of diabetes mellitus and other categories of glucose intolerance. Diabetes 28:1039–1057, 1979.

Nemchik R: Facing up to the long term complications. RN 6(7):38–44, 1983.

Silver BJ: Is diabetes inevitable with aging? Geriatric Medicine Today 4(11):44–46, 1985.

Skyler JS, Beaty CM, Goldberg RB: Managing diabetes: An updated look at diet. Geriatrics 39(7):57–68, 1984.

Maintaining the Elderly With Cardiac Problems

1. Overall cardiac performance is not affected as the elderly carry out the daily activities of living, but with aging, the heart responds more slowly and less efficiently to stress.
2. Exposure to risk factors during the aging process increases the prevalence of secondary changes in a growing percentage of the elderly.
3. Early recognition of cardiac problems followed up with appropriate treatment allows many clients with chronic heart disease to maintain an active lifestyle.
4. Astute assessment of the elderly for cardiac problems is essential, as the presentation is often atypical with absence of classic symptomatology.
5. The high susceptibility of the elderly to untoward effects of cardiac glycosides, diuretics, beta-blockers, and calcium channel blockers

requires close monitoring of the client to prevent victimization by the intervention.

6. Reduction of risk factors, prompt recognition of cardiovascular problems, appropriate treatment, rehabilitation, and compliance are essential components of a therapeutic program for promoting and maintaining cardiac function and in turn function in all dimensions.

ALTERATIONS IN THE CARDIOVASCULAR SYSTEM ASSOCIATED WITH AGING

Structural Changes

1. The aging heart does not increase in size, but there is a slight increase in left ventricular wall thickness.
2. Yellowish brown lipofuscin, amyloid, and fibrous tissue infiltrate myocardial cells.
3. Cardiac valves thicken somewhat.
4. Pacemaker cells appear to decline.
5. The aorta and its branches demonstrate increased rigidity and less elasticity.

Functional Changes

1. Cardiac output (the amount of blood ejected by the left and right ventricle per minute) and oxygen uptake decline.
2. The heart rate undergoes several changes.
   a. The average heart rate declines slightly with aging.
   b. The time to reach peak heart rate steadily lengthens with aging as contraction and relaxation of cardiac muscle are prolonged.
   c. Following a challenge, the heart rate returns more slowly to the resting state.
   d. The maximum heart rate that can be obtained during intense exercise diminishes markedly.
   e. Cardioacceleratory response to physiologic stimuli, such as postural change, cough, and the Valsalva maneuver, is blunted.
3. Stroke volume (the amount of blood ejected with each contraction of the left ventricle into the systemic circulation) falls partially as a result of the increase in afterload (resistance to left ventricular ejection).
   a. Maximal stroke volume, cardiac output, and oxygen uptake are reduced in the elderly in response to exercise.

4. Myocardial elasticity and contractility are reduced as collagen tissues become sclerotic, release and uptake of calcium are impaired, and adrenergic receptors diminish.
5. Ectopic beats and atrial and ventricular arrhythmias occur more frequently but are usually not pathologic.
6. Both systolic and diastolic blood pressures tend to rise with age.
   a. There is a greater increase in systolic blood pressure in the older person than in the young adult performing the same amount of work.
   b. Increased fatty deposits in the intima of arteries cause vessel rigidity, reduced distensibility, and increased circulatory insufficiency, which in turn increase blood pressure and workload on the heart.
7. Reduced baroreceptor sensitivity results in a decline in the moment-to-moment adjustment of variation that:
   a. Counteracts increases and decreases in arterial pressure.
   b. Prevents syncope precipitated by stresses, such as postural change, meal consumption, or defecation.

STRATEGIES FOR PRIMARY PREVENTION OF CARDIAC PROBLEMS

1. Promote a healthy lifestyle that reduces the following risk factors:
   a. Hypertension.
   b. Cigarette smoking.
   c. High cholesterol in blood.
   d. Overweight.
   e. Diabetes mellitus.
   f. Physical inactivity.
   g. Stress.
2. See Strategies for Health Promotion in Chapter 1.

COMMON PRESENTATIONS OF ALTERATIONS IN CARDIAC FUNCTION

Angina (ischemic-type Heart Pain)

1. Classic angina pectoris, characterized by substernal pain radiating to the neck, jaw, and down the inner aspect of the left arm and

lasting 5 to 10 minutes, is less frequently the presenting sign of coronary artery disease in the elderly than in younger individuals.

2. Stable angina pectoris occurs in response to a predictable degree of exertion and is characterized by a stable pattern of onset, duration, and intensity over time.

3. Unstable angina pectoris is experienced as paroxysmal chest pain triggered by an unpredictable degree of exertion or emotion during the day or night. The attacks usually increase in number, duration, and intensity over time.

4. Decubitus, nocturnal, and postprandial angina are associated with extensive trivessel coronary disease.
    a. Nocturnal angina occurs only at night and is thought to be associated with dreaming.
    b. Angina decubitus occurs when the person is supine and lessens on arising.
    c. Postprandial angina occurs after meals.

5. Variant angina (Prinzmetal's angina) is similar to classic angina, but it occurs when the client is at rest; it is thought to be related to coronary artery spasm occurring at specific times of the day.

6. Intractable angina is chronic, incapacitating, and unresponsive to intervention.

Anginal Equivalents

1. Instead of angina, the elderly often manifest anginal equivalents, such as dyspnea, acute fatigue or other atypical discomforts.

2. Silent ischemia may mimic other problems common to the elderly.
    a. Pain in the back, shoulders, elbows, or hands may seem to be arthritic.
    b. Gastric discomfort and burning usually at night are often misdiagnosed as peptic ulcer disease.
    c. Postprandial discomfort is often incorrectly interpreted as hiatal hernia.

Syncope

1. Cardiovascular syncope is characterized by the client:
    a. Experiencing abrupt onset without forewarning.
    b. Falling to the ground and sustaining injury.
    c. Returning quickly to full consciousness.
    d. Experiencing an episode lasting from 15 seconds to 2 to 3 minutes.

2. The cause of syncope should be diagnosed promptly, and appro-

priate treatment should be instituted early to prevent secondary injuries from falls.

3. Causes of cardiovascular syncope in the elderly are as follows:
   a. Atrial bradytachycardia syndrome is the most common arrhythmic cause of syncope in the elderly.
   b. Supraventricular and ventricular tachycardias are more likely to cause syncope in the elderly, who tolerate tachycardia poorly.
   c. Emotions, emesis, or pain can cause generalized vasodilatation with hypotensive syncope.
   d. Orthostatic hypotension associated with primary aging changes or untoward effects of medications may cause syncope.
   e. Nonarrhythmic cardiac conditions that interfere with aortic outflow or venous return may precipitate syncope.
4. Arrhythmic syncope may mask any associated symptoms of myocardial infarction (MI).
5. Often, the elderly ignore the first episode of syncope, especially if it is of short duration and there are no immediate sequelae.
6. Assisting the client or family to recognize and report arrhythmias and adverse reactions to drugs is vital in preventing syncope and secondary injuries.

Palpitations

1. Palpitations are reported when the heartbeat is unusually rapid, strong, or irregular enough to make a person aware of it.
2. Causes of palpitations are as follows:
   a. Common intermittent arrhythmias in the elderly that include benign arterial premature beats, episodic supraventricular tachyarrhythmias, atrial bradytachycardia syndrome with alternating slow and rapid heart rhythms, and ventricular premature beats.
   b. Consumption of alcohol or caffeinated beverages.
   c. Side effects of cardioactive drugs.
   d. Anxiety.
3. Clients frequently describe palpitations as:
   a. A disagreeable awareness of the heartbeats.
   b. Fluttering, racing, jumping, skipping, flip-flops, or strong beating.
   c. A "bird in the chest," a "fish out of water," or a "jackhammer in the neck."
4. Diaphoresis, anginal pain or dyspnea accompanying palpitations may suggest pathology.
5. During the assessment process, the client should be encouraged to

tap out the rhythm of the palpitations, as the rhythm may be helpful in establishing the diagnosis.

6. Clarification of the cause and the type of palpitations experienced by the client in the community is at times achieved by 24-hour electrocardiogram (ECG) monitoring with a Holter recorder and a diary kept by the client of any symptoms.
7. With no history of syncope or significant coexisting heart disease, subjective palpitations are for the most part benign.
8. Relief from benign palpitations is usually achieved by reassurance and withdrawal of all offending agents or conditions.

CARDIAC PROBLEMS MOST COMMON IN THE ELDERLY

The most common cardiac problems experienced by the elderly are coronary heart disease followed by hypertensive, valvular, and arrhythmic heart disease.

Coronary Heart Disease (Ischemic Heart Disease)

1. The prevalence of atherosclerotic coronary heart disease with morbidity is over 20% in persons 65 years of age and older.
2. Classic angina occurs less frequently in the elderly, but approximately 50% of elderly clients present with unstable angina pectoris. See "Angina," previously.
3. Prompt consistent relief with sublingual nitroglycerin establishes the diagnosis of angina.
4. Treatment of the elderly client with coronary artery disease is geared toward assisting the client in maintaining the lifestyle desired rather than severely limiting activities.
5. Long-term medical therapy with digitalis, nitrates, beta-blockers, and calcium channel blockers requires careful monitoring for untoward effects, particularly those on the central nervous system.
6. Coronary artery bypass graft or coronary angioplasty is selectively utilized to treat the elderly high-risk client with coronary artery disease. See "Cardiac surgery," later.
7. Acute MI occurs in approximately 10% of men over age 65 and 5% of women over age 65 as a consequence of coronary heart disease.
   a. Elderly clients with a history of angina, hypertension, and ischemic heart disease are more likely to experience MI.

    b. MI tends to occur more frequently in the elderly when at rest or asleep.

    c. MI may be present with:

       (1) Typical substernal pain.

       (2) Sudden dyspnea (may dominate).

       (3) Acute confusion.

       (4) Exacerbation of heart failure.

       (5) Lightheadedness.

       (6) Syncope.

       (7) Weakness.

       (8) Abdominal pain.

       (9) Persistent vomiting.

      (10) Cough.

      (11) Renal failure.

      (12) Pulmonary edema without chest pain in those over age 70.

    d. The client and family should be alerted to the need to promptly report the presenting symptoms of MI and the need to obtain prompt medical care for the client.

    e. The client experiencing MI requires hospitalization for medical or surgical treatment.

    f. Rehabilitation after MI is essential to return the client to an active lifestyle.

Hypertensive Heart Disease

1. The prevalence of hypertension rises with advancing years.

2. Hypertension is a major risk factor for:

    a. Coronary artery disease.

    b. Cerebral vascular events.

    c. Congestive heart failure.

    d. Renal failure.

    e. Peripheral vascular disease.

3. Because the client with hypertension may remain asymptomatic for years even though systemic damage is occurring, periodic screening for "silent" hypertension should be made available.

4. Blood pressure in the elderly should be monitored using appropriate equipment and guidelines.

    a. Cuffs should be of adequate width to avoid diagnosing elevated blood pressure falsely in those with brachial artery sclerosis.

    b. Wider cuffs are required for obese clients.

    c. Guidelines for the measurement device should be followed.

    d. Blood pressure should be taken on both arms with the client supine and then in an erect position (to check for orthostatic hypotension).

  e. The client should be comfortable with the arm bare.

  f. Both systolic and diastolic pressures should be measured. Diastolic pressure should be recorded at the disappearance of the sound.

  g. The client should be informed of the blood pressure readings, and the recommendations of the Joint National Committee on Dectection, Elevation, and Treatment of High Blood Pressure should be initiated (Table 13–1).

5. Sudden onset of diastolic hypertension, resistance to medication in a client previously well controlled, or the development of unexplained hypokalemia necessitates assessment for a secondary cause for hypertension.

6. Some authorities recommend treatment for isolated systolic hypertension (e.g., systolic blood pressure above 160 mm Hg even if the diastolic pressure is below 90 mm Hg).

7. Treatment for essential hypertension should be individualized.

  a. A nonpharmacologic regimen of sodium restriction in the diet and weight reduction is recommended for those with borderline hypertension.

  b. Pharmacologic therapy often consists of angiotensin-converting enzyme inhibitor, a beta-blocker, or a calcium channel blocker.

    (1) The aim is to reduce the diastolic pressure to less than 90 mm Hg or by at least 10 mm Hg.

Table 13–1. *Initial Blood Pressure Measurement and Recommended Action**

Measurement	Recommended Action†
Diastolic	
Below 85 mm Hg	Recheck within 2 years
85 to 89 mm Hg	Recheck within 1 year
90 to 104 mm Hg	Confirm within 2 months
105 to 114 mm Hg	Evaluate or refer promptly within 2 weeks
Above 115 mm Hg	Evaluate or refer immediately for care
Systolic (When diastolic is below 90 mm Hg)	
Below 140 mm Hg	Recheck within 2 years
140 to 199 mm Hg	Confirm within 2 months
Above 200 mm Hg	Evaluate or refer promptly to source of care within 2 weeks

*From the Joint National Committee 1984 Report on Detection, Evaluation, and Treatment of High Blood Pressure. US Dept of Health and Human Services. NIH No. 84-1088. Washington, DC: US Government Printing Office, 1984.

†If actions for follow-up of diastolic and systolic blood pressure are different, the shorter recommended time period takes precedence and a referral overrides a recheck recommendation.

(2) Therapy is initiated with low doses and is gradually increased as needed.

(3) Blood pressure readings in both arms are used to adjust dosage.

(4) Sympathetic blockers and antihypertensive agents with central nervous system depressant effects (e.g., reserpine and clonidine hydrochloride) are used cautiously, as the elderly are susceptible to postural hypotension and central nervous system depressant effects.

Sick Sinus Syndrome

1. A functional or anatomic impairment in the region of the sinoatrial (S-A) node results in intermittent failure of the sinus pacing mechanism and in subsequent arrhythmia.
2. Manifestations of sick sinus syndrome include:
   a. Periods of regular sinus rhythm alternating with bradycardia or tachycardia.
   b. Paroxysmal weakness.
   c. Fatigue.
   d. Syncope.
   e. Dyspnea.
   f. Palpitations.
3. Holter ECG monitoring for at least a 24-hour period is most helpful in establishing the diagnosis.
4. Maintenance of heart rate is usually accomplished by implantation of a pacemaker.

Congestive Heart Failure

1. Congestive heart failure (CHF) is a major complication of cardiac disease that progressively increases with age.
2. The most common causes of CHF are:
   a. Chronic hypertension.
   b. Overt coronary disease.
   c. Valvular disease.
3. As the signs and symptoms of early CHF in the elderly are often obscured by other conditions or may mimic other disease, the client and family should be alerted to report the following symptoms:
   a. Somnolence.
   b. Confusion.
   c. Disorientation.
   d. Weakness.

   e. Fatigue.

   f. Recent weight gain.

   g. Failure to thrive.

   h. Dyspnea (may or may not be present).

   i. Inspiratory rales.

   j. Peripheral edema (not a reliable sign of failure).

   k. Distended neck veins with the client reclining at a 45-degree angle.

4. Cognitive impairment, if present, may worsen and further confuse the picture.

5. Early diagnosis of CHF is frequently based on the above findings plus a history of underlying heart problems and knowledge of physical, social, or environmental factors currently experienced that can stress the circulatory system.

6. Signs of CHF should be reported early, and treatment should be instituted to prevent decompensation with progression to pulmonary edema.

7. Efforts should be made to prevent or at least be alert to the following circumstances, which lead to exacerbation of CHF:

   a. Progressive deterioration of ventricular function.

   b. Daily physical demands requiring a greater percentage of total circulatory reserve.

   c. Reduced circulatory reserve in response to stress, such as fever, infection, or anemia.

   d. Myocardial damage, including MI.

   e. Reduced renal function.

   f. Subclinical emboli.

   g. Excess sodium in the diet associated with dietary indiscretion.

8. Therapy for CHF is geared toward promoting diuresis, improving oxygenation, and reducing afterload and preload.

   a. Bed or chair rest increases diuresis, renal perfusion, peripheral tissue oxygenation, and venous tone.

     (1) Legs should be elevated while sitting to reduce edema caused by right-sided failure.

   b. Diuretics and digitalis preparations are used to increase cardiac output.

     (1) Maintenance therapy with digitalis requires close monitoring because of high risk of digitalis toxicity in the elderly.

     (2) Maintenance use of digitalis is somewhat controversial.

   c. Vasodilators alone or in combination are used to reduce preload and afterload.

   d. When the above therapeutic regimen has not been effective, adding chloroxine (Capitrol) or prazosin hydrochloride (Minipress) has been beneficial.

ASSESSMENT OF THE ELDERLY CLIENT WITH ALTERATIONS IN CARDIAC FUNCTION

In addition to a history and physical assessment, a wide range of diagnostic tests is now available for evaluating the cardiovascular status of elderly clients.

Standard Laboratory Tests

1. Blood count.
2. Blood chemistry profile.
3. ECG.
4. X-ray.

Specialized Noninvasive Cardiac Diagnostic Procedures

1. Noninvasive procedures are preferred to invasive procedures, which may carry significant risk for the elderly.
2. Holter ECG recording over 24 hours is used for detecting arrhythmias.
3. An exercise tolerance test is used to assess the adequacy of coronary perfusion and global cardiovascular performance.
   a. The treadmill is used most widely in testing the elderly, as it is easy to adjust the grade and speed of walking to the limitations imposed by musculoskeletal problems experienced by older persons.
4. Echocardiography (sonography) provides dynamic visualization of cardiac structures and information about ventricular and mitral valve function. Chest cage deformities and coexisting emphysema in many of the elderly make for less satisfactory results.
5. Radionuclide imaging is useful in assessment of cardiac performance and myocardial perfusion defects.
   a. The radionuclide ejection test is used to evaluate total and regional cardiac performance.
   b. A radionuclide ejection fraction (the stroke volume divided by

the end-diastolic volume) in normal individuals is greater than 0.6 and increases with exertion.

c. A radionuclide ejection fraction greater than 0.5 is considered favorable, an ejection fraction less than 0.35 indicates significant cardiac disease, and an ejection fraction under 0.2 suggests a poor prognosis.

Specialized Invasive Cardiac Diagnostic Procedures

1. Cardiac catheterization and coronary angiography (invasive procedures) are used for precise evaluation for surgical intervention, the extent and severity of the coronary disease process, the functional state of the ventricles, the severity of valvular lesions, and the size of an existing shunt in elderly clients with significant cardiac disease.
2. Minimal increase in morbidity and mortality risk is associated with these invasive procedures in clients over age 70.

MANAGEMENT

Pharmacologic Agents

Recent advances in the development of pharmacologic agents, such as diuretics, beta-adrenergic blockers, and calcium channel blockers, have made treatment available for chronic cardiac conditions that may sustain the elderly at a functional level in the community. See under "Cardiovascular Agents" in Chapter 6.

Pacemakers

Pacemakers are implanted in the symptomatic elderly for the treatment of arrhythmias, such as bradycardia, sinus node disease, atrial tachycardia syndrome, and refractory re-entrant tachycardias. After implantation, the pacemakers may be programmed for rate, output, voltage, sensitivity, and mode (demand or fixed-rate).

Cardiac Surgery

Cardiac surgery is gradually being extended to older clients as a therapeutic intervention.

1. The three most common surgical heart procedures performed on the elderly are:
   a. Coronary artery bypass graft (CABG) surgery.
   b. Valve replacement.
   c. Atrial septal defect repair.
2. Among the elderly, the success rate is greatly affected by the quality of the preoperative preparation, the anesthesia, the technical competence of the surgical team, and the postoperative care.
3. Severe trivessel coronary stenosis or left main stenosis, significant aortic stenosis, and atrial septal defect with greater than a two-to-one shunt are correctable.

Percutaneous Transluminal Coronary Angioplasty

Percutaneous transluminal coronary angioplasty (PTCA) is utilized as treatment for localized proximal coronary stenosis of one or two major coronary vessels in elderly clients with a success rate of 70 to 80%.

1. Calcified lesions and tortuous angulated coronary vessels diminish the probability of effective dilatation.
2. PTCA is especially appealing to older clients, as hospitalization is necessary for only 2 days after the dilatation.

STRATEGIES FOR HEALTH MAINTENANCE

1. Design a plan of care with the client or family to promote achieving optimal emotional and physiologic improvement, to attain an acceptable level of self-care, and to resume useful activity.
2. Refrain from aggressive risk modification, as it is unwarranted in the elderly except for advising cessation of smoking.
3. Include in the program:
   a. Client and family education.
   b. Progressive physical activity.
   c. Psychosocial counseling.
   d. Clear, detailed, specific instructions regarding diet, activities, and medications.
4. Review physical and psychosocial assessments for losses or physical disabilities that may interfere with performing activities of daily living.

    a. Losses may bring on depression with fatigue, anorexia, insomnia, and lack of interest in personal hygiene and appearance.

    b. Determination should be made as to whether these behaviors are related to cardiac problems or to other causes. For example, dyspnea may be caused by anemia or an inactive lifestyle rather than a cardiac problem.

5. Request parameters for an individualized exercise program from the client's physician. The benefits of an exercise program for the elderly client with a cardiovascular problem are as follows:

    a. Produces a sense of well-being that encourages the older client to continue daily living, recreational, and social activities.

    b. May modify decreased joint mobility of aging and enhance neuromuscular coordination.

    c. Counteracts effects of immobility.

    d. Helps relieve anxiety and depression.

    e. Helps in attaining and maintaining ideal weight.

    f. May reduce need for medication in which the side effects are hazardous to the elderly client.

6. Teach the elderly client initiating an exercise program to:

    a. Start with warm-up activities to ensure increase in deep muscle temperature and to prevent muscle injuries.

    b. Perform limbering-up exercises to promote more effective conditioning.

    c. Increase time walking gradually.

    d. Start with early gradual ambulation followed by progressive activities.

        (1) Walking at even 3 to $3\frac{1}{2}$ miles per hour results in significant conditioning response with improvements in joint mobility and muscular coordination.

    e. End slowly with a cool-down period after exercise. Light exercise, such as walking or easy pedaling, is appropriate for the cool-down period.

    f. Limit running and jumping because they tend to raise the incidence of orthopedic complications.

    g. Choose activity that will not increase existing physical limitations.

        (1) A client with arthritis should be guided toward aerobic exercise such as walking, swimming, or riding a stationary bike that does not put undue pressure on weight-bearing joints.

        (2) Consider activities of daily living as a form of exercise.

    h. Evaluate response to exercising.

        (1) Vital signs should increase with exercise unless the client is receiving therapy with a beta-blocker.

        (2) Falling blood pressure or failure of the heart rate to increase

with exercise suggests severe cardiac disease that should be reported to a physician.

   (3) A client who is not taking a beta-blocker and whose vital signs fail to increase with exercise should be warned to avoid unsupervised exercise.

7. Caution the client to avoid overexertion.
   a. Assist in planning activities during the day with rest periods in between.
   b. Help the elderly to learn energy-saving techniques (e.g., encourage organizing activities).
8. Teach the client to prevent hyperthermia or hypothermia when exercising by:
   a. Dressing appropriately for exercise.
   b. Checking on adequate ventilation in the exercise area.
   c. Walking in the late morning or early afternoon during the winter.
   d. Walking in the early morning and late afternoon during the summer.
   e. Avoiding walks in windy weather.
   f. Covering the mouth with a scarf to help warm inspired air in cold weather.
9. Protect against infection by advocating:
   a. An appropriate excercise program.
   b. A nutritious diet geared to reduction of risk factors. See Chapter 4.
   c. Avoidance of anyone with a respiratory infection.
   d. Development of stress-reduction techniques.
10. Advise a nutritional program that includes:
    a. Nutrient-dense foods to maintain or reduce weight as appropriate.
    b. Foods low in saturated fats.
    c. Foods containing high-density lipoproteins.
    d. Adequate protein, vitamins, and minerals.
    e. Foods with good sources of potassium to prevent hypokalemia in clients taking loop diuretics or thiazides.
    f. Exclusion of food high in sodium.
    g. Small frequent meals of high-density foods that will supply adequate bulk.
       (1) Avoiding large meals is preferable, as CHF decreases circulation to the stomach and small intestine so that food moves slowly through the gastrointestinal tract and produces a feeling of fullness and distention.
11. Discuss changes in sexuality related to cardiovascular alterations. See under "Cardiovascular Disease," Chapter 9.

12. Promote compliance with drug therapy.
   a. Monitor cardiac response to drug therapy.
   b. Monitor for adverse reactions and for toxicity of drugs detoxified by the liver. Detoxification may be reduced or delayed by alterations in cardiac function that further reduce hepatic blood flow.
   c. Advise against the use of over-the-counter (OTC) drugs.
     (1) Emphasize avoiding the use of OTC expectorants, which are more likely to interact with cardiac drugs and worsen failure.
     (2) Alert the client and family to report a dry, nonproductive cough occurring at night and clearing during the day, as it may be a symptom of fluid overload caused by CHF and not a cold.
   d. See cardiovascular drugs in Chapter 6.
13. Assist the client in making arrangements for obtaining tests for serum blood levels as needed.
14. Review appropriate care with the client utilizing a pacemaker.
   a. Review the literature that came with the pacemaker.
   b. Emphasize the importance of monitoring pacemaker function in order to identify early sensing problems, such as premature battery depletion, random electronic component failures, and electrode dislodgment.
   c. Ascertain that the client is checking his radial pulse 1 full minute every day. A pulse slower than the preset rate should alert the client to notify his physician, as the battery (usually lasts 6 to 12 years) may be running down and may need replacement.
   d. Assist the homebound client in maintaining regular monthly checkups on pacemaker function.
     (1) Monitoring for the client living far from his physician may be achieved by telephone. A small device that transmits a single-lead ECG by telephone may be bought or leased.
     (2) The equipment and phone calls are usually covered by health insurance.
   e. Advise the client that if he suspects electrical interference, he should turn off the appliance.
     (1) Most pacemakers are now well shielded against electrical interference from radios, televisions, microwave ovens, and other electrical appliances.
     (2) Large telephones or certain antitheft alarm systems have intense magnetic fields that can temporarily alter pacemaker function.
   f. Advise the client to carry an identification card that indicates the manufacturer of the pacemaker and describes its settings and programmable functions. The name and telephone number of

the client's physician and the hospital where the pacemaker was implanted should also be on the card.

(1) A copy of the card should be kept at home for easy replacement if lost.
(2) Wearing a Medic Alert tag is also desirable and advantageous, as it is more visible than the identification card. (See Fig. 6–1.)

Resources

The American Heart Association
7320 Greenville Avenue
Dallas, TX 75231

Provides a list of local chapters. Local chapters provide printed literature and sponser self-help groups for clients and families. They also offer smoking withdrawal programs and cardiopulmonary resuscitation programs.

Information Specialist
High Blood Pressure Information Center (HBPIC)
120/80 National Institutes of Health
Bethesda, MD 20205
(301) 496-1809

Provides consumer education materials, catalogues, fliers, posters, and bibliographies.

National, Heart, Lung, and Blood Institute Publication Listing (Catalogue)
Technical Information Specialist
National Heart, Lung, and Blood Institute (NHLBI)
Department of Health and Human Services
Building 31, Room 4A-21
9000 Rockville Pike
Bethesda, MD 20205
(301) 496-4236

Giant Food, Inc.
P.O. Box 1804
Washington, DC 20013

On request, will provide a 14-page pamphlet, *Calling a Halt to Salt*, which lists the sodium content and calories for a wide variety of foods and unsuspected sources of salt in food items.

References

American Heart Association. An older person's guide to cardiovascular health. Dallas, 1985.
American Heart Association. Coronary care: Rehabilitation of the patient with symptomatic coronary atherosclerotic disease. Dallas, 1981.
American Heart Association. Exercise testing and training of individuals with heart disease or at high risk for its development. Dallas, 1981.
Joint National Committee 1984 Report on Detection, Evaluation, and Treatment of High Blood Pressure. US Dept of Health and Human Services. Public Health Service, National Institutes of Health. DHEW pub. no. (NIH) 84-1088. Washington, DC: US Government Printing Office, 1984.
Luckmann J, Sorensen KC: Medical-Surgical Nursing. Philadelphia: WB Saunders Co, 1987.
Malasanos L, Barkauskas V, Moss M, Stoltenberg-Allen K: Health Assessment. St. Louis: CV Mosby Co, 1986.
Moss AJ: Cardiac disease in the elderly. In Calkins D, Davis PJ, Ford AB, eds: The Practice of Geriatrics. Philadelphia: WB Saunders Co, 1986.
Porterfield L, Porterfield JG: What you need to know about today's pacemakers. RN March 1987, pp. 44–49.
Stanley M: Helping an elderly patient live with CHF. RN September 1986, pp. 35–42.
Tarazi RC: Hypertension in the elderly. In Calkins D, Davis PJ, Ford AB, eds: The Practice of Geriatrics. Philadelphia: WB Saunders Co, 1986.
Wei J, Gersh BJ: Heart disease in the elderly. Current Problems in Cardiology 12(1):7–65, 1987.

14

Coping with Depression and Dementia

DEPRESSION
DEMENTIA

Depression and dementia are the two most common mental health disorders experienced by the elderly in the community.

DEPRESSION

1. An estimated 10 to 65% of the elderly experience depression.
2. Depression in the elderly appears to be related more to multiple real losses and environmental stresses than to anger turned inward, as it is in the younger population.
3. Although depression is prevalent among the elderly, diagnosis and appropriate treatment are often delayed because presentation of depression is frequently atypical and feelings of sadness and low spirits are accepted as being inevitable with old age.
4. As a result of the overlap of symptomatology and the erroneous belief that senility is inevitable with aging, depression, which is more treatable than organic brain syndrome and for which the prognosis is better, is often misdiagnosed as organic brain syndrome.
5. Many elderly unconsciously accept the negative stereotype that society draws of them. They lose self-esteem and, finally rejecting themselves, become depressed, despairing, and barred from work and love.
6. Case finding is particularly important, as the elderly tend to seek

help for somatic symptoms but do not seek treatment for mental health problems.

7. Associated with depression in the elderly is an increased suicide rate, which is demonstrated in all countries with reliable statistics.
8. Prevention of and treatment for depression in the elderly necessitate that the public discard the stereotype of the elderly as noncontributory and sexless and provide opportunity for the elderly to actively participate in a caring society.
9. Crisis care and ongoing mental health services are needed in the community to assist the elderly in completing grief work for losses experienced and in coping with the challenges before them.

Theories of the Etiology of Depression in the Elderly

1. Physiologic theory attributes endogenous depression to primary changes causing a deficiency in neurotransmitters, which facilitates conduction of nerve impulses at synapses. Pharmacologic therapy with tricyclic antidepressants is the treatment of choice.
2. Intrapsychic theory relates depression in the elderly to a continuation of the personality throughout the life span. Unresolved conflicts or maladaptive patterns in the early years may result in depression, or depression may be a continuation of a chronic state.
3. Environmental theories suggest that events in an individual's life or social situation may precipitate a reactive depression. Poverty, poor physical health, loneliness, or other losses, especially in those with limited coping behaviors, may trigger a reactive depression.
4. Iatrogenic depression may be caused by psychotropic drugs, antiparkinsonian drugs, or antihypertensive agents.
5. Secondary depression may occur in association with trauma or illness, such as head injury, Parkinson's disease, stroke, thyroid dysfunction, neoplasms, and alcoholism.

Presentation of Depression

1. Symptoms tend to be denied or somaticized with more socially acceptable physical symptoms and complaints (e.g., gastrointestinal upset or sleeplessness) reported than emotional symptoms.
   a. More than one third of elderly depressed clients experience masked depression (depression equivalent) with prominent somatic complaints rather than those of mood disturbances.
   b. These clients appear hypochondriacal traveling from doctor to

doctor with a multitude of somatic complaints that do not respond to treatment.

c. Persistently focusing on somatic complaints, the elderly depressed tend to deny sadness, worry, or irritability.

2. Less guilt is expressed than in earlier life depressions.
3. Apathy with loss of energy is prominent.
4. Paranoid symptoms, with suspiciousness to frank delusions, are more common in the elderly depressed than in younger persons.
5. Statements of not caring anymore and expression of feelings of helplessness or hopelessness may indicate the presence of suicidal ideas and intent.
6. See "Emotional Reactions of the Elderly in Response to Loss," in Chapter 2.

Suicide and the Elderly

PREVALENCE

1. The elderly population accounts for roughly 25% of suicides, although they constitute only 11% of the entire population.
2. White men in their eighties are the highest risk for suicide.
3. The suicide rate appears to be rising for older women.
4. Elderly black men and women do not demonstrate increased risk for suicide, as their status may have improved.
5. Suicide risk increases as the severely depressed client begins to improve but still is experiencing feelings of hopelessness or helplessness.
6. Subintentional suicides, which involve long, drawn-out destructive behavior, are not counted as part of the suicide statistics but are prevalent in the elderly population.

CONTRIBUTING FACTORS

1. Suicide in the elderly tends to be related to bereavement, physical problems, or severe loss of status, which particularly affects older men.
2. Suicide may be the final use of control.
3. Rationalized or philosophic suicide decision making is more common when health is failing.
4. Suicide may be an attempt to prevent the expenditure of funds that would drain the spouse or family of financial resources.

METHODS USED TO ACCOMPLISH SUICIDE

1. Violent lethal methods, such as drug overdose, hanging, jumping off high places, and use of firearms and explosives, are used by the elderly man.
2. Long, drawn-out destructive behavior is characterized by:
    a. Not eating.
    b. Not taking medication.
    c. Drinking excessively.
    d. Delaying treatment.
    e. Taking risks physically.

STRATEGIES FOR SUICIDE PREVENTION

1. Reduce the occurrence and persistence of depression.
2. Assess for causation and provide effective treatment when depression is present.
3. Gear treatment to alleviation of depression and restoration of a sense of control of one's life.
4. Be alert when depression seems to have lifted, as clients may then have gathered enough energy to carry out suicide.
5. Deal openly with suicidal ideation by asking about intent.
6. Recognize the fallibility of rescue fantasies (fantasy that the professional will rescue the client in time), and take immediate action to protect the client when suicidal intent is revealed.
7. Suicidal ideation or a suicidal threat should be reported, and attempts should be made to dissuade the client from using the suicide option.
8. Be alert to the subtle cues, such as paying up all bills or talk of getting affairs in order, as the elderly tend to give less warning that suicide is being contemplated before they carry out the act.
9. Recognize that the client with a well-thought-out plan and a lethal method is at higher risk.
10. Ensure the availability of outreach services, particularly for withdrawn and isolated seniors. Suicide Hot Line numbers are listed in the telephone directory.

Differences Between Reactive Depression and Major Clinical Depression

REACTIVE DEPRESSION

1. A reactive (situational) depression occurs in a mild to severe form in response to loss or to events over which one has little control.

2. Resolution of a situational depression often occurs over time, as feelings of control are restored and support is received.

MAJOR CLINICAL DEPRESSION

1. A major clinical depression immobilizes the client.
2. The cause may be related to unresolved conflicts, despair over one's past life, or changes in the central nervous system or endocrine system.
3. Medication is usually the treatment used.

Causes of Reactive Depression

1. Losses that are actual, threatened, or fantasized, such as a loss of:
   a. Mobility, diversion, or communication.
   b. Resistance to disease or trauma.
   c. Physical beauty.
   d. Orgasmic capacity.
   e. Confidence in cognitive function.
   f. First-class citizenship (i.e., becoming a member of an aged minority).
   g. Self-esteem.
   h. A spouse (most destructive loss).
2. Chronic illness causing lasting disability.
3. Societal devaluation associated with negative stereotyping.
4. Loneliness that prevents interaction with others, which would contribute to one's feeling of being accepted.
5. Powerlessness or loss of control.
6. Relocation.
7. Retirement.
8. Anniversary reactions to events in the past.

Impact of the Elder's Depression on the Family

1. Families are most disturbed by symptoms of denial of the problem, apathy, insomnia, irritability, and hostility in the elder.
2. Scapegoating by the depressed client is experienced particularly by the member of the family who provides the most care.
3. Families suffer fatigue, frustration, changing life routines, anger, and guilt that interfere with maintaining nurturing attitudes toward the elder.

Assessment for Depression

1. A client history should be obtained.
   a. Time of onset, rapidity of progression, and severity of both physical and psychic symptoms should be explored for causation, which may be related to physical illness or aging changes or may be coincidental with other depressive symptoms or situational crises.
   b. Somatic complaints must be carefully evaluated and not dismissed or attributed to aging or depression.
   c. Medication history should be reviewed, particularly for use of a drug that may have triggered depression.
      (1) Alcohol, benzodiazepines, barbiturates, corticosteroids, reserpine, propranolol, methyldopa, and haloperidol have been frequently associated with induced depression.
2. Physical assessment should be focused on identification of problems in any system that may precipitate a secondary depression.
3. Behavioral manifestations of depression should be assessed for the client's ability to function within his environment.
4. Criteria for major depression in the Diagnostic and Statistical Manual of Mental Disorders (DSM III) should be considered.
   a. Dysphoric mood (exaggerated feeling of depression and unrest). This is often not reported, as the elderly tend to have "masked depression."
   b. Poor appetite or weight loss or gain. This is not especially indicative of depression, as it accompanies the aging process and is seen in many disease conditions.
   c. Sleep disturbances, such as insomnia or hypersomnia.
   d. Psychomotor agitation or retardation with a high anxiety component.
   e. Loss of interest or pleasure in usual activities.
   f. Loss of energy with undue fatigue.
   g. Feelings of worthlessness, self-reproach, or excessive or inappropriate guilt.
   h. Complaints of reduced ability to think or concentrate.
   i. Recurring thoughts of death or suicide.
5. Assessment to differentiate *pseudodementia* (dementia caused by depression) and *true dementia* (an organic mental disorder) may be difficult, as cognitive deficits, disorientation, distractibility, and apathy may present in both conditions. Significant differences between the depressed and the demented client are as follows:
   a. The depressed client:
      (1) Exhibits no history of memory loss, disorientation, or habit

deterioration, such as self-exposure, incontinence, or lack of social tact.
- (2) Retains sense of orientation.
- (3) Demonstrates mood disturbance often accompanied by irritability and hostility.
- (4) Rejects questions angrily.
- (5) Responds positively to a therapeutic trial of antidepressants.
b. The client with organic brain disturbance:
- (1) Attempts to answer questions but replies may be irrelevant, nonsensical, or confabulatory.
- (2) Demonstrates primitive reflexes, perseveration, or actual neurologic deficit.
- (3) May react to medication with increased confusion because of anticholinergic effect of medication.
6. A mental status examination may be conducted by:
   a. Interview.
   b. Questionnaire.
   c. Observer-related tests.
   d. Psychologic and neuropsychologic testing.
   e. Tests for evaluating depression in the elderly, such as:
   - (1) The Beck Depression Inventory.
   - (2) The Hopkins Symptoms Checklist.
   - (3) The Brink Geriatric Depression Scale.

Modalities Used in Treatment of Depression

1. Individual or group psychotherapy is one method of treatment.
   a. Elderly clients seem to improve with psychotherapy.
   b. Empathetic, genuine, warm, and consistently accepting forms of psychotherapy produce the best results.
   c. Interpersonal therapy aimed primarily at supporting the client in working through issues that cause conflict and negative emotions may improve social functioning.
   d. Reality orientation, attitude therapy, reminiscing, sensory retraining, and pet therapy are modalities with the objective of reorienting the client to person, place, time, and situation; encouraging social interaction; and reinforcing acceptable behavior that raises self-esteem.
2. Behavior modification with shaping of activities promotes a sense of accomplishment and self-esteem.
   a. Shaping involves breaking down target behavior into parts and encouraging performance of each part stepwise until the target behavior is performed.

3. Activity therapy helps improve physiologic functioning and helps develop a sense of well-being.
    a. Aerobic exercise, such as walking and swimming, is recommended.
    b. Tai Chi Chuan ancient martial arts are helpful in relieving stress and depression, as they require concentration and integration of body and mind.
4. Touch therapy promotes relaxation.
    a. Massage relieves tension.
    b. A beauty make-over improves morale.
5. Rest and recreation provide for enjoyable energy expenditure alternating with periods of rest that prepare one for more activity.
6. Antidepressant medication is used primarily for severe depression.
    a. Drugs of choice are the tricyclics because they are more effective and less toxic than the monoamine oxidase inhibitors.
    b. Dosages must be reduced by one half to one third of the doses used in the younger population.
    c. The highest tolerated dose is administered for at least 4 weeks. If clinical improvement is noted, a maintenance dose is ordered for several months. Then the dosage is gradually decreased over a 2- to 3-month period.
    d. The client must be monitored for side effects of the medication ordered.
7. Electroconvulsive therapy (ECT) is the treatment of choice for suicidal clients or for severe psychotic depression.
    a. ECT seems to restore neurotransmitter secretion.
    b. Contraindications for ECT are mild myocardial infarction or a lesion within the skull.
8. Psychiatric day-care centers are usually available only for those with major psychiatric disorders.

Strategies for Care of the Depressed Client

1. Assess for cause and associated conditions, factors, or losses in the physical, psychosocial, and spiritual dimensions.
2. Consider the premorbid personality of the client and the cause of the depression when planning care.
3. Use good communication techniques: wait for the elderly client to complete interaction, listen, and identify the client by name.
4. Evaluate the sensory deficits that may contribute to depression.
5. Use direct, active intervention in psychotherapy whether in a group or individual setting.

    a. Discuss the nature of the depression, the presence of depression, the nature of symptoms, and the time limitation of depression.

    b. Be attentive, give the client choices, and provide clear feedback.

    c. State expectations of the client clearly in the form of an opinion.

6. Use a consistent approach agreed upon by all members of the health care team.

7. Include the family in the planning and therapy.

8. Assist the client in regaining control of his life by:

    a. Involving the client in the care regimen and decision-making process.

    b. Helping the client in structuring his daily life and in keeping a schedule.

9. Assess the client's ability to cope with perceived losses or stresses, and encourage the client to use past successful coping behaviors.

10. Make yourself available to the client.

    a. Listen to the client.

    b. Discuss options.

    c. Encourage routine decision making with the client, but recommend delaying significant decisions during depressive episodes.

    d. Support the client when he makes a decision.

    e. Assist the client in carrying out decisions when feasible.

11. Support the client through the grieving process when depression is related to bereavement of spouse or other significant loss. See under "Emotional Reaction of the Elderly in Response to Loss," in Chapter 2.

12. Aim to increase physical, mental, and social activity.

    a. Avoid getting into a power struggle with the client over involvement in activity.

    b. Encourage and assist in gradually increasing activity that will help in recovery and be included in the client's routine.

13. Encourage participation in activities that will foster self-esteem.

    a. Accept a small token or refreshment offered by the client, as making a contribution raises self-esteem.

14. Encourage the use of relaxation techniques.

15. Assist the client in meeting space needs.

16. Provide information about the presence and appropriate use of resources for the elderly in the community.

    a. Strengthen the client's support system by letting him know that it may be beneficial to utilize mental health professionals (which he may have refused to use in the past because of the stigma attached) and by telling him where to obtain help if he wishes.

17. Gear care to instilling hope by dealing in an empathetic, warm,

caring, and positive way with feelings of hopelessness, helplessness, and worthlessness.
   a. Encourage the client to replace thoughts that provoke sadness with ones that are pleasant.
   b. Assist in guided imagery.
   c. Offer support and validation with a realistic perspective.
18. Refer to appropriate health professionals for depression-related problems beyond the scope of the generalist nurse.

Resources

Public Inquiries Section
Science Communication Branch
National Institute of Mental Health (NIMH)
Department of Health and Human Services
Parklawn Building, Room 15c–17
5600 Fishers Lane
Rockville, MD 20857
(301) 443-4513

Prepares and distributes publications for professional and lay audiences. Answers general inquiries and provides information on mental health exhibits and films.

Mental health supportive services are provided by the Area Agency on Aging. See Appendix for State Agencies on Aging.

DEMENTIA

1. Dementia (also identified as organic brain disorder, arteriosclerosis, cerebral atrophy, or pseudodementia) is a severe global impairment of cognitive functions (thinking, memory, and personality) of the brain. Dementia can be progressive but is frequently reversible.
2. The incidence of dementia rises and the problems associated with the condition become increasingly evident as life expectancy increases.
3. Ten per cent of the population over age 65 are estimated to suffer from dementia. Whereas only 5% of those between 65 and 69 years of age are affected, 20% of those over age eighty are significantly demented.

4. As an estimated 30 to 40% of the dementias are curable, the client should be carefully assessed to rule out diseases in which treatment may reverse the dementia (e.g., depression).
5. Problems that may cause a reversible cognitive disturbance in older persons can also affect those who already have an irreversible dementia (e.g., electrolyte imbalance).
6. The client, family, and health care team need to understand the nature and course of the illness in order to make appropriate plans.
7. One to 1.5 million noninstitutionalized demented elderly cause heavy financial, physical, and emotional burdens for their families and communities.
8. The current $6 billion a year paid for the care of the demented elderly is expected to more than double by the year 2030.
9. In recognition of dementia as a growing community health problem, the Comprehensive Alzheimer's Assistance, Research, and Education (CARE) Act of 1985 (H.R. 2280) was developed and passed to provide improved care and assistance for Alzheimer's victims and their families.

Irreversible Dementias

SENILE DEMENTIA OF THE ALZHEIMER'S TYPE

1. Senile dementia of the Alzheimer's type (SDAT) constitutes 50 to 70% of the irreversible dementias in elderly Americans (2.5 million). When no reversible cause of intellectual impairment can be identified, SDAT is diagnosed but can be confirmed only by autopsy after the death of the client.
2. Pathology noted at autopsy includes:
   a. Cerebral atrophy with loss of neurons, particularly in areas essential for memory, cognition, and thought processes.
   b. Accumulations of twisted filaments (neurofibrillary tangles) and other abnormal structures within the neurons.
   c. Amorphous aggregates of protein (amyloid) adjacent to and within blood vessels.
   d. Cellular debris and amyloid forming neuritic plaques that initially occur in the hippocampus and temporal lobes and then progress to the frontal and parietal lobes.
   e. Severe reduction in the amount of neurotransmitters (chemical messengers), most notably acetylcholine.
3. Some of the above changes are seen in the brains of older people

who were not demented, but not all changes are noted in a single case nor are the changes evident in such great numbers.

4. Research under way to discover the cause and treatment of Alzheimer's disease is investigating the effects of genes, abnormal accumulations of proteins, infectious agents, environmental toxins, and inadequate blood flow.

5. Symptoms of SDAT are as follows:

    a. Early symptoms:
       (1) Failing attention.
       (2) Declining memory and mathematical ability.
       (3) Errors of judgment.
       (4) Irritability.
       (5) Personality changes.
       (6) Loss of sense of humor.
       (7) Poor orientation.

    b. Progressive symptoms:
       (1) General deterioration of mental function.
       (2) Marked memory loss.
       (3) Impairment of learned-skill movements.
       (4) Disturbance of language.
       (5) Loss of ability to recognize objects.
       (6) Partial or total disorientation as to person, place, or time.
       (7) Impaired recent memory.
       (8) Impaired number retention.
       (9) Impaired ability to abstract.

    c. Dementia dominates, but depression, hallucinations, delusions, and paranoid manifestations may also occur.

6. Cognitive deterioration is progressive, but the rate varies, depending upon neuronal integrity, physical decompensation, and adequacy of the support system.

7. With the progression of Alzheimer's disease, the immune system seems to become more impaired. The client becomes vulnerable to pneumonia (the most common cause of death) or to other infection.

8. Prognosis depends upon the age of onset, individual health status, support systems, and treatment of concurrent health problems. On the average, the life expectancy for the client with SDAT is 7 to 9 years, but the demented client may continue to live for as long as 20 years and even longer (rarely).

MULTIPLE-INFARCT DEMENTIA

1. Multiple-infarct dementia (MID), or vascular dementia, constitutes about 30% of the dementias of the aged.

2. The loss of brain tissue from a series of small insidious strokes or infarcts causes MID.
   a. The first infarct may result in a short-lasting, mild weakness of an arm or leg; slurred speech; or even dizziness. Usually the client recovers within days. One or more of these episodes may occur before intellectual decline is noted.
   b. Small arterioles in the brain are occluded by plaque build-up from atherosclerotic disease or by blood emboli that lodge in these arterioles and prevent blood flow to the parts of the brain they normally supply.
   c. Deprived of oxygen and glucose, the brain cells die and the infarcted area of cell death softens and stops functioning.
3. Progressive deterioration of the brain results in dementia that proceeds in a stepwise fashion. Decline is often more gradual than with SDAT and is usually patchy rather than uniform until finally dementia becomes dominant. See characteristics of dementia above, under "Senile Dementia of the Alzheimer's Type."
4. Focal neurologic abnormalities, dysarthria (defective speech), abnormal gait, and spastic limbs with brisk reflexes are often present.
5. Clients with MID are markedly "slowed down," often overweight, and suffer from other diseases, such as hypertension, diabetes, and symptoms of arterial disease in other parts of the body.
6. About one half of the clients with MID also have Alzheimer's disease.
7. Extension of MID is potentially preventable if it is caught early, via control of hypertension, the use of anticoagulants, or even thromboendarterectomy when bilateral carotid artery disease is present.

OTHER IRREVERSIBLE DEMENTIAS

Other irreversible dementias are caused by the following disorders:
1. Huntington's disease.
2. Pick's disease.
3. Creutzfeldt-Jakob disease.
4. Parkinson's disease.
5. Multiple sclerosis.
6. Syphilis.
7. Cerebral atherosclerosis.

8. Glioblastoma multiforme.
9. Metastatic cancer.

Potentially Reversible Dementias

Causes of potentially reversible dementias are as follows:
1. Metabolic disorders.
   a. Azotemia or renal failure.
   b. Electrolyte imbalances, including hyponatremia or hypernatremia (secondary to diuretic therapy), hypoglycemia, or hyperglycemia, and hypocalcemia or hypercalcemia.
   c. Hepatic failure.
   d. Hypothyroidism or hyperthyroidism.
   e. Cushing's syndrome.
   f. Hypopituitarism.
2. Infectious disorders.
   a. Because of problems with thermoregulation, spiking fever does not usually occur in the elderly, and dementia may present before acute and subacute systemic viral and bacterial infections are diagnosed.
3. Circulatory disorders.
   a. Cardiac conditions, including acute myocardial infarction, congestive heart failure, and arrhythmias.
   b. Vascular occlusion and pulmonary embolus.
4. Pulmonary disorders (chronic obstructive pulmonary disease [COPD]).
5. Brain disorders.
   a. Vascular insufficiency.
   b. Trauma.
   c. Tumors.
   d. Cerebral infection.
   e. Normal pressure hydrocephalus.
6. Pain related to:
   a. Fecal impaction.
   b. Urinary retention.
   c. Bone fracture.
   d. Surgical abdomen.
7. Sensory deprivation.
   a. Blindness.

   b. Deafness.
 8. Environmental changes.
   a. Isolation.
   b. Hospitalization.
 9. Alcohol.
   a. Toxic reactions related to decreased tolerance for alcohol with age.
   b. Alcoholism with acute hallucinosis or delirium tremens.
10. Nutritional deficiencies.
   a. Anemia.
   b. Avitaminosis, particularly of vitamin B_{12}, folic acid, or niacin.
11. Accidental hypothermia.
12. Chemical intoxication with heavy metals (lead, arsenic, or mercury).
13. Psychiatric disorders.
   a. Depression (often superimposed on SDAT).
   b. Mania.
   c. Anxiety.
   d. Paranoia.
14. Medications.
   a. Misuse of over-the-counter (OTC) and prescribed medications.
   b. Use of illicit and consciousness-altering agents.
   c. Untoward effects of drugs.
   d. Drug-drug interactions.

Assessment for Dementia

 1. A detailed physical and social history from the client, family, and past medical records is obtained.
 2. Physical examination is comprehensive, with particular attention to the presence of the following:
   a. Flapping tremor is frequently present in metabolic derangements but is absent in SDAT.
   b. Aphasia with an inability to communicate may be mistaken for dementia.
 3. A mental status and psychiatric evaluation is necessary.
   a. Confirmation and documentation of deterioration in intellectual function are obtained by administration and evaluation of a baseline mental status examination followed up with serial examinations.
   b. A quick mental status examination may be administered and evaluated in the field when dementia is suspected. The following abilities are assessed:
   (1) Orientation for time, place, and person.

　　　　(2) Short-term memory.
　　　　(3) Arithmetic calculation.
　　　　(4) Ability to name objects.
　　　　(5) Comprehension of spoken and written language.
　　　　(6) Ability to write a spontaneous sentence.
　　　　(7) Ability to copy simple geometric figures.
　4. Assess for the characteristic behaviors of dementia.
　　　a. See SDAT behaviors, previously.
　　　b. Early-stage symptoms, often unnoticed by the family, include forgetfulness, with concern (especially among well-educated professionals) and avoidance of groups.
　　　c. Mid-stage symptoms include:
　　　　(1) Confusion.
　　　　(2) Denial of memory problems.
　　　　(3) Rambling conversations or poverty of speech.
　　　　(4) Disorientation.
　　　　(5) Flattening of affect.
　　　　(6) Impairment in social functioning.
　　　　(7) Impairment in accomplishment of household tasks.
　　　　(8) Suspiciousness.
　　　　(9) Paranoid symptoms.
　　　　　(a) Paranoid symptoms that develop as the client tries to make sense of his world must be distinguished from those paranoid symptoms that may exist as part of a paranoid disorder.
　　　d. Late-stage symptoms include:
　　　　(1) Wandering.
　　　　(2) Impaired activities of daily living.
　　　　(3) "Living in the past."
　　　　(4) Angry outbursts.
　　　　(5) Frank delusional thoughts.
　　　　(6) Incontinence.
　5. Assessment to differentiate between pseudodementia (dementia caused by depression) and true dementia should be done, as the symptomatology overlaps. See symptoms under "Assessment for Depression," previously.
　6. Assessment for delirium, an abnormal mental state frequently superimposed on recognized or unrecognized dementia, should be included.
　　　a. Delirium usually includes intellectual impairment and other signs of disordered mental function, such as:
　　　　(1) Fluctuating alterness.
　　　　(2) Tremors.

        (3) Restlessness.

        (4) Confusion.

        (5) Stupor.

        (6) Diminished attention span.

        (7) Decrease in amount of sleep with day-night reversal.

        (8) Hallucinations (particularly visual).

        (9) Delusions.

      (10) Autonomic reactions, such as rapid pulse, flushed skin, and dilated pupils.

      (11) Intense emotional states.

  b. The onset of delirium is usually abrupt and obvious but may be insidious.

  c. The turmoil of delirium may be muted or absent when superimposed on a pre-existing dementia.

      (1) Clients doubly affected seem to experience the onset of a dementia or the worsening of an established dementia.

      (2) The superimposed delirium may be overlooked, and its reversible cause may be left untreated.

  d. The course of delirium is usually brief and may be terminated in death, recovery, or progression into another syndrome.

7. An inventory of OTC and prescribed drugs currently being taken should be obtained, and considerations should be given to:

  a. Compliance with the drug regimen (use and misuse).

  b. The possibility of side effects or drug interactions.

8. Ancillary tests, including blood hematology and chemistry tests, urine tests, tests for thyroid function, a serologic test for syphilis, a chest x-ray, an electroencephalogram (EEG) and a computed tomography (CT scan) of the brain, should complete the assessment.

Strategies for the Care of the Demented Client and the Caregiver

WORKING WITH THE FAMILY

1. Establish a cooperative and helpful relationship with the client and family.

2. Empathize with the family, educate them about the client's dementia, and make suggestions for management.

3. Provide anticipatory guidance for preventing disability that may prematurely cause functional dependency of the client.

PLANNING WITH THE CAREGIVER TO MEET HER OWN NEEDS

1. Sources of stress for the caregiver that put her at risk for stress-related mental health problems include the following:
   a. The need to be ever vigilant to the unpredictable behavior of the demented client requires the caregiver to assume a hyperalert state that causes many stress-related symptoms.
   b. The demented client's memory loss; daily fluctuation in ability to function; habit of constantly asking questions; and behavior problems, such as combativeness and agitation, are particularly stressful.
   c. Being alone with the demented client for extended periods of time increases the susceptibility to stress-related problems.
   d. Failure of other family members to help:
      (1) Reduces the time that the caregiver has for meeting personal needs.
      (2) Constricts social life.
      (3) Increases isolation.
2. Encourage the caregiver of the Alzheimer's victim to maintain her health by:
   a. Conserving energy for important tasks.
   b. Using outside help from the start.
   c. Obtaining temporary relief (respite) by:
      (1) Using adult day-care centers.
      (2) Accepting help from others.
      (3) Taking vacations.
3. Refer the family to the Alzheimer's Disease and Related Disorders Association (ADRDA) Inc., for literature, information, and referral services. (See Resources, following.) Local chapters and their affiliated family-support groups offer personalized assistance and encouragement as well as information about local resources.

WORKING WITH THE CLIENT AND FAMILY

1. Encourage continuation of medical coverage and the use of specialists for:
   a. Diagnostic work-up.
   b. Assistance with care of concurrent disorders that may be contributing to the dementia.
   c. Periodic review of medications and supervision for discontinuing nonessential medications that may contribute to the dementia.
      (1) Necessary medications should be introduced gradually when

possible, and the client should be observed closely for reaction to medication regimen.

(2) Tranquilizers may be prescribed to lessen agitation, anxiety, and unpredictable behavior.

(3) Benzodiazepines are usually contraindicated, as they tend to increase confusion and lead to paradoxical agitation.

(4) Phenothiazines may cause extrapyramidal effects, such as parkinsonian tremors and dyskinesia.

(5) Medication may be prescribed to improve sleeping patterns.

(6) Associated depression may be alleviated with medication.

(7) Treatment of hypertension may be appropriate for MID but care is needed, as cerebral blood flow may be further reduced by medications.

2. Emphasize the need for the demented client to continue mental and physical activity to:
   a. Prevent premature functional disability.
   b. Maintain function.
   c. Reduce restlessness.

3. Plan for general care of the clients, including:
   a. Personal hygiene.
   b. Good nutrition.
   c. Adequate fluids.
   d. Avoidance of alcohol (as it may contribute to confusion).

4. Stress the need for careful treatment for even minor illness.

5. Teach the family how to protect against complications, such as falls, nighttime confusion, bedsores, incontinence, and fecal impaction. These conditions may present without classic manifestations and may aggravate or cause delirium or dementia.

6. Suggest that the client wear an identification bracelet with name, phone number, and indication of memory impairment. This safeguard may provide reassurance to the client and family.

7. Encourage environmental modifications in the home for safety, such as:
   a. Night lights.
   b. A gate on the stairway.
   c. Hard-to-reach locks on outside doors and the kitchen door.
   d. Keeping doors locked at night.

8. Stress the need for ongoing appropriate reality orientation for the demented client.

9. Minimize sensory deprivation by:
   a. Providing good lighting and appropriate eyeglasses for vision-impaired clients.
   b. Facing hearing-impaired people when talking and encouraging

the use of hearing aids when appropriate. Maintenance of hearing is important because of the tendency toward interpersonal difficulties and paranoia in the deaf elderly.

10. Avoid moving intellectually impaired elderly clients to new locations, as it is difficult for marginally oriented persons to cope with new surroundings.

11. Detailed care of the Alzheimer's victim and family is beyond the scope of this book, but the following references offer practical comprehensive information for their care.

Resources

Alzheimer's Disease and Related Disorders Association, Inc.
70 E. Lake Street
Chicago, IL 60601
(312) 853-3060
(800) 621-0379
(800) 527-6037 in Illinois

Educational materials order form available on request. Alzheimer's Disease and Related Disorders Association (ADRDA), Inc., promotes research and education of health care professionals and families of victims of Alzheimer's disease. ADRDA acts as a spokesperson for the Alzheimer's client to government and social service agencies.

Information Officer
National Institute on Aging (NIA)
Department of Health and Human Services
Building 31, Room 5c-35
9000 Rockville Pike
Bethesda, MD 20205
(301) 496-1752

Publishes brochures and fact sheets on Alzheimer's disease.

Recommended Readings on Alzheimer's Disease and Related Disorders

1. Aronson MK, ed: Understanding Alzheimer's Disease. New York: Charles Scribner's Sons, 1987.*

---

*Available from ADRDA National Headquarters and chapters.

2. Cohen D, Eisdorfer C: The loss of self: A family resource for the care of Alzheimer's disease and related disorders. New York: WW Norton & Co, 1986.
3. Heston LL, White JA: Dementia: A Practical Guide to Alzheimer's Disease and Related Illnesses. New York: WH Freeman & Co, 1983.*
4. Mace NL, Rabins PV: The 36-Hour Day: A Family Guide to Caring for Persons with Alzheimer's Disease and Related Dementing Illnesses. Baltimore: The Johns Hopkins Press, 1981.*
5. McDowell FH, ed: Choosing a Nursing Home for the Person with Intellectual Loss. New York: The Burke Rehabilitation Center, 1980.*
6. McDowell FH, ed: Managing the Person with Intellectual Loss at Home. New York: The Burke Rehabilitation Center, 1980.*

References

Blazer D: Psychiatric disorders. In Rossman I, ed: Clinical Geriatrics. Philadelphia: JB Lippincott Co, 1986.

Blazer DG, Bachar JR, Manton KG: Suicide in late life. Journal of the American Geriatric Society 34:519–525, 1986.

Carnevali DL, Patrick M: Nursing Management for the Elderly. Philadelphia: JB Lippincott Co, 1979.

Carpenito LJ: Nursing Diagnosis: Application to Clinical Practice. Philadelphia: JB Lippincott Co, 1983.

Charatan FB: Affective disorders of the elderly. In Psychiatric Problems of the Aged. Symposium sponsored by the American Academy of Family Physicians and the University of Texas Medical School at Houston, 1981.

Cohen D, Eisdorfer C: Dementing disorders. In Calkins E, Davis PJ, Ford AB eds: The Practice of Geriatrics. Philadelphia: WB Saunders Co, 1986.

Cohen D, Eisdorfer C: Depression. In Calkins E, Davis PJ, Ford AB, eds: The Practice of Geriatrics. Philadelphia: WB Saunders Co, 1986.

Coping & Caring: Living with Alzheimer's Disease. Washington, DC: American Association of Retired Persons, 1986.

Dawson P, Kline K, Wiancko DC, Wells D: Preventing excess disability in patients with Alzheimer's disease. Geriatric Nursing 7:298–301, 1986.

Drachman DA: Ask the doctor. ARDA Newsletter 3:4, 1983.

Ebersole P, Hess P: Toward Healthy Aging. St. Louis: CV Mosby, 1985.

Fitzgerald M: Alzheimer's Disease: Caring for the Caregiver. The DO 8:93–97, 1986.

Gioiella EC, Bevil CW: Nursing Care of the Aging Client. East Norwalk, Conn: Appleton-Century-Crofts, 1985.

Hirst S, Metcalf BJ: Promoting self-esteem. Journal of Gerontological Nursing 10:72–77, 1984.

Levenson AJ: Organic brain syndrome. In Psychiatric Problems of the Aged. Symposium sponsored by the American Academy of Family Physicians and the University of Texas Medical School at Houston, 1981.

Luckmann J, Sorsensen KC: Medical-Surgical Nursing. Philadelphia: WB Saunders Co, 1987.

Rapoport S: Brain in aging and dementia. NIH Pub. No. 83-2625. Bethesda, MD: Clinical Center Office of Clinical Reports & Inquiries, 1984.

St. Pierre J, Craven RF, Bruno P: Late life depression: A guide for assessment. Journal of Gerontological Nursing 12:5–10, 1986.

---

*Available from ADRDA National Headquarters and chapters.

15

Chronic Problems

THE NATURE OF CHRONICITY

1. Most elderly individuals in the community suffer from at least one chronic condition, with those over age 85 (the frail elderly) most likely to suffer from multiple problems.
2. A chronic health problem may be overwhelming to both the elderly and the family, as it is persistent, distressing, and potentially disabling.
3. Reaction to chronicity depends on:
   a. Previous coping behaviors.
   b. Perception of the individual and the family as to the extent and seriousness of the illness or trauma and associated losses.
   c. Availability of resources in the home and community to support rehabilitation.
4. A state of wellness may be achieved if the elderly are able to manage or control these problems and do not allow the problems to significantly interfere with functioning.
5. The goal of the health care provider is to reduce dependency imposed by chronic conditions and to postpone or prevent further decline in function.
6. Strategies for assisting the elderly and the family in coping with chronic problems include:

    a. Postponing chronicity by promoting a healthy lifestyle (adopting health-promoting behaviors).

    b. Encouraging the reduction of risk factors.

    c. Preventing or at least minimizing the effects of risk factors.

    d. Aiming to establish informed management and, when possible, control of chronic health problems so that function is improved and common forms of disability are reversed (e.g., management and control of incontinence).

    e. Offering hope by presenting options, encouraging choices, and strengthening the coping ability of older adults and their families to assume responsibility for their own well-being.

    f. Referring both the client and family to appropriate resources in the community.

CHRONIC PAIN

1. Chronic pain is a subjective experience of distress that lasts longer than 6 months and may be limited (may stop by itself), intermittent, persistent, or intractable (cannot be controlled, relieved, or cured).

2. Because the severity of suffering is often not explained by detectable disease, the nurse must depend on the elaboration of the client as to the presence and character of pain.

3. The response of family, friends, and health care provider to chronic pain is different than their response to acute pain that is readily identified and promptly treated, as ongoing chronic pain is not perceived as life-threatening.

    a. When there is a physical cause for chronic pain, family members may show concern and empathy, but the relationship between the client and family is often characterized by guilt-ridden attentiveness and periodic angry outbursts.

    b. Friends may avoid the client and gradually fade away.

    c. Accusations of laziness or malingering and dismissal from work may occur.

4. The elderly may adapt to chronic pain with few behavioral or physical changes, but maladaptation may occur with depression, withdrawal, isolation, anger, dependency, self-focusing, frustration, limited interests, and increased drug use.

5. Palliative long-term management is the primary focus of treatment.

    a. Too often treatment involves a gradual escalation of progressively more potent analgesics, sedatives, and tranquilizers that often adversely affect the elderly.

    b. Therapy techniques involving behavior modification and noninvasive as well as invasive procedures that help the elderly successfully manage chronic pain are now available.

c. Clients with persistent chronic pain should be referred to pain clinics that specialize in providing modalities for pain reduction.

Response of the Elderly to Chronic Pain

1. Often the elderly deny the reality of the chronic nature of the pain and insist on searching for a total and complete cure. This denial delays the development of active adaptational efforts toward living with the pain.
2. The individual's ability to work, think, or sleep is impaired as the experience of pain becomes nagging and persistent. At times, the will to live is reduced and suicidal preoccupation ensues.
3. The elder may use pain for secondary gains, such as increased attention, affection, or financial reward for disability.
4. Physical dependence, sleeplessness, and fatigue may be camouflaged as combativeness, noncooperation, withdrawal, or depression.
5. Psychogenic pain may be associated with the effects of multiple losses, as the elderly more readily focus on physical symptoms rather than on the distressing feelings associated with losses of friends, loved ones, health, and status.
6. Unresolved grieving may precipitate headache, back pain, or chest pain occurring at the anniversary of a significant loss.
7. Early life experiences and cultural and religious backgrounds influence the meaning of pain and lead to expressions of different levels of pain in response to essentially the same problem.
   a. Individuals whose religious beliefs teach that pain is a means of obtaining grace or is a punishment of God that is "good for the soul" are more likely to be accepting and stoical with pain.
   b. Cultural influences may affect attitudes about pain expectancy (belief that pain is unavoidable in certain situations) and pain acceptance (willingness to accept pain).
   c. The state of anxiety provoked by pain includes the concern about the unknown, the loneliness caused by pain, the helplessness rising from pain, and the threat to self-image or body image.
   d. How readily a client complains of pain appears to be related to his culture.
      (1) Clients of a Mediterranean culture may admit to pain more readily than those of a northern European culture.
      (2) An Italian may complain verbally of his present discomfort.
      (3) A Jew may complain and cry also, but may be concerned about the threat of the pain.

(4) A so-called "Old American" or Wasp (white Anglo-Saxon Protestant) may be stoical and may tend to avoid complaining and provoking pity by minimizing pain.

Reasons for Inadequate Treatment for the Client with Chronic Pain

1. The tendency to accept pain with aging as though it were to be expected leads to failure in reporting pain and delay in treating the problem.
2. The belief that the elderly are hypochondriacal leads to failure in taking their complaints seriously.
3. The care giver may deny the pain of the chronic sufferer, who, in refusing to improve, threatens the care giver's self-image as a provider of relief, comfort, cure, and restoration.
   a. Denial of the client's pain reduces feelings of guilt or helplessness suffered by the health care provider.
4. Atypical presentation of pain in the elderly contributes to the difficulty of determining the cause.
   a. The elderly seem to be more sensitive to deep pain and less sensitive to cutaneous pain.
   b. See under "Anginal Equivalents" in Chapter 13.
5. Misjudgment in attributing less intense pain to those suffering the longest occurs.
6. The client who experiences neither relief of pain nor the satisfaction of being understood withdraws and stops complaining.

Assessment for Pain

1. Difficulties in assessing pain or factors influencing pain experience in the elderly include the following:
   a. Pain itself cannot be observed because it is a subjective experience.
   b. The health care provider must depend on the elaboration of the client as to the presence and character of the pain.
   c. Differentiating between organic pain resulting from a physical cause and psychogenic pain reflecting emotional losses is problematic.
   d. Pain presentation may be atypical in the elderly.
   e. The gravity of the cause of the pain is not necessarily correlated with the amount of pain felt.
   f. The threshold for pain differs in individuals.

2. The nurse should ask the client for the following information associated with the pain:
   a. Onset.
   b. Mode of onset.
   c. Duration.
   d. Location.
   e. Quality.
   f. Time of occurrence.
   g. Provoking factors.
   h. Relieving factors.
3. Appropriate questioning will identify severe problems and break the silence that may be associated with pain. Questions should include:
   a. Where does it hurt?
   b. When did it begin?
   c. What are the best and worst times of the day?
   d. Which treatment relieves the pain?
   e. Which activities make the pain worse?
4. The nurse should ask the client to rate pain on a scale of zero to ten, with zero representing no pain and ten representing the worst pain the client can imagine.
5. Rating of pain is helpful at the initial assessment, before and after treatments, and at different points in time to help in the evaluation of the character of the pain and the response to therapy.

Strategies for Relief of Chronic Pain

1. Help the client to identify factors contributing to pain and to deal constructively with them.
2. Recognize that pain is not inevitable, intolerable, or unmanageable, and transmit this to the client so that he will be infused with some hope and belief.
3. Help the client to understand what can and what cannot be done to relieve the pain.
4. Work with the elderly client and the family to reduce the intensity of pain and pain behavior by using measures to lessen secondary gains, anxiety, fear, and depression.
5. Refer the client to a local pain control clinic where the following options available for control of chronic pain may be explored:
   a. Medication.
      (1) Benefit and risk must be considered in long-term use of medication.

       (2) Analgesia often subjects the elderly to side effects of medication and to drug-drug or food-drug interactions.

       (3) Tolerance to a drug leads to the need for larger dosage with increased risk.

   b. Applications of heat or cold.

   c. Massage.

   d. Passive stretching exercises.

   e. Behavioral techniques.

       (1) Meditation.

       (2) Biofeedback.

       (3) Guided imagery.

       (4) Progressive relaxation training.

   f. Acupuncture or acupressure.

   g. Transcutaneous electrical nerve stimulation (TENS).

   h. Hypnosis.

   i. Nerve blocks (injection with local anesthetics).

   j. Neurosurgical procedures for pain relief (recommended mostly for intractable pain).

6. Encourage involvement in work, family, social, and recreational interests to reduce focusing on self and to lessen involvement with matters of illness and pain.

Resources

International Pain Foundation
909 N.E. 43rd Street, Suite 306
Seattle, WA 98105-6020
(206) 547-2157

   Publishes a newsletter and booklets providing information on new developments in pain research and therapy.

National Chronic Pain Outreach Association
4922 Hampden Lane
Bethesda, MD 20814
(301) 652-4948

   Provides information on local branches of support groups.

American Chronic Pain Association
257 Old Haymaker Road

Monroeville, PA 15146
(412) 856-9676

Provides information on local branches of support groups.

Commission on Accreditation of Rehabilitation Facilities
2500 North Pantano Road
Tucson, AZ 85715
(602) 886-8575

Provides a list of facilities with currently accredited pain programs on request.

OSTEOPOROSIS

1. Osteoporosis is a reduction in total bone mass that makes the individual highly susceptible to incurring fractures of the wrist, vertebrae, and hip with little or no precipitating trauma.
2. In the past, occurrence of the disease was identified predominantly in postmenopausal women; however, as the elderly live longer, osteoporosis is also prevalent in men over 80 years of age.
3. At least 25% of women over the age of 65 have back pain, deformity, or loss of height caused by vertebral fractures resulting from osteoporosis.
4. The pathogenesis of osteoporosis is not clear at this time, as the causes appear to be multifactorial.
5. Identification of important factors that predispose an individual to osteoporosis is vital for assessing risk and for planning prevention and treatment.
6. Since no therapy has been found to reverse osteoporosis, the goals of therapy are to stabilize bone mass and to prevent future fractures.
7. Prevention of osteoporosis is a major goal of health care of the elderly, as the complications of osteoporosis cause pain, deformity, and major disability; significantly reduce the quality of life; and require more than $3 billion annually for the provision of health care.

Bone Composition, Remodeling, and Aging

1. Bones are composed of differing proportions of cortical tissue (solid, dense) and trabecular tissue (porous, resembling a honeycomb).
   a. The long bones (tubular bones) are composed mainly of cortical tissue with areas of trabecular tissue at the ends.

    b. The vertebrae (cancellous bones) consist primarily of trabecular tissue surrounded by a thin layer of cortical tissue.

    c. Cancellous bone is most prone to the effects of osteoporotic changes.

2. Bones maintain themselves by remodeling, a continuous cyclical process of resorption as small parts of old bone are removed and new bone is formed.

3. This process is tightly coupled during growth, with the rate of bone formation on the outer surface exceeding resorption (breakdown of bone on the inner surface lining the marrow cavity) until a person reaches the early thirties when peak bone mass is achieved.

    a. Peak bone mass is generally 25% greater in men than in women.

4. At approximately age 35, a little more bone is lost than is remodeled.

    a. Bone loss continues at a faster rate in women than in men.

    b. Accelerated bone loss for 5 to 10 years following menopause is superimposed on the already occurring age-related loss in women.

    c. Bone loss occurs silently over a period of years.

    d. The major sites of fracture in osteoporosis are in trabecular bone tissue of the vertebral body, proximal femur, and distal radius.

Late-Life Osteoporosis Syndrome

1. Type 1 (postmenopausal) osteoporosis occurs in women between the ages of 60 and 80 as postmenopausal estrogen deficiency accelerates vertebral (trabecular) bone loss and spontaneous fractures occur most commonly of the eight to 12 thoracic vertebrae and the first three lumbar vertebrae.

2. Type 2 (senile) osteoporosis occurs as a result of the small but steady decline in bone mass (trabecular and cortical) with age that makes the elderly (especially those who started out with a relatively low bone mass) more susceptible to fractures with falls.

Risk Factors for the Development of Osteoporosis

1. Genetic background and body characteristics.

    a. White women with a northwestern European background are at especially high risk, while women of Mediterranean background are at lower risk.

    b. Thin, slender women with fair skin, light hair, and light eye color are at high risk.

       (1) Overweight women are at lower risk, as estrogen is available

to them from adrenal androgens converted to estrogen in fatty tissue, and they experience more load-bearing with mechanical stress that helps maintain bone mass.

   c. Black women have a greater bone mass and are not at high risk for development of osteoporosis.
2. Diet.
   a. Low calcium intake increases the risk of developing osteoporosis.
      (1) Women generally consume less calcium than recommended from adolescence on.
      (2) Absorption of calcium is reduced in the elderly.
      (3) Lactose intolerance results in reduced calcium intake.
   b. Vitamin D deficiency interferes with the absorption of calcium by the intestines.
   c. High amounts of protein in the diet may cause excessive excretion of calcium via the kidney.
3. Early onset of menopause, which appears to result in an earlier accelerated reduction in bone mass.
   a. Cigarette smoking is associated with an earlier than normal menopause.
4. Lack of exercise that allows for further bone loss.
   a. Regular exercise helps maintain bone mass and even stimulates formation of new bone.
   b. Immobilization is associated with bone loss from the lumbar vertebrae, which the elderly may not be able to restore.
5. High intake of caffeine and alcohol.
6. Use of certain drugs, such as corticosteroids, isoniazid, tetracycline, some anticonvulsants, aluminum-containing antacids, thyroid supplements, furosemide, and heparin.
7. Endocrine, kidney, and vitamin D–related disorders; multiple myeloma; rheumatoid arthritis; diabetes mellitus; advanced alcoholism; and cirrhosis of the liver associated with a higher risk of developing secondary osteoporosis.

Strategies for Prevention

1. Ensure adequate calcium intake. The diet should contain foods high in calcium (Table 15–1).
   a. If the daily diet does not include at least 800 mg of calcium for the premenopausal woman and at least 1500 mg for the postmenopausal woman and older man, supplementation with elemental calcium should be used.
   b. Calcium carbonate, 40% elemental calcium, is well tolerated, inexpensive, and even well absorbed with achlorhydria.

Table 15–1. *Calcium Content of Some Common Foods**

Food†	Weight or Measure	Calcium (mg)
Plain skim and low-fat yogurts	1 cup	
Low-fat flavored and fruited yogurts	1 cup	
Dry nonfat milk	¼ cup	350–450
Sardines, with bones	3 ounces	
Some fruited yogurts	1 cup	
Skim and low-fat milks	1 cup	
Whole milk, chocolate milk, and buttermilk	1 cup	250–350
Swiss and Gruyère cheeses	1 ounce	
Hard cheeses, such as Cheddar and Edam	1 ounce	
Processed cheeses	1 ounce	
Cheese spreads	1 ounce	150–250
Salmon, with bones	3 ounces	
Collards	½ cup	
Cheese foods	1 ounce	
Soft cheeses, such as mozzarella, blue, and feta	1 ounce	
Cooked dried beans, such as navy, pea, and lima	1 cup	
Turnip greens, kale, dandelion greens	½ cup	
Ice creams and ice milks	½ cup	
Evaporated whole milk	1 ounce	50–150
Cottage cheeses	½ cup	
Sherbets	½ cup	
Broccoli	½ cup	
Orange	1 fresh	
Dates, raisins	¼ cup	
Egg	1	
Bread, whole wheat or white	1 slice	20–50
Cabbage	½ cup	
Cream cheese	1 ounce	

*From Health and Human Services Pub. No. 85-2198 (FDA).

†The foods within each grouping are generally listed in order of decreasing calcium content. Calcium content falls within the ranges shown in the right-hand column.

    c. Elemental calcium content, rather than total weight of the supplement, should be noted. An antacid, e.g., Tums, is probably the least expensive form of supplementation that provides 40% of elemental calcium carbonate in a 500-mg tablet.

    d. Calcium supplements are best taken on an empty stomach.

    e. Bone meal and dolomite (a rock mineral resource) should be *avoided,* as these two forms of calcium supplement may contain lead in levels high enough to pose a health hazard.

    f. Because calcium supplements may interfere with other medications, such as tetracyclines, iron, phenothiazines, and levodopa, they should not be taken within 1 to 2 hours of other drugs.

    g. Calcium supplements containing vitamin D should be avoided, as their use may lead to excessive toxic intake of vitamin D.

    h. Use of calcium in those who have nephrolithiasis or hypercal-

cinuria must be carefully monitored and may even be contraindicated.

2. Ensure that 400 IU of vitamin D are obtained daily. See "Vitamin
   D" under "Nutritional Recommendations" in Chapter 4.
3. Avoid high levels of protein in the diet. See "Protein" under "Nutritional Recommendations" in Chapter 4.
4. Restrict excessive use of alcohol and caffeine-containing beverages.
5. Do not smoke cigarettes.
6. Perform regular exercise that places moderate stress on the spine
   and long bones of the body, such as walking, dancing, and bicycle
   riding, at least several times a week.
   a. As little as 1 hour a week of weight-bearing exercise appears to
      reduce bone loss and may even stimulate increased growth of
      new bone.
   b. High-risk clients should exercise daily.
   c. The exercise program should begin slowly and build up to three
      to five sessions a week.
   d. Women should include more walking in their daily activities. For
      example, parking the car a short distance from a destination and
      then walking provides an opportunity for exercise.

Presentation of Osteoporosis

1. Most clients with osteoporosis are symptom-free until they experience a fracture.
2. The precipitating factor may be minimal trauma resulting from
   activities such as opening a window, making a bed, stepping off a
   curb, coughing, stooping, or receiving a hug.
3. As osteoporosis progresses, the collapse of the anterior side of the
   vertebra (a wedge fracture) is followed with collapse of the posterior
   side of the vertebra. Collapse of both the anterior and posterior
   sides is termed a compression fracture, a crush fracture, or a totally
   collapsed vertebra.
4. A client with a new vertebral fracture may complain of a sudden,
   sharp, severe pain over a vertebral process, worsened by motion
   and accompanied by localized tenderness and muscle spasm.
   a. Acute pain usually subsides in 1 to 3 months after the bone heals
      into a new collapsed form.
   b. During the chronic phase, the client is more likely to complain
      of chronic dull back pain from paravertebral muscle spasm re-
      lated to the mechanical stress on ligaments, muscles, and joints.
   c. There is no correlation between the severity of the damage pres-

ent and the degree of pain perceived by the client. Even with totally collapsed vertebrae, some clients do not report pain.

d. New compression fractures occur at a variable rate.

5. Increased lumbar lordosis, progressive dorsal kyphosis ("dowager's hump"), loss of height (1 to 3 inches), and a protruding abdomen result from multiple vertebral fractures over time and present body image problems.

6. Decreases in both chest and abdominal volume occur.

a. Reduced pulmonary capacity leads to exercise intolerance.

b. Reduced abdominal capacity leads to early feelings of satiety.

7. A fracture in the distal radius often results in a deformed wrist.

8. Abnormal gait may be related to a previous fracture of the proximal femur.

9. Periodontal disease may be a manifestation of osteoporosis.

Diagnostic Studies

1. Osteoporosis is difficult to diagnose because the usual diagnostic tests do not reveal bone loss until substantial damage is done or a fracture has occurred.

2. Laboratory studies of serum and urine chemistries are generally normal.

3. X-ray demonstrates the presence of fractures but does not quantify bone mineral content and unequivocal changes until 20 to 25% of mineral content of the bone has been reduced.

4. Single-beam photon absorptiometry is used to measure the mineral content of the forearm. This method may miss bone abnormality because only one third of the clients with clinical osteoporosis demonstrate decreased bone mass in the bones of the limbs (appendicular skeleton).

5. Computed tomography and dual-photon absorptiometry are screening and follow-up techniques used to measure both the trabecular and cortical bone in the vertebrae.

a. Dual-photon absorptiometry is not available in many centers.

b. Tomography is widely available, but the exposure to radiation and errors caused by fat content of the bone marrow are disadvantages.

6. Differentiation between primary osteoporosis and secondary osteoporosis is important for determining appropriate treatment.

7. Bone biopsies are used for ruling out other pathology.

Treatment

1. The previously detailed measures for prevention are also applicable for treatment of osteoporosis.

2. Calcium supplementation aids in the treatment of osteoporosis.
   a. Oral calcium supplementation is recommended for the elderly
      based on:
      (1) The decline in the ability of the intestines to adapt to low
          calcium intake with age.
      (2) Some evidence indicating that calcium may reduce the rate
          of bone loss and the incidence of fractures.
      (3) The inability of many older people to tolerate enough milk
          or eat enough other foods for adequate calcium intake.
   b. Calcium supplementation to 1500 mg/day is recommended to
      correct negative calcium balance, reduce bone loss, and possibly
      decrease the frequency and number of fractures.
3. Vitamin D is needed to increase calcium absorption and utilization.
4. Treatment for acute pain related to a recent vertebral fracture may
   be managed at home, provided that the client is cooperative and
   has sufficient assistance available.
   a. Bed rest for 1 to 3 weeks provides the most effective relief.
      (1) A hard mattress, with a board between the mattress and box
          spring for firm support and a sheepskin covering over the
          mattress to provide soft contact with the spine, is recom-
          mended.
      (2) The client may lie on her back with a thin pillow under her
          head and a pillow under the knees to avoid undue strain on
          the spine.
      (3) The client may lie on her side rather than on her back with
          a pillow to support the back and a pillow between the bent
          knees until the pain subsides enough to allow turning freely
          with minimal discomfort.
      (4) Long periods of immobilization are to be avoided, as further
          loss of bone mass may occur with the risk of new fractures.
   b. Common analgesics, such as aspirin or acetaminophen, and mus-
      cle relaxants generally provide relief of pain, but codeine or
      propoxyphene hydrochloride may be required to relieve pain.
   c. A laxative may be needed to maintain bowel movements.
   d. Careful use of a heating lamp or pad and gentle massage are
      often helpful.
   e. Persistent pain after 2 to 3 weeks may require provision of a back
      support to enable ambulation.
      (1) At first, the client is to sit for short periods (15 minutes) that
          are increased in frequency to about eight times daily.
      (2) After sitting becomes comfortable, progressive ambulation is
          started with short, frequent periods of walking that are grad-
          ually lengthened.

   f. For at least 2 to 3 months after the fracture, an intermittent rest regimen should be followed with the client lying in a horizontal position for 15 to 20 minutes every 2 to 3 hours during the day.

5. Treatment for pain in the lumbosacral area that occurs when the client is ambulatory most of the day (1 to 3 months following the vertebral collapse) is applicable.
   a. Increased lumbar lordosis that compensates for the collapsed vertebrae causes pain that is greater with activity but is alleviated by horizontal rest.
   b. Treatment with continuation of the intermittent rest regimen, rather than the use of analgesia, is preferable.
   c. The pain passes within 3 to 9 months when local structural adaptations take place.

6. Treatment for chronic dull pain related to paravertebral muscle spasm consists of the use of acetaminophen (e.g., Tylenol), propoxyphene hydrochloride (e.g., Darvon), and gentle massage. Use of narcotics should be avoided.

7. Long-term treatment involving exercises to improve posture, increase muscle tone, and loosen stiff joints is best designed for the individual client by a physiotherapist.
   a. Daily walking with rubber-soled shoes is helpful.
   b. Extension exercises of the spine are recommended.
   c. Flexion exercises of the spine are contraindicated, as they increase the vertical compression forces on the vertebrae.

8. Avoidance of a high-protein diet, excessive alcohol and caffeine ingestion, and cigarette smoking is recommended.

9. The use of estrogen therapy in the treatment of primary osteoporosis remains somewhat controversial.
   a. By preventing rapid bone loss, estrogen may prevent osteoporotic fractures after menopause; however, it does not restore bone loss or reduce fractures in those with osteoporosis.
   b. Because bone loss may accelerate after discontinuing estrogen, lifelong therapy may be necessary.
   c. Therapy with estrogen increases the risk of endometrial cancer and gallbladder disease.
   d. Cyclic therapy with the use of progestin in addition to the estrogen seems to protect against endometrial cancer but increases the risk of hypertension, coronary artery disease, fluid retention, and thromboembolic phenomena.

10. Therapy with sodium fluoride is used with calcium and vitamin D primarily for clients who continue to experience vertebral crush fractures.
    a. Fluoride tends to increase trabecular bone mass, but by concur-

rently decreasing cortical bone mass, fluoride places the client more at risk for femoral fracture.

   b. Fluoride therapy takes about 1 year before it affects progression of the disease.

   c. Therapeutic doses of 40 to 50 mg/day are required, often resulting in arthralgia, epigastric pain, and nausea.

11. Calcitonin has stimulated increased trabecular bone volume, but, because it is expensive and is associated with severe toxic effects, it has not found wide acceptance and use.

Strategies for Coping with Osteoporosis

1. Reassure the client that some improvement in chronic back pain is likely to occur with an intermittent rest regimen.
2. Advise the client to follow strategies for prevention of osteoporosis, as detailed previously.
3. Stress the importance of measures to prevent fractures. Teach the client to:
   a. Avoid lifting heavy weights, stooping, or bending to pick up objects.
   b. Avoid sports with risk of trauma, such as horseback riding and basketball.
   c. Improve safety of the environment by removing loose rugs and avoiding stairs without sturdy banisters.
   d. Use a cane for balance to reduce the chance of falling.
   e. Wear low rubber heels and cushioned soles to reduce trauma to the back when walking.
   f. Avoid immobilization to prevent further bone loss.
   g. Avoid twisting the body to the side when sitting in and rising from a chair.
   h. Get into a car by sitting sideways with both legs outside the car, then lifting both legs together and swinging them into the car. Use the same process in reverse when getting out of a car and then stand up.
   i. Participate in a regular planned exercise program recommended by a physician or a physiotherapist.
   j. Reduce the use of drugs that impair balance, such as barbiturates, or drugs that increase bone loss, such as glucocorticoids, when possible.

Resource

Osteoporosis Prevention Program
University of Connecticut
Health Center
Farmington, CT 06032
(203) 679-2129
Boning Up: A Guide to Osteoporosis Prevention (1985)

DIGESTIVE PROBLEMS

1. The elderly are increasingly susceptible to digestive problems associated with primary aging changes that reduce appetite, interfere with absorption of nutrients, and cause them discomfort and embarrassment.
2. A better understanding of the nature and causes of primary digestive changes enables the elderly to choose strategies that minimize their impact.
3. Recognition and reporting of the warning signals of serious secondary changes, often erroneously attributed to aging, are essential for appropriate diagnostic studies and treatment to promote wellness.

Causes of Digestive Problems in the Elderly

1. Primary aging changes, such as:
   a. Disturbed motility of the esophagus causes a disorganized response to swallowing and delayed transit time.
   b. The lower esophageal sphincter often becomes incompetent, and reflux esophagitis occurs.
   c. Impaired gastric motility delays gastric emptying.
   d. A decrease in gastric production of hydrochloric acid and pepsin interferes with digestion of protein and iron.
   e. Atrophy of the lining of the small intestine with broadening and shortening of the villi results in subclinical degrees of malabsorption of amino acids, carbohydrates, and fats.
   f. Reduced tone and motility of the colon may result in constipation.
2. Seondary changes, such as:
   a. Peptic ulcer.
   b. Gallbladder disease.
   c. Gastritis.

    d. Viral gastroenteritis.
    e. Cancer of the stomach.
    f. Pancreatic disease.
3. Lifestyle changes, such as:
    a. Increased use of medications.
    b. Reduced exercise.
    c. Changes in eating habits.
4. Indigestion may occur for no apparent reason.

ASSESSMENT FOR CAUSES OF DIGESTIVE PROBLEMS

1. A health history should be obtained first.
2. Physical and psychosocial assessment should follow.
3. Check for presence of the following warning signs of secondary changes:
    a. Severe stomach pains that last a long time; are recurring; or come with shaking, chills, and cold, clammy skin.
    b. Bloody or recurrent vomiting.
    c. Sudden change in bowel habits and consistency of stools lasting more than a few days (e.g., diarrhea lasting longer than 3 days) or the sudden onset of constipation.
    d. Overt blood in stools or black stools.
    e. Jaundice of the skin, eyes, or dark or brown-colored urine.
    f. Pain or difficulty in swallowing food.
    g. Prolonged loss of appetite or unexplained weight loss.
    h. Diarrhea that wakes the client at night.
4. Diagnostic procedures, such as gastrointestinal series, sonogram, tomography, X-rays, endoscopy, and routine blood and urine tests, are indicated if the above warning signs occur or if the indigestion is severe enough to interfere with daily routine.

Common Digestive Problems

CONSTIPATION

For a complete discussion of constipation, see Chapter 3 under "Constipation."

DIVERTICULOSIS

1. Small pouchings or sacs in the wall of the colon sometimes produced by chronic constipation.

2. Usually is asymptomatic, but occasionally may cause pain in the left lower quadrant of the abdomen.
3. A diet high in fiber and liquids recommended.

DIVERTICULITIS

1. Diverticulitis is an inflammation of the diverticula of the colon with collection of bacteria and other irritating material in the pouches.
2. Muscle spasms and cramplike pain in the abdomen occur, especially in the lower left quadrant.
3. Mild attacks are treated at home with a bed rest, liquid diet, anticholinergics, nonopiate analgesics, and antibiotics.
4. Hospitalization is required for management of a severe attack.

INDIGESTION (DYSPEPSIA)

1. Symptoms of indigestion are as follows:
   a. Nausea.
   b. Regurgitation (backwash of stomach contents into the esophagus or mouth).
   c. Vomiting.
   d. Heartburn.
   e. Prolonged upper abdominal fullness, or bloating after a meal.
   f. Stomach discomfort and pain.
2. Causes of indigestion are those noted earlier for digestive problems.
3. Treatment is instituted after diagnostic studies are completed.
   a. Specific therapy is instituted for a secondary change.
   b. In the absence of a specific illness, the following dietary precautions are recommended:
      (1) Avoid greasy foods or solid foods containing meat.
      (2) If the client is lactose-intolerant, use only milk and milk products treated for lactose (Lactaid).
      (3) For severe symptoms, follow a liquid diet or eat soft foods in small amounts until symptoms subside.

GAS

Gas (flatus) is normal in the gastrointestinal tract and is usually eliminated by belching or by expelling the gas through the rectum.
1. Gas may collect in some portion of the gastrointestinal tract and lead to pain, distention, and bloating.
   a. Bloating after eating is thought to be due to gas, but no con-

nection has been demonstrated between the symptoms and total amount of gas in the abdomen.
  b. Some people (especially after eating) experience intestinal spasm with pain with normal amounts of gas.
  c. Upper abdominal pressure and pain after eating may be relieved by belching.
  d. Gas that accumulates on the right side of the colon may cause pain similar to that caused by gallbladder disease.
  e. Gas in the upper left portion of the colon may precipitate splenic flexure syndrome, with pain spreading to the left side of the chest that may be confused with angina of heart disease.
  f. Abdominal distention may occur during the day and is most severe after the largest meal.
    (1) Distention occurs more frequently in women who have been pregnant or in those individuals who have lax abdominal rectus muscles as a result of age or disease.
    (2) Distention present during sitting or standing but absent when lying down is probably due to muscular weakness rather than gas. Exercises to improve tone of abdominal muscles or a support garment are then indicated.
2. Causes of extra gas in the gastrointestinal tract include:
  a. More frequent swallowing that occurs when a person has a post-nasal drip or chews gum.
  b. Rapid eating.
  c. Poorly fitting dentures.
  d. Drinking carbonated beverages.
  e. Eating gas-producing foods, such as cauliflower, Brussels sprouts, brown beans, broccoli, bran, or cabbage.
  f. Increasing fiber intake too rapidly.
  g. Ingestion of milk and milk products when lactase-deficient.
3. Recent research suggests that if the electrical impulses that govern the motion of the gastrointestinal tract are disrupted, disorganization occurs with a variety of symptoms, including pain, diarrhea, constipation, bloating, and a sensation of too much gas in the system.
4. Persistent, troublesome increase in the frequency or severity of belching or flatus requires assessment for secondary changes by a physician.
5. Teach the client the following strategies for reducing gas in the digestive tract:
  a. Eat meals slowly, and chew food thoroughly.
  b. Check with a dentist to make sure that dentures fit properly.
  c. Avoid chewing gum or sucking on hard candies.

d. Eliminate carbonated beverages like beer and soda from the diet.
e. Avoid milk and milk products if there is lactose intolerance unless the food has been treated with lactase.
f. Eat fewer gas-producing foods.
g. Try exercises, such as sit-ups, to increase tone if abdominal distention is a problem, unless such exercises are contraindicated by another condition.

HEARTBURN AND ESOPHAGEAL REFLUX

Heartburn and regurgitation of acid reflux may reflect the presence of hiatal hernia or incompetency of the lower esophageal sphincter.

1. Heartburn is experienced as a burning pain behind the breast bone that occurs after meals and may last from minutes to hours.
2. Hiatal hernia may produce mild heartburn after dietary indiscretion, but the condition is not clinically significant.
3. Strategies for preventing heartburn and regurgitation are geared toward reducing the frequency and volume of acid reflux. Teach the client to:
   a. Avoid the use of the following in the diet:
      • Tomato products
      • Juices
      • Fats and fried foods
      • Peppermint
      • Coffee
      • Tea
      • Chocolate
      • Cola drinks
   b. Avoid the use of anticholinergics, female hormones, alcohol, and nicotine in cigarettes, as these agents potentiate lower esophageal dysfunction.
   c. Avoid overdistending the stomach by eating excessively or by drinking large quantities of fluids with meals.
   d. Use antacids, cimetidine, or ranitidine as ordered for relief.
   e. Avoid eating for several hours before going to bed.
   f. Avoid the use of tight corsets or body braces when possible.
   g. Raise the head of the bed 4 to 8 inches or elevate the shoulders with a support or pillow at an angle of at least 30 degrees when sleeping to prevent reflux.

    h. Follow appropriate diet and exercise guidelines when weight loss is advisable.

    i. Not smoke.

IRRITABLE BOWEL SYNDROME

Irritable bowel syndrome (IBS) accounts for about 31% of gastrointestinal disorders in those over age 65 and is the most common gastrointestinal problem of the elderly.

1. IBS is also known as functional bowel disease, spastic colon, colitis, and mucous colitis. IBS does not cause inflammation and is not to be confused with ulcerative colitis.
2. The signs and symptoms of IBS may be continuous and long-standing or recurrent over years, but are not associated with any demonstrable organic disease.
   a. Clients with IBS usually have some combination of constipation and diarrhea as well as pain, gas, and abdominal bloating.
3. Diet and stress seem to be the factors that trigger abnormal colon function in those who suffer from IBS.
   a. An urge to defecate within 30 to 60 minutes after eating may normally occur. In people with IBS, the urge often occurs within a shorter period of time and is accompanied by cramps and sometimes diarrhea.
   b. The severity of the response depends on the number of calories in a meal and especially on the amount of fat, the strongest stimulus of colonic contractions after a meal.
   c. In the elderly, recent onset of IBS is often correlated with the stress of illness or death of a family member, poverty, estrangement from children, relocation, or recognition of mortality.
4. A conservative approach with reassurance and diet therapy is first initiated.
5. Treatment for the elderly includes reassurance; supportive psychotherapy; diet regulation; and judicious administration of medication, such as antacids, antispasmodics, bulk agents (e.g., Metamucil), and if needed, psychoactive drugs.
6. Teach the client the following strategies for preventing the discomforts of IBS:
   a. Avoid those foods that cause distress.
   b. Include whole-grain breads and cereals, fruit, and vegetables, as high-fiber diets keep the colon mildly distended and help prevent spasm. Some fiber, by keeping water in the stool, prevents constipation.
   c. Increase fiber in diet slowly initially to minimize gas and bloating.

These symptoms tend to dissipate over time as the gastrointestinal tract becomes used to increased fiber intake.
  d. Eat smaller portions of each food at mealtimes, and eat more frequently if necessary.
  e. Eat foods low in fat and rich in carbohydrates and protein.
     (1) Foods high in carbohydrates and low in fat include:
        • Pasta
        • Breads
        • Fruits
        • Rice
        • Cereals
        • Vegetables
     (2) Foods high in protein and low in fat include:
        • Chicken and turkey (without skin)
        • Skim milk
        • Lean meats
        • Most fish
        • Low-fat cheeses
  f. Use antacids as prescribed to relieve heartburn or epigastric discomfort after eating.
  g. Be alert to side effects if antispasmodics, such as phenobarbital-belladonna mixtures or donnatal, are used. If side effects occur, report to the physician for decrease or withdrawal of medication.
  h. Learn to regulate diet.

Lactose Intolerance

Lactose intolerance occurs more frequently in the elderly than in the younger population, as older individuals are increasingly unable to digest milk and milk products properly as a result of a deficiency of the enzyme lactase needed to digest lactose.
  1. Cramps, gas, bloating, and diarrhea may occur 15 minutes to several hours after milk or a milk product is consumed.
  2. Teach the client the following strategies for managing lactose intolerance:
     a. Use dairy products commercially treated with lactase or add lactase enzyme (sold in health food stores) to regular milk when possible.
     b. Eat smaller servings of dairy products.
     c. Eat fewer dairy products, but add other foods that contain calcium to the diet (see Table 15–1).

Resources

American Digestive Disease Society (ADDS)
7720 Wisconsin Avenue
Bethesda, MD 20814
(301) 652-9293

Provides materials on digestive diseases.

Information Specialist
National Digestive Diseases Education and Information Clearing-house
1555 Wilson Boulevard, Suite 600
Rosslyn, VA 22209
(301) 496-9707

Provides fact sheets on digestive diseases, a directory of professional and lay digestive disease organizations, and reports on research.

URINARY INCONTINENCE

1. Urinary incontinence may range from slight to severe involuntary losses of urine during the day or night.
2. Incontinence occurs whenever the pressure in the bladder equals or overcomes sphincter resistance.
3. At least one in ten persons aged 65 or older has a problem with loss of urinary control that threatens self-esteem, socialization, and skin integrity.
4. The most frequent causes of incontinence in the elderly are related to neurogenic, anatomic, or infectious problems.
5. Isolation and depression ensue, as the incontinent elderly often withdraw from social life in an attempt to hide the problem of loss of urinary control from family, friends, and even physicians.
6. Lack of knowledge about possibilities for treatment and the belief that nursing-home care is the only choice available are common and all too frequently lead to institutionalization of the incontinent elderly.
7. Following assessment, incontinence can be treated, controlled, and possibly cured in many elderly.

The Mechanism of Micturition (Voiding)

1. The process by which the urinary bladder empties itself is a reflex act subject to learned voluntary control.
2. When the bladder fills to about 150 ml, the first urge to void is felt, and fullness is experienced around 400 ml.
3. When the bladder contains about 200 to 300 ml of urine, the detrusor muscle (outer wall of the bladder) is stimulated to send impulses to the sacral portion of the spinal cord, where the micturition reflex is initiated.
4. The sensory impulses also travel to the brain, where the sensation of a full bladder and a desire to void arise.
5. Unless inhibited, the detrusor muscle of the bladder begins to rhythmically contract and force the urine out through the relaxed internal and external sphincter of the urethra until the bladder is completely empty.
6. The adult may voluntarily inhibit the emptying reflex for a length of time, but as the bladder fills and pressure increases, inhibition of the emptying reflex is impossible and the bladder empties itself completely.

Assessment for Causes of Urinary Incontinence

1. A health history is obtained.
2. Physical, neurologic, and psychosocial examinations follow.
3. A urinalysis is performed.
4. A urine culture is obtained.
   a. An elderly woman must be instructed how to obtain a "clean catch" in midstream. Aseptic technique must be emphasized to prevent contamination.
      (1) If the initial clean catch is abnormal, a sterile catheterization is indicated.
   b. After retracting the prepuce, a man must cleanse the glans and meatus to obtain a clean catch.
5. A catheterization is done if there is a question of residual urine in order to measure the postvoid residual.
6. The simplest tests for diagnosis are used rather than more complex tests, which are reserved for complicated or unexplained incontinence.

Transient Urinary Incontinence

1. Transient urinary incontinence occurs in conjunction with:
   a. Acute medical illness.

    b. Urinary tract infection.

    c. Constipation.

    d. Diarrhea.

    e. Atrophic vaginitis.

    f. Clouding of the sensorium, as with metabolic derangement and electrolyte imbalance.

    g. Side effects of medication.

    h. Episodes of cardiovascular crisis.

2. Treatment requires identifying the precipitating condition and treating it aggressively. For example, treating atrophic vaginitis with an estrogen preparation (e.g., Premarin cream), applied with an applicator usually one to two times a week for 6 weeks, usually resolves transient incontinence caused by the vaginitis.

3. Strategies for care of the client experiencing transient incontinence include the following:

    a. Explain that this incontinence is only temporary and should resolve itself with aggressive treatment of the precipitating condition.

    b. Review the recommended treatment with the client for understanding and ability and intent to comply.

    c. Urge the establishment of regular toileting as soon as possible to prevent incontinence from becoming established.

Established Urge Urinary Incontinence

1. Urge incontinence is characterized by an urge to void preceding an uncontrolled loss of urine, with failure to hold urine long enough to reach a toilet.

2. Cause of urge incontinence is related to infection of the lower urinary tract, neurologic damage, or bladder spasms.

3. There is usually a history of urinary frequency and loss of urine during the day and at night.

4. Treatment is directed toward reducing bladder spasm or increasing bladder capacity.

    a. Medication, such as anticholinergic drugs or anticholinergic antispasmodic drugs, is effective in controlling 85% of cases of urge incontinence.

    b. Behavioral management techniques may be used in conjunction with medication.

    c. Surgery involving bladder denervation or augmentation usually is not indicated for the elderly.

5. Strategies for care of the client experiencing urge incontinence include the following:

a. Teach bladder-training techniques to improve perception of bladder fullness, and to delay voiding in conjunction with prescribed medication.

b. Instruct the client to:
   (1) Establish regular voiding habits compatible with the client's lifestyle.
   (2) Try to void at least every 2 hours and to be sensitive to feelings of fullness.
   (3) Use a means for protection in cases of an accident, but avoid using diapers.
   (4) Maintain fluid intake at 1500 to 2000 ml daily spaced during the day with limited fluid intake in the evening. Adequate fluids are needed to produce sufficient urine to maintain the micturition reflex.
   (5) Avoid strenuous exercise.
   (6) Use relaxation techniques to manage stress.
   (7) Reduce dietary irritants, such as caffeine, spiced foods, carbonated drinks, and highly acidic foods.

c. Teach the client how to perform Kegel (pelvic floor) exercises when there is a need to improve the tone of the pelvic musculature.
   (1) To perform Kegel exercises, teach the client to:
       (a) Initially urinate a small amount and then start and stop the stream to gain an awareness and feeling of control of muscles involved in contracting the pelvic floor. (Then the client is ready to start with Kegel exercises.)
       (b) Assume a standing, sitting, or lying down position.
       (c) Tighten the anal sphincter as if to keep from having a bowel movement and then release.
       (d) Alternate tightening the anal sphincter for a count of five with relaxing the muscles of the pelvic floor for a count of five.
       (e) Increase the Kegel exercises to at least ten times four to six times a day.
   (2) Encourage the client to persist with Kegel exercises, as significant improvement may be slow (about 3 months).
   (3) Explain to the client that some pelvic discomfort and sexual stimulation may occur with Kegel exercises.

d. Teach the client to monitor for side effects of anticholinergic or antispasmodic drugs, such as dry mouth, blurred vision, nervousness, and constipation. (The elderly are sensitive to these medications.)

Established Overflow Urinary Incontinence*

1. Overflow incontinence is characterized by:
   a. Periodic or continuous dripping of small amounts of urine from a constantly filled bladder.
   b. Continuous wetness because of a small urinary leakage day and night.
   c. Lack of response to bladder filling.
   d. Long periods between voiding.
   e. Large volume of morning voiding.
   f. Hesitancy and straining to void.
   g. Weak interrupted urinary stream.
   h. Incomplete bladder emptying.
   i. Increased risk of urinary tract infection.
2. Overflow incontinence is usually secondary to:
   a. Obstruction of an enlarged prostate.
   b. Urethral stricture.
   c. A neurogenic or hypotonic bladder with loss of normal contraction.
   d. Chronic use of tranquilizer drugs.
3. Treatment is directed toward the cause of inadequate bladder emptying.
   a. Drug therapy with cholinergics (e.g., bethanecol chloride) and alpha-adrenergic blockers to stimulate the bladder and release the urethral internal sphincter may be used when the cause is not due to obstruction.
   b. Surgery is performed to relieve the obstruction of prostatism and urethral stricture. (Urethral obstruction is rare in females.)
   c. When surgery is not feasible or the cause is a nonobstructive hypotonic bladder, clean intermittent catheterization is preferable to an indwelling Foley catheter for the alert, competent, ambulatory elderly client.
   d. An indwelling urethral or suprapubic catheter is least preferable. Teach the client daily catheter care, and arrange for replacement of the indwelling catheter every 4 weeks.
   e. Medications in a drug regimen should be changed for those experiencing overflow related to drug side effects.
4. Strategies for care of the client experiencing overflow incontinence include the following:
   a. Discuss surgery (if recommended) with the client, and assist him in making appropriate arrangements for care.

---

*Paradoxical because of overflow nature.

b. When surgery is not feasible to remove obstruction or when the cause of incontinence is neurogenic, teach the client to:
   (1) Try to void every few hours regardless of whether or not the bladder feels full.
   (2) Tighten the abdominal muscles, and with the hand apply gentle pressure downward (Credé's maneuver) to help empty the bladder completely.
   (3) Perform clean intermittent self-catheterization as ordered.
   (4) Provide catheter care for an indwelling catheter daily, and arrange for catheter change every 4 weeks.
   (5) Report early signs of urinary tract infection to ensure prompt treatment.
   (6) Use cholinergic drugs as ordered, such as bethanecol chloride (Urecholine), to stimulate contractions strong enough to empty the bladder, and observe for side effects of cholinergic drugs. (This applies to clients with a hypotonic bladder.)

Established Stress Urinary Incontinence

1. Stress urinary incontinence is characterized by sudden loss of urine associated with physical activity or exertion, such as coughing, sneezing, laughing, lifting, or other body movements that increase intra-abdominal or intravesicular pressure.
   a. Stress incontinence does not occur at night when the client is in bed unless the client coughs or engages in strenuous movements, such as sexual intercourse.
   b. The amount of urine lost may vary considerably.
   c. Stress incontinence is not associated with other voiding complaints.
2. The causes of stress urinary incontinence are as follows:
   a. Trauma from infection or surgery.
   b. A paralytic external bladder sphincter.
   c. More frequently in women as a manifestation of reduced urethral resistance with relaxation of the pelvic musculature, usually as a result of childbirth.
3. Assessment for stress urinary incontinence should include the following:
   a. In addition to routine testing, a pelvic examination for inflammation, infection, prolapse, anal tone, pelvic relaxation, and presence of a cystocele or urethrocele is essential for diagnosis and appropriate treatment.
   b. Assessment should be made for loss of urine in relation to activity

to distinguish between stress or urge incontinence, as treatment differs for each condition.

(1) In stress incontinence, urine loss occurs simultaneously with exercise.

(2) In urge incontinence, urine loss occurs several seconds after exertion or stress and at night in the absence of exercise.

4. Treatment should include the following:

a. Kegel exercises are recommended to retrain and improve tone of the pelvic musculature.

b. Alpha-adrenergic agents to stimulate the receptors in the trigone and internal sphincter area have achieved a 75% success rate in mild to moderate cases of stress incontinence.

c. Surgery for incontinence caused by pelvic relaxation is a bladder suspension. This is associated with an 85 to 90% success rate.

d. Artificial urinary sphincter implantation procedures for clients with severe urinary incontinence caused by a paralytic urinary sphincter or a fibrous or traumatized urethra or for clients with postprostatectomy incontinence are associated with a success rate of 70 to 80%.

(1) The silicone rubber semiautomatic device, composed of a pressurized balloon, the deflate bulb, and the cuff, is surgically implanted (Fig. 15–1).

(2) The pressurized balloon is placed in the bladder, the cuff is placed around the bladder neck or bulbous urethra, and the deflate bulb is placed in the labia or hemiscrotum.

(3) The device automatically pressurizes the cuff and occludes the urethra. The cuff is opened periodically by the client by squeezing the deflate bulb, which causes transfer of the fluid in the cuff to the balloon.

(4) After the bladder empties, the fluid from the balloon returns to inflate the cuff.

(5) The device is contraindicated for those unable to empty the bladder completely and for those with memory problems.

5. Strategies for the client experiencing stress urinary incontinence include the following:

a. Teach the client Kegel exercises when there is a need to improve the tone of the pelvic musculature. (See under "Established Urge Urinary Incontinence," previously.)

Functional Incontinence

1. Functional incontinence occurs with normal bladder and urethral function and appears related to inability to recognize the need to

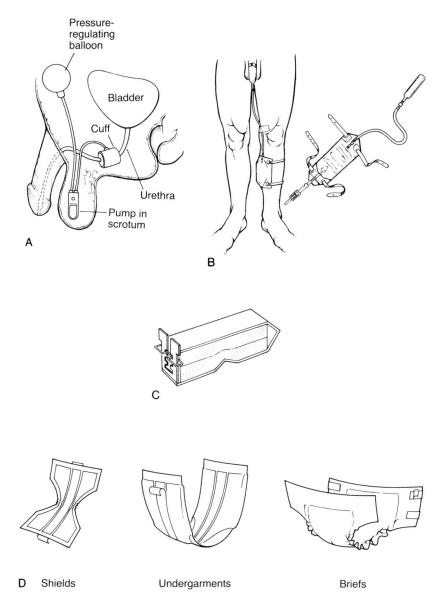

Figure 15–1. Equipment for the management of urinary incontinence. A, *Artificial urinary sphincter.* B, *Urine collected in a condom-like sheath attached to an external urinary drainage system.* C, *Penile clamp that compresses the male urethra to prevent incontinence.* D, *External sanitary protective devices. (Courtesy of American Medical Systems, Inc, Minnetonka, Minnesota.)*

void in an appropriate place or an inability to communicate a sense of urgency or immediacy of needing to void.

    a. Large amounts of urine are voided in inappropriate situations and environments.

    b. The client may be unaware or insensitive to the event.

2. Functional incontinence occurs most often with clients experiencing dementia or closed head injuries.

3. A diagnosis of functional incontinence is made after tests have ruled out other causes.

4. Strategies for care of the client experiencing functional incontinence are as follows:

    a. Contingency management, a behavioral method using reinforcers to establish continent behaviors, has shown some success with clients suffering from organic brain syndrome or senile dementia.

    b. If the client remains incontinent after standard treatment and leakage continues, pads, external devices, and catheters may be used to keep the client dry and to prevent embarrassment and low self-esteem (see Fig. 15–1).

Complex Urinary Incontinence

1. Combined urge and stress incontinence may occur in the elderly, with symptoms of both present.

2. Treatment is directed first toward relief of the most prominent type of incontinence.

    a. Treatment is then provided for both urge and stress incontinence as needed.

    b. Ultimately, if incontinence persists in spite of surgery or medication, an indwelling urethral catheter or a suprapubic catheter may be used.

3. Strategies for the client experiencing complex urinary incontinence include:

    a. Assisting the client in complying with the therapeutic regimen prescribed.

    b. Teaching daily catheter care if the client has an indwelling catheter, and arranging for change of drainage device every 4 weeks.

    c. Monitoring for side effects of cholinergic drugs.

Behavioral Measures for Controlling Urinary Incontinence

1. Kegel exercises.

    a. Used to treat stress incontinence in clients with intact cognitive function.

    b. Six to 8 weeks usually required for success.
2. Habit training (bladder training or bladder drill).
    a. Teaches person to void at predetermined times to avoid accidents.
    b. By gradually increasing the time intervals between voiding, corrects the habit of frequent voiding and attempts to improve voluntary control over the micturition reflex and to increase bladder capacity.
3. Contingency management.
    a. Behavioral method that has been successful with incontinent elderly suffering cognitive impairment, as in dementia.
    b. Uses reinforcers to establish continent behavior.
4. Biofeedback.
    a. Useful in treating stress urinary incontinence alone or in conjunction with habit training or contingency management.
    b. Provides client with visual feedback of bladder pressure, abdominal pressure, and internal and external sphincter activity.
    c. Information used to teach the client to inhibit bladder contractions voluntarily or to control sphincter muscles while relaxing abdominal muscles.

Resources

Continence Restored
785 Park Avenue
New York, NY 10021
(212) 879-3131

A nonprofit support group.

Help for Incontinent People
Department RBC
PO Box 544
Union, SC 29379

Functions as a clearinghouse for information and services; publishes *Resource Guide of Continence Products and Services.*

References

Chey WY: What is dyspepsia? A Digestive Diseases Clearinghouse Fact Sheet. Rosslyn, Va: National Digestive Diseases Education and Information Clearinghouse, 1983.

Clearfield HR: Gas in the Digestive Tract. NIH Pub No. 85-883. Washington, DC: US Government Printing Office, 1985.

Cohen S: The Irritable Bowel Syndrome. NIH Pub No. 85-693. Rosslyn, Va: National Digestive Diseases Education and Information Clearinghouse, 1985.

Coralli CH, Raisz LG, Wood CL: Osteoporosis: Significance, risk factors, and treatment. Nurse Practitioner 1(9):16–32, 1986.

Diokno AC: Urinary incontinence in the elderly. In Calkins E, Davis PJ, Ford AB, eds: The Practice of Geriatrics. Philadelphia: WB Saunders Co, 1986.

Garfinkel R: Pain management in the elderly: A cross cultural perspective. Center for the Study of Aging Newsletter 6(5):5, 8, 1984.

Grainger S: No cause, no cure—but he's still in pain. RN February 1987, pp 43–46.

Hallal JC: Osteoporotic fractures exact a toll. Journal of Gerontological Nursing 11(8):13–18, 1985.

Heidrich G, Perry S: Helping the patient in pain. American Journal of Nursing 82(12):1828–1831, 1982.

Jarvis L: Community Health Nursing. Philadelphia: FA Davis Co, 1985.

Jennings J, Baylink D: Osteoporosis. In Calkins E, Davis PJ, Ford AB, eds: The Practice of Geriatrics. Philadelphia: WB Saunders Co, 1986.

Kirkpatrick MK: A bladder retraining program in a long-term care facility. Nursing Homes July–August 1987, pp 29–31.

Kwentus JA, Harkins SW, Lignon N, Silverman JJ: Current concepts of geriatric pain and its treatment. Geriatrics 40(4):48–54, 1985.

Malthie A: Pain management. In Covington TR, Walker JI, eds: Current Geriatric Therapy. Philadelphia: WB Saunders Co, 1984.

McCormick KA, Burgio KL: Incontinence: An update on nursing care measures. Journal of Gerontological Nursing 10(10):16–19, 22, 23, 1984.

Moore DE, Blacker HM: How effective is TENS for chronic pain? American Journal of Nursing 83(8):1175–1177, 1983.

Olsson G, Parker G: A model approach to pain assessment. Nursing May 1987, pp 52–57.

Portenoy RK: Optimal pain control in elderly cancer patients. Geriatrics 42(5):33–40, 1987.

Sklar M: Gastrointestinal diseases. In Calkins E, Davis PJ, Ford AB, eds: The Practice of Geriatrics. Philadelphia: WB Saunders Co, 1986.

Weinstein RS: Osteoporosis. In Rakel RE, ed: Conn's Current Therapy. Philadelphia: WB Saunders Co, 1986.

White JE: Osteoporosis: Strategies for prevention. Nurse Practitioner 11(9):36–47, 1986.

Accident, Crime, and Abuse Prevention

ACCIDENTS AND THE ELDERLY
FALLS
BURNS
ASPHYXIA
DRUG POISONING
MOTOR VEHICLE–RELATED ACCIDENTS
CRIME AND THE ELDERLY
ABUSE AND THE ELDERLY

The impact of accidents, crime, and abuse on the elderly is usually greater than in the younger population, as elders are more vulnerable to the consequences of these events.

ACCIDENTS AND THE ELDERLY

1. Each year about 600,000 elderly are treated in emergency rooms for home injuries.
2. In 1984, accidents were the eighth leading cause of death for people over 65 years of age.
3. Medical care for injuries to persons 65 years of age or older totals more than $3 billion a year.
4. Although the elderly suffer accidental injuries less frequently than younger people do, when an injury occurs it is much more likely to result in immobility and shock, with disability and death occurring from cardiac or respiratory complications.

5. The elderly most at risk for multiple accidents are those who are weak, confused, or chronically ill.
6. The most frequent accidents in the home are falling in the bathroom and on stairs, burns with smoke inhalation, and scalds from tap water.
7. A large percentage of accidents may be preventable by reducing environmental hazards and by providing adequate medical evaluations and appropriate treatment for disabling conditions.
8. Teaching clients with chronic irreversible medical problems adaptive behavior and how to use assistive equipment reduces susceptibility to accidents and their sequelae.
9. Emergency telephone numbers for reporting crime and fire and requesting ambulance assistance should be posted by the telephone. These numbers are available in the front page of the local telephone directory.
   a. If the victim cannot dial the emergency number, he should dial "0" (operator) and stay on the line. If the victim cannot stay on the line, he should give the operator the street address and community where help is needed.
   b. If an elder does not have a telephone, he should be assisted in working out a means of communication with others in his community.
10. Use of a personal medical emergency response system (PERS) (Fig. 16–1) can help an elderly individual meet his need for security and independence. At the time of an accident, an elder may use his PERS to call for assistance, report his condition, save time, reduce complications, and possibly save his life.
    a. The PERS may be rented or purchased by the individual.
    b. Some home health and social agencies rent PERS to clients at a fee lower than that charged by vendors.
    c. A resource for information about a PERS is "Meeting the Need for Security and Independence with Personal Emergency Response Systems," PF 3986 (1187)-D12905, published by the:
       Consumer Affairs Program Department
       American Association of Retired Persons
       1909 K Street, N.W.
       Washington, DC 20049

Causes of Accidents in the Elderly

1. Primary aging changes that result in weakness, incoordination, impaired hearing, and alterations in gait, in vision, and in homeostatic functions increase the risk of accidents.

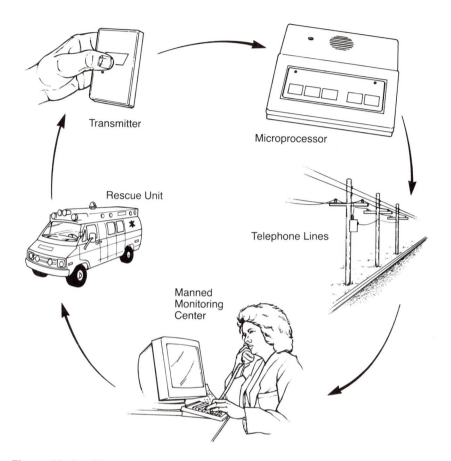

Figure 16–1. *Personal emergency response system. The client in need of emergency assistance presses the button on the transmitter (hand-held, pendant, or attached to the wall) that activates the microprocessor. The signal is transmitted via telephone wires to a computerized monitoring center (may be local or national) where information on the client is stored. With some personal emergency response systems, voice contact is possible. The appropriate nearest ambulance service, police department, or fire department designated by the client in the memory bank is then notified by the monitoring service, and help is promptly on the way.*

 a. A tendency to deny the limitations of aging as a defense against anxiety and the frequent depression that accompanies bereavement and disengagement increase the risk of accidents occurring.

2. Secondary changes associated with alterations in the central nervous system, neurosensory deficits, cardiovascular disease, metabolic imbalances, and musculoskeletal deficits contribute to the risk of accidents.

  a. Accidents among the elderly are often attributable to the effects of superimposed disease on the physical and mental changes of aging.
  b. The first manifestation of the onset of an acute illness may be an accident, as decreased appreciation of pain and reduced febrile response may mask symptoms of acute disease.
  c. Conditions predisposing the elderly to accidents may be acute or chronic, such as:
     (1) Dementia, depression, parkinsonism, or somnolence.
     (2) Cerebrovascular insufficiency associated with anemia, strokes, small cerebral infarcts, transient ischemic attacks (TIAs), or loss of patency of carotid or vertebral vessels.
     (3) Arrhythmias, including Stokes-Adams disease with heart block.
     (4) Postural hypotension.
     (5) Hyponatremia, hypovolemia, hypoglycemia, hypokalemia, hypercalcemia, hypomagnesemia, and azotemia.
     (6) Loss of proprioception (awareness of posture, movement, and changes in equilibrium and the knowledge of position, weight, and resistance of objects in relation to the body, associated with diseases of the spinal cord or peripheral nerves, such as cervical spondylosis and peripheral neuropathy).
     (7) Arthritis and osteoporosis.
  d. Chronic disease fosters apathy and a sense of detachment from the environment, resulting in diminished alertness and reduction in self-care.
3. Inappropriate use of drugs and alcohol can cause an existing condition to remain uncorrected or can cause somnolence, postural hypotension, or confusion to precipitate.
4. Environmental conditions can be hazardous or can fail to meet the needs of the elderly.
5. Emotional stress, e.g., boredom, loneliness, preoccupation, anxiety, aggression, frustration, and fear, make the elderly more vulnerable to accidents.
6. Lack of appropriate adaptive behaviors or lack of use of assistive equipment that would compensate for loss of function increases the risk of accidents.

Strategies for Prevention of Accidents

1. Optimal health care is essential to prevent the contribution of primary and secondary changes to the occurrence of accidents.
2. Correction of environmental hazards and environmental adjust-

ments to better meet the needs of the elderly individual reduces risk and improves the quality of life.

3. Accurate reporting of all accidents, whether followed by injury or not, is essential, as accidents may serve as warnings of malfunction and guides to appropriate prevention.

FALLS

1. According to the National Safety Council (1985), falls are the leading cause of accidental death in those over 65 years of age and account for 35% of all deaths in those elderly.
2. It is estimated that one third of all persons 60 years of age and older suffer falls each year.
3. The incidence of falls is greater in women, with higher mortality and morbidity, than in men because women are more likely to suffer osteoporosis, to live alone, and to experience longer periods of disability.
4. More than one third of the time for those over age 74, these falls are reported to cause fractures (especially those with hip involvement) that lead to restriction of activity and often terminal complications.
5. The elderly individual who suffers repeated falls may be unaffected for a while; if falls persist, however, there is a loss of confidence, reduction in activity, increasing weakness, and, finally, immobility that often necessitates placement for long-term care.

Causes of Falls in the Elderly

ENVIRONMENTAL CONDITIONS

Environmental conditions, such as the following, predispose the elderly to falling.
1. Slippery, smooth, and wet floors.
2. Surfaces with miscellaneous clutter, such as that created by rugs, pets, toys, and grandchildren.
3. Bathroom hazards, such as slippery tub, wet surfaces, or a low toilet seat.
4. Low beds.
5. Staircase hazards, such as:
   a. Poor visibility and poor lighting that cause the elderly to miss

the last step or group of steps. (The older person cannot catch himself and continues to fall.)
   b. Steep steps and inadequate handrails.
   c. Poor marking of steps.
   d. Poorly designed stairs or walkways.
   e. Absence of railings and handles.
   f. New, unfamiliar stairway.

PRIMARY AGING CHANGES

Primary aging changes may increase susceptibility to falling.
1. Reduction in control over body and movement, associated with slowed central processing and reduction in proprioceptive signals, predisposes the elderly to loss of balance and falling.
2. The ability to avoid a fall following an unexpected trip or to respond to environmental hazards is impaired with diminished muscle strength and control, increased muscle tone (rigidity), weaker muscle cushioning, slowed righting reflexes, arthritic joints, and inelastic tendons or ligaments.
3. The knowledge of where the feet are when descending a staircase is affected as body-orienting reflexes are reduced (this occurs more commonly in women). The sensitivity to illusions of disequilibrium may be unrelated to the state of visual acuity in general, but there is greater need for visual information as proprioception declines.
4. Vestibular dysfunction, manifested by dizziness, is more likely to occur when one is looking down a stairway, but is most dangerous when one is climbing up a stairway.
5. Alterations in gait, deformed feet in ill-fitting shoes, and poor judgment associated with resistance to advice increase the likelihood of tripping.
   a. Those who are advanced in age do not pick up the feet as high when stepping.
   b. Men tend to acquire a bent posture and a wide-based and small-stepped gait.
   c. Women tend to acquire a narrow-based, "waddling" gait.
6. Impaired vision and hearing interfere with ability to avoid obstacles.
7. Reduction in short-term memory predisposes to tripping over forgotten objects.

SECONDARY CHANGES

Conditions associated with secondary changes may cause falls.
1. Syncope in the elderly usually results either from decreased cerebral blood flow or from metabolic causes.

    a. The association between syncope and falls is often not clearly made by the client. The fall is often attributed to environmental causes or "bad luck."

2. Drop attacks (sudden falls without loss of consciousness) may occur without apparent cause, but usually are related to any of the following:
   a. Postural hypotension.
   b. Weakness of the quadriceps muscle, especially in clients with rheumatic disease. The weakness leads to easy fatigability and falling as the muscle gives out.
   c. Extension and rotation of the neck by a client with osteoarthritis of the cervical spine and some shortening of the neck with spondylosis that may result in vertebrobasilar insufficiency and that may inhibit the function of antigravity muscles.
      (1) In the client with cervical osteoarthritis, because the vertebral arteries may have a winding course with less elasticity in the arterial wall, sudden movements of the head and neck precipitate momentary blood loss from the medulla.
      (2) The antigravity muscles (quadriceps) may be temporarily paralyzed until some nervous pathway is re-established.
      (3) Associated leg weakness is transient but may persist for hours.
      (4) Transient flaccid paralysis affecting the legs and some trunk muscles may persist for hours if the individual is not helped to brace the feet against a hard object.

3. Orthostatic (postural) hypotension, defined as a drop of 20 mm Hg of systolic pressure between lying and standing, is prevalent among 20 to 30% of well elderly individuals as homeostatic mechanisms of blood pressure are decreased.
   a. Postural hypotension may result from autonomic dysfunction related to age, diabetes, central nervous system damage, hypovolemia, parkinsonism, metabolic and endocrine disorders, and use of antihypertensive and antidepressant medications.
   b. The condition is suspect in persons who become faint or experience dizziness following a sudden change of position or who experience syncope after eating or defecation.
   c. When blood pressure levels are checked while the client is lying down and then rechecked after 2 minutes when the client is sitting or standing, a drop of 20 mm Hg is considered evidence of significant orthostatic hypotension.
   d. The orthostatic drop may be greater on arising, as blood volume tends to decrease at night.
   e. Postural hypotension results in few falls, as elderly individuals

are often warned by becoming light-headed and sit down before actually falling.

4. Dizziness or vertigo, a common complaint of those who fall, occurs when there is impairment of several of the visual, vestibular, proprioceptive, tactile, and auditory orienting functions.

   a. The client complains of dizziness or lightheadedness; the complaints are vague, but reflect an uncertainty of position or motion in space.

   b. Vague lightheadedness may be cardiovascular or may reflect hyperventilation, orthostasis, anxiety, or depression.

   c. Symptoms described as imbalance on walking often reflect a gait disorder.

   d. Spatial disorientation and dizziness may occur when the elderly client is using supplementary lenses after cataract extraction.

   e. Transient orthostatic hypotension may predispose the client to dizziness.

   f. *True vertigo,* a sensation of true rotary movement, may indicate a disorder of the vestibular apparatus *(peripheral vertigo),* such as benign positional vertigo, acute labyrinthitis, or Ménière's disease.

   g. The elderly client complaining of dizziness tends to walk with a broad-based, unsteady gait and experiences difficulty turning or walking on uneven ground.

   h. The client falls to one side or the other as the room seems to spin.

   i. Nystagmus occurs with the vertigo.

   j. If vertigo cannot be attributed to peripheral vertigo, computed tomography (CT scan) is performed to rule out central vertigo caused by brain pathology.

   k. Usually upon experiencing vertigo, the client prevents falling by grasping something or sitting down as quickly as possible.

   l. Vertigo is most dangerous when it occurs in an individual standing on stairs or looking down from a height.

5. Dehydration caused by diarrhea, fever, inadequate fluid intake, or excessive use of diuretics causes syncope, drop attacks, and postural hypotension.

6. Impaired gait associated with hemoplegia (following a stroke), arthritis, and Parkinson's disease places the elderly client at greater risk for falling.

INAPPROPRIATE PATTERNS OF CARE

Falls may result from:

1. Excessive use of restraints.

2. Prolonged immobilization, leading to muscular weakness, loss of bone mass, and lack of practice of ambulatory skills.

Assessment for Cause of a Fall

1. A systematic search for the cause of the fall is made after stabilization of injuries.
2. The history is directed toward identifying the circumstances surrounding the fall, such as:
   a. Sequence of events.
   b. Symptoms experienced.
   c. Associated activities and stresses.
   d. Potential predisposing factors in the environment.
3. Physical examination, assessment of mental status, and neurologic examination are done.
4. Laboratory work includes a complete blood count, chemistries, electrocardiogram, and a thyroid function test.
5. Ambulatory cardiac Holter monitoring is performed. The client must keep a diary of activities and symptoms during Holter monitoring to evaluate for a relationship between syncope and suspected arrhythimas.

Management After a Fall

1. Treatment is directed toward specific etiologic or predisposing factors believed to be present.
2. Reversible physiologic problems, such as arrhythmias, dehydration, and TIAs, are treated.
3. Careful evaluation for other contributing factors, such as visual and hearing problems, is completed.
4. The client's drug regimen is reviewed, and dosages are adjusted to minimize their contribution to falling. Drugs more likely to predispose clients to falls are those that induce:
   a. Somnolence, such as hypnotics.
   b. Postural hypotension, such as diuretics, nitrates, antihypertensive agents, and tricyclic antidepressants.
   c. Confusion, such as cimetidine and digitalis.

Strategies for Prevention of Falls

SYNCOPE

1. Encourage male clients who are subject to micturition syncope to sit while urinating.

2. Advise clients who are subject to carotid sinus syndrome to avoid tight collars or extreme neck rotation.

Orthostatic Hypotension

1. Monitor the client for hypotensive side effects of diuretic therapy.
2. Advise the client to:
   a. Sleep in bed with the head elevated to minimize sudden drop in blood pressure on rising.
   b. Avoid walking after eating.
   c. Sit up and stand up slowly and wait a moment before making the next move.
   d. Try wearing support stockings to prevent venous pooling in the legs.

Vertigo

1. A very careful history is essential to establish the cause of dizziness or vertigo.
2. Prior to an extensive work-up for dizziness or vertigo, the ear canal should be checked for cerumen, which may cause vertigo.
3. Labyrinthitis with low-pitched tinnitus and hearing loss is self-limited but may be treated with meclizine hydrochloride or an antihistamine.
4. Otolaryngologic consultation is required in the case of Meniérè's disease.
5. Teach the client to:
   a. Avoid positional vertigo by not assuming those positions that result in vertigo.
   b. Avoid sudden turning on the heel. Making a small circle to make a turn helps maintain balance and helps to prevent vertigo.
   c. Carry a cane or hold someone's arm to improve balance.

Drop Attacks

1. Advise the client:
   a. Wearing a cervical collar often abolishes drop attacks.
   b. Avoid looking up when on a ladder, as when changing bulbs and adjusting drapes.
   c. Working with the arms over the head should be avoided.
   d. A headrest in the car to prevent sudden backward movement of the head may prevent vertebrobasilar insufficiency.

    e. Tilted mirrors and high sinks help to avoid movement of the head upward.
2. How to manage should a drop attack occur.
    a. If a person who has fallen is helped back on his feet, as soon as the feet touch the ground the nervous pathway may be reconnected and the person may walk away as though nothing has happened.
    b. Tone and strength may be restored by the client pushing his feet against a wall or some other solid object.
    c. A person who has fallen may use the arms to hold on to a chair or other large object and pull himself to his knees and then upright.

MUSCULOSKELETAL DEFICITS

1. Recommend for clients with a musculoskeletal deficit a trial of short-term rehabilitation in consultation with a physiotherapist to improve safety and diminish long-term disability.
2. For clients with irreversible problems, residual limitations should be explained and assistance provided in developing coping methods.
3. Quadriceps-muscle strengthening by a systematic program with the knee at full extension at least three times a day often leads to significant improvement over 2 to 3 months.
4. Assistive devices help with gait disturbances; the devices include walkers, crutches, canes, and shoe modifications.
    a. Check in the Yellow Pages of the telephone book for local distributors of surgical appliances and supplies.
    b. Request catalogues of equipment from these local suppliers to determine what equipment is available to meet the client's needs.
    c. Check for the proper fitting of shoes and appropriate height of walkers and canes.
5. A program of gait training is particularly helpful to clients following a stroke, following hip surgery, or experiencing Parkinson's disease.
    a. For the client with impaired gait who cannot swing the affected limb high enough, prevention of falls includes removal of thresholds, extension cords, low couches, chairs on casters, rickety tables, and sharp-cornered furniture. The floor plan should be simplified.
    b. Refer the client with Parkinson's disease and his family to:
    The American Parkinson Disease Association
    116 John Street
    New York, NY 10038
    (Publications: *Parkinson's Disease Handbook: A Guide for Patients*

and Their Families; Home Exercises for Patients with Parkinson's Disease; Aids, Equipment, and Suggestions to Help the Patient with Parkinson's Disease)

6. Advise clients with balance problems to stop and wait until somebody in a hurry has passed by.
7. Advise the client to slow down when passing through doorways from a less well illuminated area to a brightly illuminated room.
8. Check that wheelchairs are maneuverable and that the client is able to get from room to room and into closets. The edges of the seat should not interfere with circulation.
9. Advise the client to avoid drinking alcohol. (Refer the client to Alcoholics Anonymous if he is an alcohol abuser.)
10. Over-the-counter (OTC) drugs should be used only with the agreement of the physician.
11. Be alert to side effects of drugs, such as somnolence, postural hypotension, and confusion.

HOME SAFETY

See Resources at the end of the discussion of accidents. Recommend that the client:
1. Discard small sliding mats and frayed rugs.
2. Eliminate trailing electrical cords.
3. Tack down carpeting on stairs and use nonskid treads (Fig. 16–2).
4. Remove throw rugs that tend to slide.
5. Tack down the ends of rugs.
6. Rearrange furniture to provide supports rather than obstacles.
7. Use a raised toilet seat.
8. Have the top and bottom steps of stairways painted a bright color that shows contrast with the other stairs, flooring, and carpet.
9. Be sure both sides of stairways have sturdy handrails (Fig. 16–3).
10. Check that handrails are sturdy and optimally contoured for a good grasp with the ends shaped so that he will know by touch alone when the top and bottom steps have been reached.
11. Keep outdoor steps and walkways in good repair.
12. Use rubber-backed nonskid rugs and nonskid floor waxes.
13. Wear corrugated or rubber soles on slippery surfaces.
14. Use grab bars on bathroom walls and nonskid mats or strips in the bathtub (Fig. 16–4).
15. Arrange furniture and other objects so that they are not obstacles.
16. Watch out for grandchildren, toys, and pets.
17. Provide adequate illumination by:
    a. Lighting all stairways and landings.

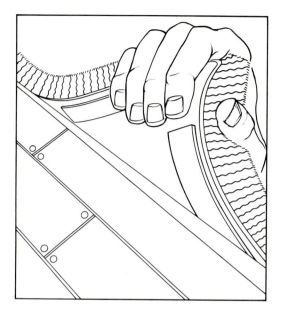

Figure 16–2. *Secure carpets and runners. (Courtesy of U.S. Consumer Product Safety Commission, 1986.)*

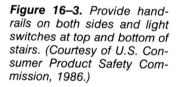

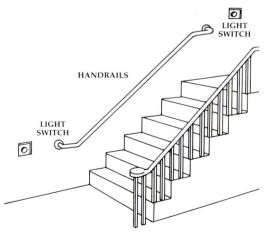

Figure 16–3. *Provide handrails on both sides and light switches at top and bottom of stairs. (Courtesy of U.S. Consumer Product Safety Commission, 1986.)*

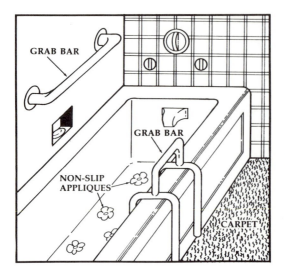

Figure 16–4. *Provide grab bars and nonslip appliqués in bathtubs and showers. (Courtesy of U.S. Consumer Product Safety Commission, 1986.)*

b. Providing light switches at both the bottom and the top of stairways.

c. Providing night lights or bedside remote-control switches.

d. Installing baseboard lights and adequate lighting at the bedside and from bed to bathroom at night.

e. Making switches easily accessible.

f. Having flashlights available for emergencies.

Resource

U.S. Consumer Product Safety Commission
Washington, DC 20207
Safety for Older Consumers: Home Safety Checklist

BURNS

1. House fires account for 75% of all deaths from fires (typically as a result of burns and smoke inhalation).

2. The highest fatality rates from house fires occur in young children and the elderly because of their difficulty in escaping from house fires and their reduced likelihood of survival after receiving fire-related injuries.

3. Although there have been recent advances in fire safety, such as widespread use of fire-resistant building materials, increased use of

smoke detectors, improved fire and emergency medical responses, and improvement in burn treatment, these gains are partially offset by fire hazards created by cigarette smoking, alcohol use, and lack of smoke detectors in the homes of the poor.

Risk Factors for Burns by the Elderly

1. Alterations in vision.
2. Inability to maintain erect posture.
3. Reduction in short-term memory.
4. Slowed reflexes for interpreting pain and withdrawing from pain.
5. Smoking in bed or in an easy chair and falling asleep with a lit cigarette.
6. Hot water or gas jet turned on and forgotten.
7. Loose clothing catching in gas jet.
8. Touching or dropping kettles containing hot water.
9. Confusion about the use of dials and controls on heating appliances.

Strategies to Prevent Burn Injuries

Teach the client to:
1. Obtain, install, and maintain smoke detectors with batteries and bulbs according to manufacturers' directions. Some fire departments and local governments will assist in obtaining and installing smoke detectors.
2. Make emergency exit plans and review them periodically.
3. Check the condition of electrical and telephone cords and electric appliances for correct usage and appropriate placement.
   a. Unplug and check wiring of outlets and switches that are unusually warm or hot to the touch.
   b. Do not use frayed electrical cords.
   c. Check that extension cords are not carrying more load than recommended by the ratings labeled on the cord and on the appliance.
4. Use light bulbs of the correct type and wattage. If the correct wattage is not known, use a bulb no stronger than 60 watts.
5. Set controls on tubs and showers with a preset temperature no higher than 49°C (120°F) or use a bath thermometer to check temperature of water. The temperature should be no higher than 46°C (115°F).
6. Maintain a safe area around the cooking stove.
   a. Mark "On" and "Off" clearly on the dials of the stove.
   b. When cooking, do not wear loosely fitting, flammable clothing

or bathrobes. Wear noninflammable cotton pajamas or night-gowns rather than polyester or nylon.

   c. Remove towels, curtains, and other items that might catch fire away from the stove.

   d. Keep handles of pots turned in while cooking.

   e. If the food that is cooking flares up, cover the pot to extinguish the fire or douse it with readily available sodium bicarbonate.

7. Use caution when using space heaters.

   a. Plug space heaters with a three-pronged plug into a three-hole outlet or use with an adapter for a two-hole receptacle, and attach the ground wire to the outlet to prevent the risk of shock.

   b. Place space heaters where they cannot be knocked over and away from furnishings and flammable materials, such as curtains or rugs.

   c. Review installation and operating instructions.

   d. Use unvented heaters with room doors open, or leave windows slightly open for ventilation.

   e. Frequently check venting systems of vented heaters for proper ventilation. (Lack of venting is the most common cause of carbon monoxide poisoning.)

   f. Have wood-burning stoves installed by a qualified person.

   g. Keep areas around heat sources free of papers and trash.

8. Improve visual environment. (See Chaper 7.)

9. Never smoke in bed or when drowsy.

10. Locate ash trays, smoking materials, heaters, hotplates, and teapots away from the bed and bedding.

11. Avoid tucking in electric blankets, putting anything on top of them when in use, or setting them so high that a burn could result.

12. Avoid using multiple door locks. Install one good lock that can be opened from the inside quickly.

13. Cap containers of flammable liquids, paints, and solvents tightly and store away from areas near heat or ignition sources, such as heaters, furnaces, water heaters, ranges, and other gas appliances.

14. Keep at least one operating dry-powder fire extinguisher available in the home.

ASPHYXIA

The elderly are at particular risk for asphyxia associated with gas, as reduced acuity of the sense of smell makes elders less sensitive to leaking gas lines, unignited taps, or taps put out by boiling over.

Strategies to Prevent Asphyxia

Teach the client to:
1. Use spring safety caps for gas jets when available.
2. Provide for adequate ventilation but avoid air currents that will extinguish the flame on the gas cooker.

DRUG POISONING

The elderly are vulnerable to drug poisoning as a result of overdosage; ingestion of mistaken drugs; and mistakes in dosage, sequence, and timing.

Strategies to Prevent Drug Poisoning

Teach the client to:
1. Label by name each drug and indicate whether it is intended for external or internal use.
2. Discard unused drugs.
3. Provide good lighting where drugs are stored for use.
4. Use a magnifying glass or wear prescribed glasses when reading labels, and follow directions for use.

MOTOR VEHICLE–RELATED ACCIDENTS

1. Motor vehicle accidents are a significant cause of accidental death and disability among individuals in the 65 to 74 age group.
2. More fragile bones and reduced ability to withstand the trauma of an accident place the elderly at greater risk as drivers and pedestrians for injury and death.
3. Older drivers have fewer total accidents than their younger counterparts; however, elderly drivers have a higher accident rate per mile driven.

Risk Factors

1. Increased sensitivity to glare.
2. Poorer adaptation to darkness.
3. Diminished coordination. Fine coordination is required to use power brakes.
4. Slowed reaction time.
5. Arthritic changes of the cervical spine causing cerebral ischemia.
6. Medications that may cause confusion or drowsiness or may impair reflexes.

7. Reduced ability to do quick problem solving and to estimate the speed of a moving object.
8. The need for training for the meaning of new laws and traffic signs.

Strategies to Reduce Motor Vehicle Accidents

1. Teach the client as a driver to:
   a. Have regular vision and hearing check-ups and to correct deficits.
   b. Schedule taking medications when they will not affect driving.
   c. Recognize limitations and know when to stop driving.
   d. Compensate for changes by driving fewer miles, driving less often, and driving more slowly.
   e. Curtail driving at night, in bad weather, and during rush hours.
   f. Reduce the risk of injury by wearing a safety belt. (Risk of injury is reduced by half.)
   g. Take a driving course to refine existing skills and to develop safe defensive-driving techniques. The American Association of Retired Persons (AARP) offers the program, "55 Alive/Mature Driving." Volunteers provide instruction to anyone over 50 years of age. Those interested in taking the course should write to
   55 Alive/Mature Driving
   AARP
   1909 K Street N.W.
   Washington, DC 20049
2. Teach the client as a pedestrian to:
   a. Allow extra time to cross streets, especially in bad weather.
   b. Wear light-colored or fluorescent clothing at night and carry a flashlight.
   c. Cross corners with others.
   d. Look from side to side because peripheral (side) vision is reduced.
   e. Be careful of curbs especially when wearing bifocals.
3. Teach the client on public transportation to:
   a. Remain alert and brace himself when the bus is turning or slowing down.
   b. Watch for slippery pavements and other hazards when entering or leaving a vehicle.
   c. Have fare ready to prevent losing balance while fumbling for change.
   d. Avoid carrying too many packages and to leave one hand free to grasp railings.

CRIME AND THE ELDERLY

1. The incidence of crimes against the elderly is not higher than in the general population, but the impact of the crime is usually greater because the elderly are more vulnerable to serious consequences of the crime, as they are more frail and often have economic problems.
2. The elderly are more susceptible to crime, as they often live in inner-city neighborhoods where crimes are more common and their physical handicaps and diminished strength make them easy prey.
3. The elder's best defenses against crime are being informed and employing strategies for crime prevention.
4. When a crime occurs, the elder should be directed to services available for the victimized elderly.
5. Crimes should be reported to the police, as this encourages better protection in the future.
6. Fear of crime may be useful by encouraging appropriate protection, but fear continued over a long period of time can become detrimental to mental and physical health as stress and limitation of activity take their toll.

Types of Crime Experienced by the Elderly

1. The most common crimes experienced by the elderly are:
   • Purse snatchings
   • Fraud
   • Theft of checks from the mail
   • Vandalism
   • Harassment
2. The more serious crimes of rape, murder, and assault are suffered less frequently by the elderly.

Strategies to Prevent Crime

IN THE HOME

Provide the client with the following instructions:
1. Lock doors and windows with good security equipment.
2. Obtain and use a 180-degree peephole.
3. Do not admit strangers without identification. Ask them to slip identification and credentials under the door.
4. Do not open the door a few inches while relying on a chain lock to keep out intruders.

5. Mark valuable property by having it engraved with driver's license or state identification number (available from the state motor vehicle administration).
6. Keep photographs of hard-to-engrave items.
7. Store small, rarely used valuables, such as jewelry, in a bank safe-deposit box when possible.
8. Make a list of valuables in the home and keep it in a safe-deposit box at a bank or give a trusted other a duplicate list.

ON THE STREET

Teach the client to:
1. Know that crime can happen, and maintain a constant attitude of prevention, practicing crime-prevention strategies.
2. Be careful in crowded places and avoid distraction.
3. Plan a route and stay alert to surroundings.
4. Walk with companions when possible.
5. Stay away from areas where crimes tend to occur, such as dark parking lots or alleys.
6. Avoid wearing good or flashy jewelry and furs when on the streets.
7. Use the following purse strategies:
   a. Avoid carrying a purse when possible and keep money and credit cards in a wallet in an inside pocket.
   b. Carry little cash and hand it over without question if attacked.
   c. If a purse must be carried, keep it close to the body with a hand over the clasp.
   d. Use a shoulder bag, as it is harder to steal than a large bulky hand-bag.
   e. Do not carry a purse in such a way that it can be opened away from the body.
   f. If carrying packages, keep a purse between body and packages.
   g. Beware of strangers who start meaningless conversations, as they may be removing a wallet or money from the purse.
   h. Arrange to have a monthly pension or social security check sent directly to the bank for deposit, when possible, to avoid carrying checks in purse.
8. Walk along busy, well-lit streets at night.
9. Stay away from buildings and walk close to the curb or even in the middle of the street, but be alert for oncoming traffic.

10. Have the key ready when walking to the front door.
11. Ask a taxi or other driver to wait until he has entered his home.

Shopping

Provide the client with the following instructions:
1. Do not show much cash.
2. Do not leave a purse on a counter or in a shopping cart.
3. Concentrate and avoid becoming distracted.

Con Games

Provide the client with the following instructions:
1. Beware of con artists who promise a windfall often contingent upon paying some money.
2. Do not withdraw money from the bank to give it to a stranger.
3. Be alert to consumer fraud in advertising, by telephone, or by mail.
4. Avoid victimization by checking out the legitimacy of claims with an appropriate source of information, such as the Better Business Bureau, a lawyer, a physician, or a bank representative, before subscribing to insurance, buying "miracle cures," contributing to charity, making investments, having home repairs done, or buying from a door-to-door salesperson.
5. Evaluate product use, including quality, safety, and warranty, before making a purchase.

Robbery

Provide the client with the following instructions should a robbery occur:
1. Give up money or jewelry; do not resist.
2. Never try to fight unless attacked.
3. Avoid provoking the robber.
4. Try to remember unusual distinguishing characteristics for later identification.
5. Report the crime to the police.
6. Apply to existing agencies that assist victims of crime. (Addresses may be obtained from the local Area Agency on Aging [see Appendix] or from the National Organization for Victim Assistance [see Resources, next].)

Resources

Law Enforcement Assistance Administration
U.S. Department of Justice
Washington, DC 20531
How to Crime Proof Your Home: Take a Bite Out of Crime

American Association of Retired Persons
National Retired Teacher's Association
215 Long Beach Boulevard
Long Beach, CA 90801
Your Retirement Anticrime Guide

National Organization for Victim Assistance
717 D Street, N.W.
Washington, DC 20004

Provides information on victim assistance programs; helps victims; and works with local programs to improve services, such as victim counseling, witness management, reparations, and so on.

Food and Drug Administration
Bureau of Medical Devices
Consumer and Regulatory Affairs
Branch (HFK-131)
8757 Georgia Avenue
Silver Springs, MD 20910

Provides information on quack products and devices.

The Crime Prevention Coalition
Box 6700
Rockville, MD 20850
Senior Citizens Against Crime

Council of Better Business Bureaus
1515 Wilson Boulevard
Arlington, VA 22209
Consumer Problems of the Elderly (Send a stamped, self-addressed envelope.)

ABUSE AND THE ELDERLY

1. Elder abuse (geriatric abuse, parent abuse, "granny battering," or "gram slamming") threatens the mental and physical health of an estimated one out of 25 elderly in the United States each year.
2. Because hospital stays are shortened with enforcement of diagnostic-related group guidelines (DRGs), more elderly are returned earlier and weaker to the community where they require care from families frequently already burdened with problems.
3. The nurse must be alert to cues of elder abuse in the home setting and in ambulatory care clinics because the elderly are often fearful or ashamed of reporting abuse.
4. A society that does not see abuse of the elderly as shocking or as wrong as it views abuse of a spouse or child provides inadequate protection for the abused elder.
5. A comprehensive federal law requiring uniform mandatory reporting, backed by enough funds to guarantee enforcement and provide support services, criminal sanctions against abusers, tax breaks for families supporting elderly members, or priority status for those families in the allotment of state services and funds, is urgently needed.

Types of Elder Abuse

FINANCIAL OR MATERIAL ABUSE

Financial or material abuse denotes the stealing of money or property.
1. Some caretakers have good intentions, but do not understand how to manage money.
2. It is easier for the caretaker to justify misuse of money when the elderly person is confused.
3. The possibility of abuse should be investigated when an elderly person decides to sign over the deed to a house or when he states he cannot financially manage any longer. The elder should be asked with whom he is living, who handles the money, and what circumstances now make it impossible for him to manage as before.
4. Violation of rights should be investigated when an elder is forced out of his home into a nursing home.

PSYCHOLOGIC ABUSE

Psychologic abuse occurs when the caretaker isolates the elder and is chronically verbally abusive and threatening.

PHYSICAL ABUSE

Physical abuse includes corporal punishment, injury, beatings, sexual assault, constraint, and deprivation of food and water.

NEGLECT

Neglect is the most common form of elder abuse.
1. Active neglect occurs when food, hygiene, medication, and other basic elements of care are deliberately withheld and when frail or senile elderly are left alone and unsupervised.
2. Passive neglect occurs when the care giver, as a result of ignorance or inability, cannot meet the needs of the elder and fails to assist in personal care, to provide mental health care, or to protect the elder from safety hazards.

Elder Abuse in the Community

1. The majority of abuse occurs in homes in which the elderly live with the abusers, who are relatives.
2. It is not unusual to find intrafamily violence with more than one type of abuse in a home in which elder abuse occurs.
3. The abused elder is often brought to the emergency department when deprivation or assault finally creates a critical physical problem. A variety of excuses for the illness or injury are offered.
4. Abuse is rarely reported by the elder because of fear of retaliation or strong feelings of kinship with the abuser.
5. Abuse is difficult to detect, as some elders decide that they would rather stay in a relationship even if they are beaten up at times because the rest of the time there is someone to help them.
6. The most difficult cases of elder abuse involve a mentally competent victim who refuses to protect himself from further abuse and who has lost subtle skills to assess others' motives.

The Abused Elder

1. Characteristically, the abused elder is a widowed woman in her mid-seventies with an income of less than $500 a month; however, older men are also abused.
2. The majority of abused elders suffer from chronic illness, while about 25% have acute illness or a history of mental illness.
3. Elderly individuals in poor health with a high incidence of dependency needs, such as medication, hygiene, and meals, are three to four times more likely to be abused than those in good health.
4. Maltreatment seems unrelated to socioeconomic status, race, religion, or educational attainment.
5. A parent providing economic support to a dependent, troubled adult child is at higher risk for financial or physical abuse from the child.
6. Elders physically or psychologically incapable of stopping the abuse are more at risk.
   a. Some elders have a poor self-image and feel that they deserve poor treatment.
   b. Many elderly are ashamed to report abuse by the family, which they perceive is supposed to be a smiling, happy unit.

The Abuser of the Elderly

1. The abuser is most commonly the family member with whom the elder lives.
   a. A son who is an abuser is more likely to physically abuse.
   b. A daughter who is an abuser is more likely to mentally abuse.
   c. Elderly spouses who serve as care givers have also been identified as abusers.
2. The abuser frequently is a well-intentioned individual laboring under the constant strain of caring for a chronically ill, confused, dependent parent or spouse.
3. The abusive care taker, already overburdened and wrestling with his own problems, perceives the addition of responsibility for the dependent elder as the "last straw."
4. The abuser is often the sole care giver, burdened with tremendous demands, no support system, no financial aid, and no practical help from other family members.
5. The care giver may be unaware of the elder's physical and mental limitations and may be ignorant of how and where to obtain outside help.

6. The care giver may be older and may have problems caring for himself.
7. There may be a history of a poor interpersonal relationship between the individuals or mental illness or drug or alcohol dependence of the abuser. There is a high correlation between elder abuse and substance abuse by the person who abuses.
8. The transgenerational cycle of violence theory suggests that the adult child is repaying the parent for abuse suffered as a child. The adult child with unresolved negative feelings may use role reversal to enact some of these negative feelings by rough, abusive behaviors.

Strategies for Prevention of Elder Abuse

1. Teach nonviolent coping behavior earlier in life.
2. Educate families about the normal aging process and the needs of the elderly.
3. Teach self-care to the elderly, or teach care needed to care givers.
4. Assist the family in making arrangements for support services in the community that can reduce family stress by addressing the needs of the elder and the family.
   a. Referral to support services is an essential part of discharge planning especially with shortened hospital stays associated with DRGs.
5. Expand neighborhood watch programs to check on those elderly with limited social contacts.
6. Advocate training for members of the criminal justice system to increase awareness of the signs of abuse and the dynamics of family violence.
7. Foster a federal approach to the problem, with enforceable, adequately funded laws that will protect the aged from abuse, absolve from liability those who report abuse, and make provision for comprehensive community support services for the elderly and their families.

Assessment for Elder Abuse

1. Bear in mind when performing assessment for elder abuse that all families have problems and that every complaint and argument is not a sign of abuse. Many children willingly and successfully assume the responsibility of caring for elderly parents.
2. The history should be directed toward physical or behavioral signs that may indicate abuse.
   a. Try to obtain privacy for the elderly client to reduce fears of

retaliation, and ask specific questions about how injuries occurred.

   b. Because injuries in the elderly may be attributed to falls or other accidents, ask the care giver about the origins of injuries and interpret carefully the explanation offered by the care giver.

3. Assess family relationships for:

   a. The elder's fear of an adult child, which may be manifested by eyes darting continuously, by sitting as far as possible from the child, and by acting as though expecting to be struck.

   b. Hostile aggressive behaviors, indications of little concern, lack of interest in suggestions, and exaggerated concern or defensiveness about issues of control by the care giver.

   c. Past and present social relationships for possible role reversal, family cohesiveness, social isolation, and lack of a support system.

   d. Role expectations of all and the family's perception of how the expectations are being met.

4. Assess for:

   a. The elder's clarity of thinking and memory.

   b. The care giver's knowledge of the elder's condition and needs and the level of commitment to meeting the elder's needs.

   c. The degree of dependency of the elder.

   d. How the dependent needs of the care giver are being met.

5. Assess whether spiritual values are enabling the family to transcend problems of aging and stress on the care giver. If spiritual values do not sufficiently support losses experienced by aging and the demands of the care giver's role, the abusive situation may be accepted more readily as justified and abuse is more likely to occur.

Strategies to Assist the Abused Elder and Family

1. Provide immediate treatment for any acute physical problem.

2. Develop a trusting, nonjudgmental, and nonthreatening relationship with the abused and, when possible, with the abuser.

3. Work with the family and community agencies to introduce appropriate support services, such as home health care, respite care, chore services, and senior day-care centers.

4. Aim toward restoring some degree of hopefulness and control about the situation.

5. Help families plan together for sharing responsibilities, for handling finances, and for learning about community resources.

6. Provide the elder and family with the number for a local 24-hour hot line for abuse.

7. Refer the family to self-help and local support groups.

8. Encourage family counseling to clarify role expectations and to strengthen the family's ability to assume new roles.
9. Document conditions observed to better identify and distinguish areas of intentional and unintentional neglect, misinformation, ignorance, or abuse.
10. Become familiar with the state law for reporting abuse, and pay particular attention to the professional responsibility mandated for reporting abuse and the freedom from liability provided both to the reporter and to the abuser.
11. Encourage the abused elder to work with a community organization that will assist:
    a. In working through fear of retaliation or loss of a preferred living situation.
    b. In filing criminal charges (when necessary), which only the elder can do himself unless judged incompetent by the courts.
    c. By providing back-up services, such as emergency transportation, relocation, assistance, and court advocacy.
    d. In obtaining an injunction, eviction, or civil commitment to remove the abuser from the home and away from the victim.
    e. In selecting and arranging for an alternative living arrangement when needed.

Resources

For the abused:
Hot line number listed for Violence and Victimization under Community Service numbers in the local telephone book.

The local Legal Aid Society.

For the care giver:
Local Area Agency on Aging (see Appendix) offers support services.

Children of Aging Parents
2761 Trenton Road
Levittown, PA 19056

Offers materials to help people interested in forming support groups.

References

Cape R: Aging: Its Complex Management. New York: Harper & Row, 1978.

Drake VC: Therapy with victims of abuse. In Beck CM, Rawlins RP, Williams SR: Mental Health Psychiatric Nursing. St. Louis: CV Mosby Co, 1984.

Rodstein M: Accidents among the aged: Incidence, cause, and prevention. Journal of Chronic Diseases 17:515–526, 1964.

Rubenstein LZ, Robbins AS: Falls in the elderly: A clinical perspective. Geriatrics 39(4):67–70, 75–76, 78, 1984.

Safety for Older Consumers: Home Safety Checklist. Washington, DC: US Consumer Product Safety Commission, 1986.

Sanders FV, Plummer EM: Assault on the aged: Is your patient a secret victim? RN July 1983, pp 21–25.

Take a Bite Out of Crime. Law Enforcement Assistance Administration, US Dept of Justice, GPO 914-072. Washington, DC: US Government Printing Office, 1979.

Thobaben M, Anderson L: Reporting elder abuse. American Journal of Nursing 85(4):371–374, 1985.

Whiteside-Yim C: Syncope in the elderly. Geriatrics 42(4):37–41, 1987.

Wieman HM, Calkins E: Falls. In Calkins E, Davis PJ, Ford AB, eds: The Practice of Geriatrics. Philadelphia: WB Saunders Co, 1986.

Winter A: The shame of elder abuse. Modern Maturity October–November 1986, pp 50–51 53–54, 56–57.

Your Retirement Anticrime Guide. Long Beach, Calif: American Association of Retired Persons and National Retired Teachers Association, 1978.

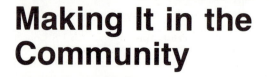

Making It in the Community

ALTERNATIVE LIVING ARRANGEMENTS
  FOR THE ELDERLY
COMMUNITY RESOURCES
FINANCIAL CONCERNS
WORK OPPORTUNITIES
LEGAL CONCERNS
CULTURAL, EDUCATIONAL,
  AND RECREATIONAL OPPORTUNITIES
SENIOR POLITICAL ACTION

1. At the same time that the elderly experience changes in the physical and psychosocial dimensions, they are in need of services that will promote the quality of their lives.
2. In recognition of these needs of the elderly, the Older Americans Act (OAA) was passed in 1965 to coordinate existing resources and to assist states in developing new programs for the elderly.
   a. The OAA established the U.S. Administration on Aging in the Department of Health and Human Services for funding, training, and research in gerontology.
   b. At the local level, the Area Agency on Aging (AAA) assumes responsibility for the coordination and planning for services to the elderly.
   c. Amendments to the OAA through the years have further recognized the rights of older Americans and have provided entitlements for improved and increased programs to better meet their needs in the following areas:

- Housing
- Nutrition
- Employment
- Health care
- Transportation
- Legal aid
- Social, recreational, and educational opportunities

3. When an elder can no longer independently manage personal and health care needs, community resources may help the client to maintain autonomy or to be cared for by family at home rather than be forced to enter a nursing home.

4. The nurse works with the client and family to assess their needs and to refer them to appropriate community resources.

5. In order for the client and family to make informed choices, data on availability of services, eligibility of the client, and sources of payment are necessary.

6. The local AAA (listed under Community Service Numbers in the local telephone directory) is a major resource for information on programs available to seniors.

ALTERNATIVE LIVING ARRANGEMENTS FOR THE ELDERLY

1. Most elderly prefer to make environmental adjustments and to utilize support services to meet their needs within their own home close to family, friends, and the community to which they are accustomed.

2. These elderly need to be connected with support services that will assist them and their family in making necessary environmental changes and in obtaining needed services.

3. Changing needs and lack of supports to assist in maintaining a preferred lifestyle may necessitate consideration of alternative living arrangements.

4. Too often, the elderly and family are unaware of the multiplicity of alternative living arrangements available that may meet the client's needs and provide opportunity for a desired lifestyle.

5. The nurse works with the client or family to assess their needs, to refer them to support services, or to assist in planning and successfully accomplishing relocation.

6. Exploration of living arrangements should best be accomplished and arrangements planned before a crisis occurs that may precipitate an uninformed decision.

7. The client or family should be encouraged to thoroughly research any prospective alternative in living arrangements for services provided, condition of the facility, financial costs, and attitude of residents and staff.
8. The chosen housing should provide good shelter within the individual's financial capability and opportunities for socialization and health care while allowing for privacy and the continuation of a positive lifestyle.

Criteria for Assessing the Adequacy of the Home Setting

1. How physical needs for food, clothing, and shelter are met.
2. The comfort, convenience, and safety of the physical environment.
3. The presence of psychologic safety.
4. The quality of life of the client.
5. Opportunities for continued socialization.
6. Roles and relationships of client, family members, other residents, neighbors, and pets.

Criteria for Assessing the Adequacy of the Community

1. Environmental characteristics.
2. Population characteristics.
3. Availability of acceptable community support services.

Priorities of Elderly Clients in Choosing Housing

1. Good shelter within financial capability.
2. Living in a homelike environment with companionship, pets, own furnishings, and personal items.
3. Privacy and the need for living space.

4. Public transportation in the community.
5. Support services in the community.

Housing Options*

1. *Accessory Apartment.* A second, completely private living unit built within the extra space of a single family home.
2. *Boarding Home (Rooming House).* Residential accommodation that usually consists of a bedroom/sitting room, private or shared bathroom, and common dining area. This housing is open to persons of all ages.
3. *Condominium.* Housing in an apartment building or townhouse complex in which individuals hold title to their living unit but share ownership of the common areas with other owners in the development.
4. *Cooperatives.* Non-profit corporations that own and operate a living facility for the benefit of the occupants who buy shares in the corporation in exchange for the right to occupy a specific living unit.
5. *Congregate Housing (Sheltered or Enriched Housing).* Specially planned, designed and managed multi-unit rental housing, typically with self-contained apartments. Supportive services such as meals, housekeeping, transportation, social and recreational activities are usually provided.
6. *Conventional Home Ownership.* Traditional ownership of a single family home, townhouse or manufactured (mobile) home.
7. *Conventional Rental Housing.* Traditional rental or leased housing in which tenants lease the right to occupy property—apartment or house—for a specific time at a specified cost.
8. *Domiciliary Care Home (Personal Care, Residential Care).* Group living arrangements that provide staff-supervised meals, housekeeping and personal care and private or shared sleeping rooms. These facilities are generally licensed and must meet design and operating standards, including minimum staff requirement.
9. *ECHO Housing (Elder Cottage, Granny Flat).* A self-contained, free-standing, removable living unit occupied by a relative on the same property and adjacent to a single-family home.
10. *Elderly Housing Project (Housing for Independent Elderly).* Rental housing planned, designed, and managed to meet the needs and interests of older tenants with services to support independent living.
11. *Federally Assisted Housing (Public Housing).* Rental housing built and operated with financial help from the federal government and designed for low-income families of all ages. Some buildings have been specifically designed to meet the needs of low-income persons age 62 and over.
12. *FHA/Veterans Administration/FmHA Home Loans.* Federally insured home loan programs for the public and eligible veterans who want to purchase approved residential property.
13. *Foster Care Homes.* Single family homes in which nonrelated older persons live with a foster family. The family provides meals, housekeeping and personal care.
14. *Homes For The Aged.* Accommodations for people with health limitations.

*Copyright 1988 American Association of Retired Persons. Reprinted with permission.

They range from private homes that offer only custodial care to skilled nursing facilities. At a minimum, such homes provide private or shared sleeping rooms, meals, housekeeping, personal care and supervision.

15. *Life Care Complex (Life Care Community, Continuing Care, Campus Complex).* Housing development planned, designed and operated to provide a full range of accommodations and services for older adults, including independent living, congregate housing, and medical care. Residents may move from one level to another as their needs change. Financial arrangements usually include a substantial entrance fee plus monthly charges.

16. *Mobile Homes (Manufactured Housing).* Compact, self-contained, factory-assembled housing units available for purchase or rental.

17. *Rental Assistance (Housing Assistance, Section 8).* Federal government program that provides financial assistance to older people and others with qualifying low incomes. No more than 25 to 30 percent of the individual's income goes toward rent in suitable housing.

18. *Retirement Village (Retirement Community).* Developments that typically offer home ownership and rental units for older people. Support services are often available for a fee.

19. *Reverse Mortgage.* One of the new financial plans designed to enable older homeowners to get cash for the equity in their homes while they continue to occupy them. Money is received in monthly payments or in lump-sum loans. The debt is outstanding for an agreed upon number of years, sometimes until the house is sold.

20. *Sale Leaseback.* Another home equity conversion plan. A home is sold to an investor who immediately leases it back to the seller (older homeowner) for life.

21. *Shared Home (Group Living).* Arrangement in which three or more unrelated people share a house or an apartment. Usually private sleeping quarters are available; the rest of the house is shared.

Nursing Homes

1. Although it is beyond the scope of this book to discuss all alternative living arrangements, choosing a nursing home is detailed to enable the nurse to better guide the client or family considering this option.

2. Although only 5% of the elderly live in homes for the aged, it is estimated that 20 to 30% of individuals will at some time in their lives require care in a nursing home.

3. Nursing homes provide continuous health care for a long period of time for those who require extensive support services and for those for whom community options are not available. Nursing care, rehabilitation programs, social activities, supervision, and basic room and food services are provided in state-licensed nursing homes.

4. The home health team, the older person (as far as is possible), and the family should be involved in the decision to enter a nursing home. Family members who make the decision alone often are overwhelmed with guilt and despair.

5. The search for a suitable nursing home should begin well in advance of seeking admission, as the best homes will have no vacancies and long waiting lists.

6. There are three levels of nursing home care:
   a. A residential-care facility (custodial-care facility) provides room and board and assistance with personal care. In addition, this type of home may offer social, recreational, and spiritual programs.
   b. An intermediate-care facility is for those clients who do not require 24-hour nursing care but need some nursing assistance and cannot live alone. Room and board, personal and health care, and social activities are provided.
   c. A skilled nursing facility (SNF) provides intensive 24-hour care and supervision by a nurse working with a doctor, who is available for emergencies.

7. Criteria to consider in choosing a nursing home include:
   a. Vacancies, length of waiting list, admission requirements, and level of care provided.
   b. Participation in Medicaid and Medicare programs. (See under "Sources of Financial Assistance" for explanations of Medicare and Medicaid.)
   c. Current state licensure of the home and the administrator.
   d. Meeting or exceeding of the state fire regulations with plans for evacuating the frail elderly, a sprinkler system, and fire-resistant doors.
   e. Availability of nursing and medical services and arrangements for emergencies.
   f. Types of rehabilitation and social programs offered to the residents.
   g. Quality and character of the food service (provisions for special health diets and ethnic preferences).
   h. Environmental design that promotes independence of the elderly with sensory and motor deficits and mental impairment:
      (1) Aids in the environment, such as handrails, low elevator buttons, easy-to-use furniture, call buttons in bedrooms and bathrooms, and wide doorways and ramps accessible to wheelchairs.
      (2) Color-coded hallways and directional signs that help residents, particularly those with poor vision or mental impairment, to manage independently.
      (3) Placement of furniture in common areas to promote interaction among the residents.
   i. Opportunities for exercise and social activity.

    j. Staff that is well trained and displays an empathetic attitude while encouraging independence and yet providing assistance when needed.

    k. Arrangements for provision of personal privacy and safety of possessions.

8. Referral by agencies, opinions of residents and families, and unannounced on-site visits can be helpful in determining the suitability of a nursing home in meeting the client's needs.

9. The legal contract or financial agreement is best reviewed with a lawyer to ascertain that it is understood.

10. Encourage the family to be actively involved in assisting the client in his transition to a nursing home by:

    a. Attending pre-admission group sessions with a social worker or nurse specialist.

    b. Assisting the elder in choosing familiar personal items, such as family photographs or favorite personal care items, to take along.

    c. Accompanying the elder to the home on moving day.

    d. Visiting regularly, as family visits are reassuring and usually lift the morale of the resident and ensure better care by the staff.

11. In 1981, an amendment to the OAA mandated that there be a state ombudsman program that acts as a liaison between the nursing home residents and their families and the nursing home administrator.

    a. A state-appointed ombudsman investigates any problems or complaints reported to him involving the residents.

    b. The problems may involve mistreatment, poor dietary services, or possible inappropriate acts of the staff.

    c. The administrator of the nursing home usually works cooperatively with the ombudsman to resolve problems.

12. For financing long-term care, it is important to remember that:

    a. Government programs and private insurance cover some health care costs of the elderly, but the largest share may have to be borne by the consumer and family.

    b. Because funding for long-term care services varies from state to state, the client or family should be encouraged to explore alternative long-term care services and funding with the local AAA.

Resources

American Association of Retired Persons
Health Advocacy Services
1909 K Street N.W.
Washington, DC 20049

Your Home Your Choice: A Workbook for Older People and Their Families
Housing Options for Older Americans
The Right Place at the Right Time: A Guide to Long-Term Care Choices
Making Wise Decisions for Long-Term Care

National Institute on Aging
Information Center
2209 Distribution Circle
Silver Spring, MD 20910
When You Need a Nursing Home

Consumer Information Center
Department 152-M
Pueblo, CO 81009
How to Select a Nursing Home ($4.75)

COMMUNITY RESOURCES

1. Programs that provide community services are funded by the government, religious groups, and the private sector.
2. Services most acceptable to the ethnic elderly are those within their community whose staff is able to communicate in their language and is sensitive to the dominant beliefs, values, and practices of their culture.
3. Programs for the elderly have experienced reductions in financial support during the 1980s, as government funding has been reduced for domestic programs.
4. The following is a brief description of some of the more established programs and services for the elderly and their families in the community.

Information and Referral Services
of the Area Agency on Aging

1. Information and Referral Services provide information and referral to community services for the elderly and their families.
2. Telephone directories with numbers regularly called and toll-free emergency numbers (often in large print) are provided.

3. Information and Referral Services are often located in multipurpose senior centers.

Personal Care Assessment Program of the Area Agency on Aging

1. The goal of the personal care assessment service is to assist the elderly in remaining as independent as possible by assessing the client's needs and referring the client or family to appropriate resources.
2. Referrals are made for personal care assessment by welfare departments, hospitals, churches, neighbors, and even clients themselves.
3. The Personal Care Assessment Program works closely with the Information and Referral Services.

Emergency Services

1. Emergency service numbers are listed in the front pages of the telephone book under community service numbers and in the Silver Pages (or Blue Pages, depending on region) under community resources guide.
2. Most local hot line numbers are made available by government and volunteer agencies for:
   • Police Emergency
   • Electric and Gas Emergency
   • Fire Emergency
   • Food and Hunger Hot Line
   • Poison Control Center
   • Emergency Ambulance
   • Protective Services for Adults
   • Sex Crime Hot Line
   • Suicide Hot Line
   • Crime Victims Hot Line
3. The American Red Cross provides:
   a. Heat kits for lack of heat in the home, weatherization of the home, and temporary lodging when the home is too cold for residence.
   b. Short-term emergency housing and emergency home-care services.
   c. Emergency transportation when a client is discharged from a hospital or emergency room.
4. The Emergency Assistance Program of the Department of Human

Resources provides cash assistance for unexpected and essential bills.

Nutrition Services

1. Congregate (group) meals are served at multipurpose senior centers and nutrition sites. Transportation may be provided to the low-cost, nutritious meals. The meals are government-funded, but donations are accepted.
2. Home-delivered meals (Meals on Wheels) are provided by privately funded and public agencies that deliver meals to elderly unable to prepare their own meals or to attend congregate meals.
3. The Commodity Food Distribution Program arranges for the free distribution of foods, such as cheese, honey, and butter, to low-income persons.
4. The Food Stamp Program provides for low-income persons to buy coupons that are worth more at the time of food purchase in the store. The program is under the auspices of the Human Resources Administration.

Transportation and Escort Services

1. Scheduling information for available transportation for various programs in the community, visits for health supervision, and personal errands (e.g., shopping) may be obtained from the AAA or local senior centers.
2. The AAA may provide van service without charge (though donations are encouraged) or may contract with a local taxi company to provide transportation at a discount rate to senior citizens.
3. In some municipalities, a reduced-fare program provides half-fare on mass transit, buses, and subways for those aged 65 or older, working or retired. The half-fare may be available on a 24-hour basis or may be restricted to non–rush hours. A Medicare card enables an elder to ride at half-fare, or a Reduced Fare Card may be obtained from the AAA or the local transportation coordinator.
4. Ambulette service may be provided by Medicaid for wheelchair-bound persons to attend medical appointments.

Pharmaceutical Insurance Coverage

Individual states have enacted bills to help eligible seniors receive assistance in paying for prescriptions. Seniors should be alerted to such programs and assisted in registering for benefits.

Programs for Isolated Seniors

1. The Friendly Visitor Program matches a volunteer visitor with an isolated senior. The volunteer meets with the elder frequently and provides friendship and help with personal or household problems, such as writing letters, running errands, or just listening and talking to the elder.
2. Telephone reassurance programs provide personal contact by daily phone calls at a prearranged time by volunteers to elderly living alone.
3. Emergency response systems are available that provide reliable contact by telephone or electronic device to police and rescue squads in time of emergency.

Multipurpose Senior Centers

1. The goal of a senior center is to provide a central location where seniors can grow, learn, relax, be creative, and socialize with other people.
2. Multipurpose senior centers provide a central location for:
   a. Luncheon programs and home-delivered meals.
   b. Socialization.
   c. Recreational activities, such as arts and crafts, physical fitness classes, or field trips.
   d. Health counseling and health screenings.
   e. Information and referral services to legal, financial, and counseling services as needed.
   f. Assistance in obtaining senior benefits.

Adult Day-Care Centers

1. The adult day-care center provides a structured program for older dependent seniors living in the community who are having difficulty carrying out activities of daily living (ADL) or who need attention and support during the working hours when the significant others with whom they live are away.
2. Day-care centers often provide enough support for these frail, dependent elders to remain in the community.

3. Health assessment and physical care are provided in addition to recreational, legal, and financial counseling services.
4. Transportation is usually provided to the program.

Home Care Services

1. Home care services include a variety of services provided by trained professionals, suh as a physician, nurse, or physical therapist, in addition to homemaker or chore services provided by housekeepers, home attendants, and home health aides.
   a. Homemaker or chore services provide personal care services (assistance with ADL), house cleaning, shopping, and administration of oral medication by a homemaker or an aide under the supervision of a registered nurse.
   b. Contact with the health care worker may provide some socialization, especially for isolated seniors.
   c. Handyman services are funded to provide elders aged 60 and older help in home repair that may enable them to maintain and remain in their own home.
   d. Home care may offer nonmedical services, such as home-delivered meals, friendly visiting volunteers, emergency response systems, and telephone reassurance.
2. There are both nonprofit and proprietary agencies that provide home care services.
   a. The Human Resources Administration provides needed home care services to those who are eligible through Medicaid.
   b. The AAA may provide housekeeping services and limited personal care for clients aged 60 and older who need assistance in maintaining themselves at home, are without live-in family, and do not qualify for Medicaid assistance.
   c. Medicare pays for a limited amount of home care after hospitalization.
   d. Local social service agencies may share the expense of home care with the elderly.

Hospice Care

1. Hospice care provides physical, psychologic, social, and spiritual care to the terminally ill person and family by a team of physicians, nurses, social workers, clergy, and volunteers.
2. The objective of hospice care is to maintain the terminally ill indi-

vidual as comfortable and pain-free or as long as possible in the care of their families, usually in the home setting.
3. Medicare will pay for hospice care in the community.

Respite Care

1. Respite care provides short-term relief either in the home or in another care setting for family members who care for an elderly person at home. While the family is away (may be for an afternoon or for a week), care is provided for the elderly client.
2. Adult day-care centers may provide respite services for the day.
3. Arrangements for respite care may be made with a nearby nursing home or through the Information and Referral Service of Area Agency on Aging.

Support Groups

There are a variety of national organizations that offer programs relevant to seniors, their families, and to health professionals working with them.

Resource

Self-Care and Self-Help Groups for the Elderly:
   A Directory
The National Self-Help Clearinghouse
33 West 42nd Street
Room 1227
New York, NY 10036

Provides information on support groups.

FINANCIAL CONCERNS

1. Frequently, the elderly need assistance in meeting the ever-spiraling costs of housing, clothing, transportation, utilities, and health care on a relatively fixed and unchanging retirement income.
2. In response to this need, a variety of entitlement programs provide income, medical care, and assistance for obtaining food, housing, transportation, and recreation at reduced cost.

Sources of Financial Assistance

SOCIAL SECURITY

Social Security is a national retirement income supplement that provides a continuing income to former workers and their families when the worker's earnings are eliminated or reduced because of retirement, disability, or death.
1. Social Security payments are available to individuals who are 62 years of age and have the necessary "earnings record."
2. Workers disabled before age 65 may be eligible for monthly payments.
3. Spouses at age 62 may receive an additional monthly payment, except when spouses and dependents can receive higher social security benefits in their own right as retired or disabled wage earners.
4. A surviving spouse is eligible for monthly payments as early as age 60 or at any age if he or she is caring for a dependent child.
5. A widow or widower who remarries at age 60 or later may be able to claim either a survivor's or a spouse's benefits. (They are eligible for whichever benefit is higher.)
6. Clients may obtain information on how to file a claim at least 3 months before becoming eligible for benefits by writing to or telephoning their local social security office.
7. For security and convenience, arrangements may be made to send social security checks directly to the recipient's bank account.
8. At age 65, individuals become eligible for Medicare (Title XVIII of the Social Security Act), a federal health insurance that helps pay the cost of many medical expenses.
   a. Persons eligible who plan to continue working should apply for Medicare benefits at a social security office at least 3 months prior to their 65th birthday.
   b. Medicare starts automatically at age 65 for those who are receiving social security or railroad retirement checks.
   c. Medicare Part A, Hospital Insurance helps pay the cost for:
      (1) Inpatient hospital care.
      (2) Inpatient care in a skilled nursing facility.
      (3) Home health care.
      (4) Hospice care.
   d. Medicare Part B, Medical Insurance (monthly premium required) helps pay the cost for:
      (1) Physician's services.
      (2) Outpatient hospital services.
      (3) Home health visits.

(4) Some other medical expenses, such as ambulance transportation, home dialysis equipment, supplies, periodic support services, independent laboratory tests, oral surgery, outpatient physical therapy, speech pathology services, x-ray tests, and radiation treatments.

(5) Some psychiatric expenses.

  e. The *Guide to Health Insurance for People with Medicare* is available at all local social security offices.

9. The elderly may purchase supplemental health insurance privately but should examine the policy carefully to ensure that the plan provides health insurance wanted and needed and does not duplicate coverage already provided by Medicare.

OTHER SOURCES

1. Supplemental Security Income (SSI) is a means-tested program that ensures a minimum monthly income to elderly aged 65 and older with limited income and resources.

  a. Information about the program, applications, and help in filing the claim are available at local social security offices.

  b. If the benefit received from social security is less than the SSI benefit and the older person is classified as financially needy, the difference between the two amounts is paid to the person in the form of an SSI benefit.

2. Medicaid (Title XIX of the Social Security Act) is a health care program for low-income persons jointly financed by federal and state governments that provides medical services to those financially eligible. An elder may be eligible for Medicaid as well as Medicare.

3. Information on a variety of benefits available to veterans may be obtained by calling the Veterans Administration Regional Office, Veterans Benefits Information as listed in the local telephone directory.

4. Housing programs for the elderly include the following:

  a. Senior citizen housing is available, with rents based on 30% of the tenant's income.

  b. Subsidies by the Department of Housing and Urban Development on the behalf of eligible tenants (aged 62 or older or disabled) may be available to make up the difference between the rent the tenant pays (approximately 30% of net income) and the rent charged by the landlord. Section 8 housing applications may be obtained from local housing authorities or community organizations.

  c. Senior citizen rent increase exemptions (SCRIE) may be available for persons aged 62 and older living in rent-controlled or rent-stabilized apartments, hotel rooms, or Mitchell-Lama apartments (government subsidized) if their income is $12,025 or less and their rent is more than one third of their income.

d. Real estate property tax reduction by as much as 50% is available in some communities for homeowners aged 65 and older or some elderly veterans (with limited income). The local Department of Taxation and Finance should be contacted about information on this yearly grant.

5. Local energy assistance programs help low-income elderly meet the cost of utilities. Emergency funds may be available to avoid utility disconnections.
6. Federal, state, or local tax credits or benefits are available to older persons. Information about these benefits may be obtained from the Federal Income Tax Information Service of the American Association of Retired Persons (AARP) Tax Aide.
7. Senior citizen benefit discounts for goods and services are offered in many communities for prescription drugs, transportation services, restaurant meals, recreation facilities, bank services, and so on. See your local community resources guide in the colored pages of telephone directories.

WORK OPPORTUNITIES

1. Many workers aged 55 and older indicate that they would prefer to continue to contribute and improve their own limited resources by working part-time in the community.
2. Community work raises self-esteem and offers a sense of purpose, as the elderly share the benefit of a lifetime of experience and provide services that enhance the lives of the recipients as well as their own.

Employment Programs

1. Senior Employment Service (Title V of the OAA) authorized the establishment of programs for part-time community service employment of low-income individuals aged 55 and older with "poor employment prospects," such as unskilled workers and women.
   a. This program subsidizes public and private nonprofit organizations to hire unemployed, low-income elders for part-time work that does not displace regular workers or eliminate regular jobs.

    b. The program employs elderly in hospitals, day-care centers, and nutrition sites.

    c. Under Title V, communities design individual programs for employment of seniors.

2. Senior Community Service Employment Program (SCSEP) is funded by the U.S. Department of Labor to provide employment for low-income individuals aged 55 and older.

    a. The seniors must not displace regular workers or eliminate regular jobs.

    b. The seniors are paid for part-time community jobs at about minimum wage in public or private nonprofit organizations, such as parks, hospitals, senior centers, schools, and day-care centers.

    c. Workers may receive an annual physical examination, on-the-job training, and related services.

    d. SCSEP allows many organizations to hire the elderly and to expand services to other elderly, particularly in nutrition sites and senior citizen centers.

    e. Project "Green Thumb" is a branch of SCSEP involved in conservation and restoration projects in rural areas.

3. The Foster Grandparent Program is designed to benefit low-income elderly and disadvantaged children.

    a. The elderly are paid to spend a certain amount of time each week in a public or private school or hospital with disadvantaged children.

    b. The foster grandparent may assist with homework, provide advice about problems, and assist in speech and physical therapy.

4. The Senior Companion Program employs low-income elderly to assist older persons in need, such as the sick, the bedridden, and the infirm.

    a. Seniors provide companionship, concern, housekeeping, cooking, letter writing, and bill paying.

    b. The program is designed to help the infirm elderly remain at home.

5. Union programs exist that employ retired workers in the service of their fellow retirees. For example, there is the Friendly Visitors Program of the International Ladies' Garment Workers' Union. After training, the friendly visitors assist retirees in advocacy matters, such as benefit application procedures, nursing home placement, and linkage to community resources.

Senior Volunteer Programs

1. The Friendly Visitors Program (Title 20 of the Social Security Act) matches a volunteer visitor with a lonely isolated elderly person.

    a. A visitor meets with the elder frequently and provides friendship and help with personal or household problems. The visitor may write letters, bring small gifts, run errands, or just give the senior someone to talk with.

    b. A telephone call may be made if the volunteer is unable to visit.

    c. The volunteer visitor prevents long periods of isolation for the infirm senior.

    d. The only reimbursement received by the volunteer is transportation.

2. The Retired Senior Volunteer Program (RSVP) is for elders aged 60 and older who want to use their experience and talents to serve or improve the community.

    a. Several hundred projects exist throughout the United States employing more than 50,000 seniors.

    b. The seniors work in a variety of activities in schools, libraries, correctional institutions, hospitals, nursing homes, telephone reassurance programs, and government agencies.

    c. Volunteers receive no pay, but they are reimbursed for travel and the cost of a meal if they are volunteering during a meal period.

3. A Volunteer Talent Bank under the auspices of the AARP matches volunteers with the right job. A senior may register with the Volunteer Talent Bank by writing for a registration form:

    AARP Volunteer Talent Bank
    1909 K Street N.W.
    Washington, DC 20049

LEGAL CONCERNS

1. Affected by complex statutory, regulatory, and decisional law, the elderly often are in need of counseling or legal services to help them protect their own rights and property and to gain access to statutory programs for which they are eligible.

2. The elderly may obtain referral from the AAA to community agencies that provide legal services to older persons and families.

Legal Issues of Concern to the Elderly

1. An elder may decide to delegate power of attorney.

    a. Delegation of power of attorney is a legal device that allows the "principal" to give to another person, called the "attorney-in-fact," the authority to act in his behalf in services, such as banking, managing real estate, incurring expenses, paying bills, and handling a wide variety of legal affairs, for a specified period of time.

  b. The *power of attorney* may continue indefinitely during the lifetime of the principal as long as the person is competent and capable of granting power of attorney.

  c. If the principal becomes comatose or mentally incompetent, the power of attorney automatically expires just as it would if the principal died. Thus, the power of attorney may expire just when it is needed most.

2. The principal may indicate intent concerning the durability of the power of attorney to survive disability or incompetency by delegating durable power of attorney, an authorized legal device that is an alternative to guardianship, conservatorship, or trusteeship.

  a. Durable power of attorney puts a significant amount of power in the hands of the attorney.

  b. The designation of durable power of attorney should be drawn up by an attorney licensed to practice in the state in which the client resides.

  c. Durable power of attorney is used to compensate for the period of time when an individual becomes incompetent to manage personal affairs appropriately.

3. Guardianship, or conservatorship, is a legal mechanism in which the court judges a person incompetent and unable to care for himself and appoints a guardian to ensure a continuum of protective services.

4. A well-prepared will provides explicit instructions for the distribution of property and, if appropriate, how that property is to be used after the person dies.

  a. Information about burial or cremation can also be included in a will.

  b. A will designates an individual or individuals to serve as the executor(s) responsible for carrying out the instructions of the will.

  c. Generally, a will makes it easier to settle affairs more quickly and with less legal expense.

5. "Right to die" bills have been enacted in several states that enable terminally ill clients (if they desire to do so) to sign a so-called "living will" that instructs their physicians to withdraw or withhold life-sustaining procedures when those efforts serve no purpose except to artificially delay death.

  a. In some states, living wills provide a legal means that enables others to carry out a person's wishes regarding the use of extreme measures to delay death.

    b. A living will is a signed, dated, and witnessed document that allows a person to state wishes in advance regarding the use of life-sustaining measures during a terminal illness.

    c. This document appoints someone else to direct care if the patient is unable to do so.

    d. The living will should be signed and dated by two witnesses who are not blood relatives of the client or beneficiaries of property bequeathed by the client.

    e. A living will should be discussed with the physician, and a signed copy should be added to the individual's medical file. Another copy should be given to the person who will make the decision in the event the individual is unable to do so.

    f. A living will should be reviewed yearly to make changes as needed.

6. Property, estate, and trust issues are governed by state laws and sometimes by local ordinances. If finances do not permit hiring a private attorney to deal with these issues, there are programs that provide legal advice and representation in court to elderly and low-income persons.

7. Tenant/landlord issues regarding leases, services, and rental rights and obligations may be referred to local housing agencies, a lawyer, or a local AAA.

8. Questions about family responsibility for financial support for health care, medical, or long-term care cause the elderly to seek legal advice about obligations.

9. Some elderly may prefer to make and prepay their own funeral arrangements so that they may choose the type of funeral and cemetery they desire.

    a. Collection of information on the cost of desired arrangements and preplanning can help avoid hasty and expensive decisions.

    b. Funeral arrangements should be made with the informed choice of the client or family.

    c. Consumers have the right to choose only those funeral and cemetery arrangements they desire.

    d. The law specifies that funeral providers must disclose the cost of all goods and services upon the request of the consumer. A written price list must be provided on request.

    e. Traditional funeral services, direct interment, cremation, or memorial services may be chosen.

    f. Arrangements for body or organ donation may be considered.

    g. Availability of death benefits should be ascertained before making the arrangements. Benefits may be obtained from the Social Security Administration, the Veterans Administration, life and casualty insurance, and other sources, depending upon the circumstances at the time of death.

　h. Specific wishes about how the funeral is to be conducted and burial arrangements should be put in writing where they can be easily found.

10. Additional issues that require some understanding of the law and professional assistance include:
　a. Making a contract.
　b. Attempting to obtain consumer credit.
　c. Setting up a business.
　d. Questions or problems involving pension rights.
　e. Entering into a late or second marriage.
　f. Arranging for an ill or incompetent person.
　g. Becoming incapacitated.

Sources for Legal Advice

1. The Human Resources Administration, which provides adult protective services for individuals who, because of physical or mental limitations, are unable to act in their own behalf. The services offer protection from exploitation, abuse, or neglect.
2. Legal Service Programs from the local Department of Aging.
3. Local Legal Aid Society.
4. Local Association of the Bar, Legal Referral Service, which makes referrals to practicing attorneys for those elderly who need assistance, who are unable to appropriately manage their own legal affairs, or for whom protective services may be needed.
5. The District Attorney's office.
6. A legal clinic in a local law school, where students under appropriate supervision provide legal assistance to seniors.
7. Local government agencies that oversee the particular area of concern.
8. Local and state consumer protection agencies.
9. Agencies involved in protecting the rights of older people and minority groups.
10. A practicing lawyer hired for 1 hour when financially feasible, who may advise about alternatives.
11. Small claims court, if necessary.

CULTURAL, EDUCATIONAL, AND RECREATIONAL OPPORTUNITIES

1. The AAA is a source for information on opportunities for enrichment in the psychosocial area available to seniors often without charge or at a reduced rate.

2. Multipurpose senior centers provide activities. See under "Multi-purpose Senior Centers," previously.
3. Many museums, educational institutions, and nonprofit organizations provide reduced or special rates for their activities.
4. Public libraries provide information, books, magazines, music tapes or records, audiovisuals, and special programs.

SENIOR POLITICAL ACTION

1. Seniors make up only 11% of the population of the United States, but they demonstrate significant political power because they consist of 20% of the voting population.
2. Senior political action groups work independently and in coalition with other movements to promote a more humane society and legislation that recognizes and protects the rights of older Americans.

Resources

Information on senior political action groups may be obtained by writing to:

Gray Panthers Project Fund
311 South Juniper Street
Suite 601
Philadelphia, PA 19107

American Association of Retired Persons
1909 K Street N.W.
Washington, DC 20049

Advocates Senior Alert Process (ASAP)
134 G Street N.W.
Washington, DC 20005

Provides at no charge information on issues such as health, social security, and the OAA programs in return for commitment to act on important issues by writing letters, making phone calls, and taking other action on a legislative issue. Special reports will be supplied to give background information needed for advocacy work.

References

Clemen-Stone S, Eigisti D, McGuire S: Comprehensive Family and Community Health Nursing. New York: McGraw-Hill, 1987.

Cox H: Later Life: The Realities of Aging. Englewood Cliffs, NJ: Prentice-Hall, 1984.

Dobelstein A, Johnson AB: Serving Older Adults: Policy, Programs, and Professional Activities. Englewood Cliffs, NJ: Prentice-Hall, 1985.

Gelfand DE: Aging: The Ethnic Factor. Boston: Little, Brown & Co, 1982.

Housing Options for Older Americans. Washington, DC: American Association of Retired Persons, 1984.

Making Wise Decisions for Long-Term Care. Washington, DC: American Association of Retired Persons, 1986.

Monk A: Handbook of Gerontological Services. New York: Van Nostrand Rheinhold, 1985.

Raukhorst LM, Stokes SA, Mezey MD: Community and home assessment. Journal of Gerontological Nursing June 1980, pp 319–327.

Stanhope M, Lancaster JL: Community Health Nursing. St. Louis: CV Mosby, 1984.

The Right Place at the Right Time: A Guide to Long-Term Care Choices. Washington, DC: American Association of Retired Persons, 1985.

When You Need a Nursing Home. Silver Spring, Md: National Institute on Aging, 1986.

Your Home Your Choice: A Workbook for Older People and Their Families. Washington, DC: American Association of Retired Persons, 1985.

Appendix

STATE AGENCIES ON AGING*

ALABAMA
State Capitol
Montgomery, AL 36130
(205) 261-5743

ALASKA
Pouch C-Mail Station 0209
Juneau, AK 99811
(907) 465-3250

ARIZONA
1400 West Washington Street
Phoenix, AZ 85007
(602) 255-4446

ARKANSAS
Donaghey Building, Suite 1428
7th and Main Streets
Little Rock, AR 77201
(501) 371-2441

CALIFORNIA
1020 19th Street
Sacramento, CA 95814
(916) 322-5290

COLORADO
1575 Sherman Street, Room 503
Denver, CO 80203
(303) 866-3672

CONNECTICUT
175 Main Street
Hartford, CT 06106
(203) 566-3238

DELAWARE
1901 North DuPont Highway
New Castle, DE 19720
(302) 421-6791

DISTRICT OF COLUMBIA
1424 K Street, N.W., 2nd Floor
Washington, DC 20005
(202) 724-5622

FLORIDA
1317 Winewood Boulevard
Tallahassee, FL 32301
(904) 488-8922

GEORGIA
878 Peachtree Street, N.E.
Room 632
Atlanta, GA 30309
(404) 894-5333

HAWAII
1149 Bethel Street, Room 307
Honolulu, HI 96813
(808) 548-2593

IDAHO
Statehouse, Room 114
Boise, ID 83720
(208) 334-3833

ILLINOIS
421 East Capitol Avenue
Springfield, IL 62706
(217) 785-3356

INDIANA
115 North Pennsylvania Street
Suite 1350, Consolidated Building
Indianapolis, IN 46204
(317) 232-7006

IOWA
Suite 236, Jewett Building
914 Grand Avenue
Des Moines, IA 50319
(515) 281-5187

KANSAS
610 West Tenth
Topeka, KS 66612
(913) 296-4986

KENTUCKY
DHR Building, 6th Floor
275 East Main Street
Frankfort, KY 40601
(502) 564-6930

LOUISIANA
PO Box 80374
Baton Rouge, LA 70898
(504) 925-1700

---

*On request the state agency on aging will provide the telephone number of the Area Agency on Aging in the local community.

MAINE
State House, Station #11
Augusta, ME 04333
(207) 289-2561

MARYLAND
301 West Preston Street
Baltimore, MD 21201
(301) 383-5064

MASSACHUSETTS
30 Chauncy Street
Boston, MA 02111
(617) 727-7750

MICHIGAN
101 South Pine, North Tower
3rd Floor, PO Box 30026
Lansing, MI 48909
(517) 373-8230

MINNESOTA
Metro Square Building, Room 204
Seventh & Robert Streets
St. Paul, MN 55101
(612) 296-2544

MISSISSIPPI
802 North State Street
Executive Building, Suite 301
Jackson, MS 39201
(601) 354-6590

MISSOURI
Broadway State Office
PO Box 570
Jefferson City, MO 65101
(314) 751-3082

MONTANA
PO Box 4210
Helena, MT 59604
(406) 444-3865

NEBRASKA
PO Box 95044
301 Centennial Mall, South
Lincoln, NB 68509
(402) 471-2306

NEVADA
505 East King Street
Kinkead Building, Room 101
Carson City, NV 89710
(707) 885-4210

NEW HAMPSHIRE
14 Depot Street
Concord, NH 03301
(603) 271-2751

NEW JERSEY
Box 2768
363 West State Street
Trenton, NJ 08625
(609) 292-4833

NEW MEXICO
224 East Palace Avenue
La Villa Rivera Building
Sante Fe, NM 87501
(505) 827-7640

NEW YORK
New York State Plaza
Agency Building 2
Albany, NY 12223
(518) 474-5731

NORTH CAROLINA
708 Hillsborough Street
Suite 200
Raleigh, NC 27603
(919) 733-3983

NORTH DAKOTA
State Capitol Building
Bismarck, ND 58505
(701) 224-2577

OHIO
50 West Broad Street
Columbus, OH 43215
(614) 466-5500

OKLAHOMA
Box 25352
Oklahoma City, OK 73125
(405) 521-2281

OREGON
313 Public Service Building
Salem, OR 97310
(503) 378-4728

PENNSYLVANIA
231 State Street
Harrisburg, PA 17101-1195
(717) 783-1550

RHODE ISLAND
79 Washington Street
Providence, RI 02903
(401) 277-2858

SOUTH CAROLINA
915 Main Street
Columbia, SC 29201
(803) 758-2576

SOUTH DAKOTA
700 North Illinois Street
Pierre, SD 57501
(606) 773-3656

TENNESSEE
703 Tennessee Building
535 Church Street
Nashville, TN 37219
(615) 741-2056

TEXAS
210 Barton Springs Road
5th Floor
P.O. Box 12768, Capitol Station
Austin, TX 78704
(512) 475-2717

UTAH
150 West North Temple
Box 2500
Salt Lake City, UT 84102
(801) 533-6422

VERMONT
103 South Main Street
Waterbury, VT 05676
(802) 241-2400

VIRGINIA
101 North 14th Street, 18th Floor
Richmond, VA 23219
(804) 225-2271

WASHINGTON
OB-43G
Olympia, WA 98504
(206) 753-2502

WEST VIRGINIA
Holly Grove, State Capitol
Charleston, WV 25305
(304) 348-3317

WISCONSIN
One West Wilson Street
PO Box 7851
Madison, WI 53702
(608) 266-2536

WYOMING
401 West 19th Street
Cheyenne, WY 82002
(307) 777-7986

Other Offices on Aging

(AMERICAN) SAMOA
Office of the Governor
Pago Pago, AS 96799
011 (684) 633-1252

GUAM
Government of Guam
Agana, GU 96910
(011) 671-4361

NORTHERN MARIANA ISLANDS
Civic Center, Susupe
Saipan
Northern Mariana Islands 96950
9411 or 9732

PUERTO RICO
PO Box 11398
Santurce, PR 00910
(809) 722-2429

TRUST TERRITORY OF THE PACIFIC
Government of TTPI
Saipan, Mariana Islands 96950
9335 or 9336

VIRGIN ISLANDS
6F Havensight Mall
Charlotte Amalie
St. Thomas, VI 00801
(809) 774-5884

Index